New Developments in
Ophthalmology

Documenta Ophthalmologica
Proceedings Series volume 7

Editor H. E. Henkes

Dr. W. Junk bv Publishers The Hague 1976

New Developments in
Ophthalmology
Nijmegen 16-18 October 1975

edited by A.F. Deutman

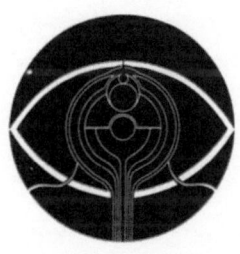

Dr. W. Junk bv Publishers The Hague 1976

ISBN-13:978-90-6193-147-8   e-ISBN-13:978-94-010-1569-1
DOI: 10.1007/978-94-010-1569-1

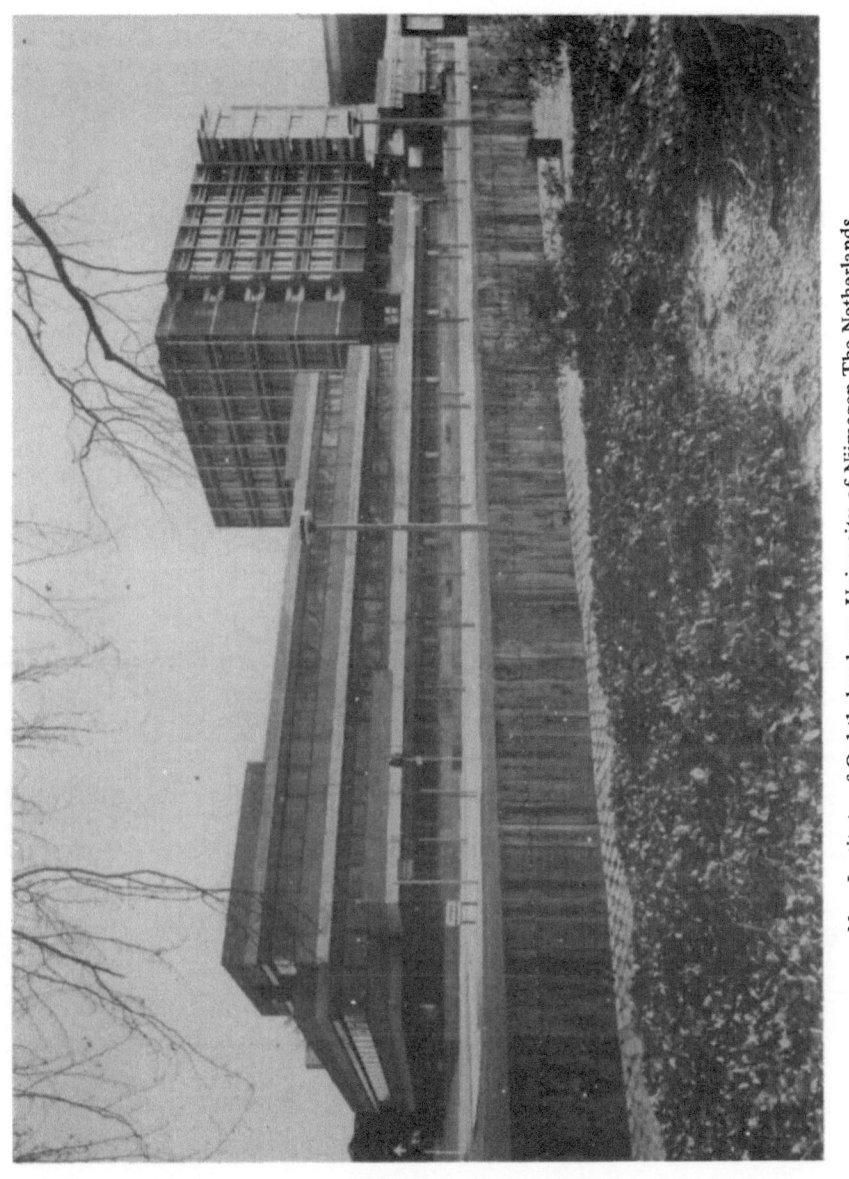

New Institute of Ophthalmology, University of Nijmegen The Netherlands.

CONTENTS

INTRODUCTION

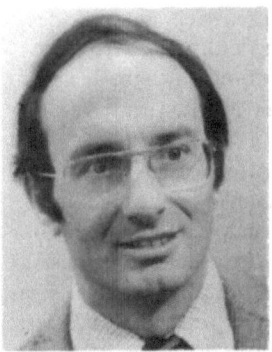

AUGUST F. DEUTMAN, M.D.

From October 16-18, 1975 many distinguished ophthalmologists visited Nijmegen to inaugurate the new Eye Institute of the University of Nijmegen with a symposium on New Developments in Ophthalmology. The meeting was held under the auspices of the Netherlandish Ophthalmological Society (NOG) and had a high attendance of over 300 ophthalmologists from The Netherlands and from abroad.

Many new and some controversial surgical techniques regarding corneal transplantation, phako-emulsification, intra-ocular lensimplantation, local excision of melanomas of the choroid and ciliary body, pars plana vitrectomy, laser treatment in disciform macular degeneration and treatment of giant retinal tears were discussed. Since new surgical techniques have to be based on profound knowledge of the anatomy and physiology of the eye, many new basic and important data regarding the cornea, the vitreous body, the retinal vessels, the choroid and the orbit were presented by some of the foremost authorities.

Technical advances in corneal transplantation were discussed, while the modern treatment of corneal ulcers and bacterial infections of the eye was presented.

New findings such as computerized tomography, facilitate the diagnosis of underlying disease in exophthalmus enormously. The treatment of retinal detachment has improved considerably over the last ten years and we feel that in particular the safe non-drainage methods deserve attention. Cryo-coagulation and photocoagulation have certain advances over diathermy and the radial placement of indenting suprascleral material may have consider-able advantages over the limbus-parallel placement in horseshoe tears.

Prophylaxis in retinal detachment is nowadays of paramount importance and when properly done without high risks. Giant tears and massive vitre-oretinal retraction (MVR) still constitute major problems in retinal detach-ment surgery. So far the intraocular injection of silicone oil seems to be the best method to combat MVR but possibly pars plana vitrectomy and SF6-gas injection may become of more value in the treatment of this still insufficiently understood condition.

Pars plana vitrectomy, the new concept developed by the Miami school, in which we gained only limited experience so far was discussed by two American surgeons with a large experience and it appears that this fascinat-ing technique is there to stay in ophthalmology.

1

Modern glaucoma surgery has gained by procedures such as trabeculectomy, which we prefer to do and the Elliot trephining with scleral flap.

The only way to influence subretinal neovascularisation is by light- or laser-coagulation and encouraging results have been seen in disciform macular degeneration.

The diagnosis of melanoma of the choroid has improved by examinations methods such as good direct and indirect and binocular ophthalmoscopy, diaphanoscopy, fluorescein angiography, P-32 test and echography. When the diagnosis of melanoma has been made we know now that local excision of melanomas of the choroid and ciliary body is technically possible. The question that is left is if it ought to be done and if so, in what kind of cases.

Exciting developments such as lensectomy and intra-ocular lemsimplantation were discussed on the last day.

Apart from the symposium papers we present in this issue a few papers from staffmembers of our Institute.

It was a very happy symposium where many good friends met. Many new ideas were brought forward and lots of experience was exchanged.

We hope to have our next symposium in about three years time and we wish to thank all the guests and participants for their outstanding job in making this symposium so successful.

Institute of Ophthalmology   A.F. Deutman.
University of Nijmegen
Nijmegen
The Netherlands

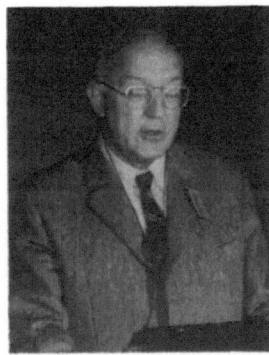

PREFACE

J.E.A. VAN DEN HEUVEL

(Nijmegen, The Netherlands)

Ladies and Gentlemen,

At this opening ceremony, in which the Institute of Ophthalmology of the University of Nijmegen is introduced into the scientific world, it seems to be an obvious choice for me to give you some insight into the genesis of this Institute.

In 1956 the Board of the University set me the task of founding a department of ophthalmology. Four years previously the Faculty of Medicine had taken up the training of medical students, and the first clinic of the Academic Hospital was opened in 1956.

When I entered the faculty grounds for the first time I saw a beautiful park which had once been in the possession of a captain of industry. But I did not see the faintest trace of any premises in which an ophthalmology department could possibly be established. The building of a nurses home, in the basement of which the ophthalmological clinic was to be housed, had not even begun yet.

I was asked what were the prospects of setting up a University Clinic of Ophthalmology in Nijmegen. The extremely peripheral geographical position of the city immediately came to my mind. Only a few miles to the East stretches the German border, to the North a wide river, the mainstream of the river Rhine, and to the South-East, again only a few miles away, runs the Maas. Reminding myself of the time-honoured reluctance of the Dutch to seek help from beyond the river – and in those days it even held good for such simple things as shopping! – I felt that, for the time being, a modest policlinic with a small ward of 22 beds would be sufficient.

In Juli 1958 the building of the provisional facilities had progressed so far that we could start our activities. It soon appeared that our prognostication had been wrong. As early as two weeks later our 22 beds were already occupied; there has been no lack of patients ever since.

One year after the beginnings of our department we were able to set up a small histological laboratory for the first junior staff member, who was working on a thesis. The activities increased very rapidly.

The small number of four junior staff members soon turned out to be *too* small. After two years, the facilities that were at our disposal, too, proved insufficient to deal with the considerable stream of patients. In 1960, already, we applied for a large extension. That was hard to obtain, because university building activities in the Netherlands, then as now, showed all the symptoms of chronic disease: life does go on, but only marginally so. We had to wait till 1964 before we could find provisional shelter in the paediatrics building, which had been finished with a year's delay owing to a fire. We could now, first of all, extend the library. I had donated my private library of medical books to the University, because it was extremely difficult in those days to buy back volumes of magazines. We could now make a beginning with the establishment of modest laboratories for biochemistry and physics, because it had become obvious by then that a University clinic could not function without a solid base of laboratories that housed the sciences I just mentioned, although with a decidedly clinical direction of research.

We were fortunate in finding highly qualified personnel to man the laboratories. Without derogating the great number of workers who have been doing an excellent job in the past seventeen years, I cannot but mention the names of the biochemist Dr. BROEKHUIJSE and, a few years his junior, the biophysicist Dr. THIJSSEN, both by now renowned scientists, who developed their departments in a way that cannot be surpassed.

Our problems concerning the policlinic and clinic were the same as with most University clinics: understaffing and lack of funds. The clinical staff worked night and day to meet the demands from both their patients and their teaching task. In 1967 it became clear that only by raising a completely new building could we comply with the requirements of the clinical department and the already undersized laboratories.

I will only make a passing remark here on the obstacles we had to surmount, the time-consuming discussions, and the delay due to other building projects being given priority. In the last five or six years prior to the completion of the new institute that you will be visiting, all staff members found it very hard to deal with the problems that arose from the growth of the department as well as that of our particular field of medicine.

Personally, I felt my activities to have become such a strain by 1971 that I requested the faculty to appoint a lecturer so that I could be relieved of a number of my tasks. Finally, in 1973, Professor Deutman could take up his share. The organisation of this symposium testifies to his energetic approach.

I am delighted that so many well-known ophthalmologists have been so kind as to grant their cooperation for this symposium. I want to extend a hearty welcome to them and thank them for all the pains they have taken for us.

When I compare ophthalmology with internal medicine and surgery, it strikes me that it shows the same development that in internal medicine and surgery has led to divisions into sub-specialisms. To a large extent these divisions occurred in the wake of technical methods, either in the field of diagnosis of treatment, which necessitated the spreading of know-how over more individuals. At the same time, scientific research into the value of those methods led to new developments.

Those who want to practise their clinical job to the full extent may find this hard to bear. Yet, in the interest of ophthalmology as a science, it should be promoted. But when the whole range of methods has been surveyed the question urges itself upon us, which of them can still be considered to be part of the normal task of an ophthalmologist. I am certainly not the first to ask this question. It is pretty obvious that many of the issues raised here are no longer 'general ophthalmology', and it might well be that we shall have to draw a clear dividing line between practical and special qualifications. This is a controversial matter, however, which I therefore defer to the board of the Nederlands Oogheelkundig Gezelschap, whom I also bid a hearty welcome and at the same time wish to thank for the special assistance they gave us.

To end with, ladies and gentlemen, I extend a very hearty welcome to all of you at the opening ceremony of the Institute that I have been looking forward to for so long a time. I hope you will all have a useful and pleasant time.

Author's address:
J.E.A.VAN DEN HEUVEL
Institute of Ophthalmology
University of Nijmegen
The Netherlands

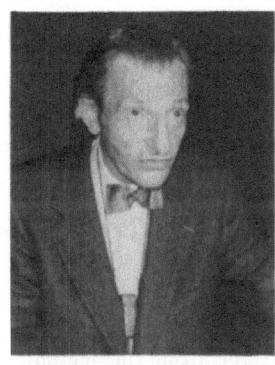

CORNEAL COLLAGENASES AND THEIR INHIBITION

J. FRANÇOIS & E. CAMBIE

(Ghent, Belgium)

Collagenases are, by definition, *enzymes* which are able to dissolve insoluble, non denatured connective tissue at the level of a well-defined place on the collagen molecule, under physiological conditions of pH and temperature. No enzymes are, therefore, included which further break down denatured collagen. In other words, collagenases are the enzymes which break down connective tissue not affected by the enzymatic action of trypsin. Still in other words, collagenases are the enzymes which develop under physiological conditions the first enzymatic cleavage process (MANDL, 1972).

We have to distinguish:

1. The *bacterial collagenases* (GALLOP et al., 1957) (clostridium histolyticum as prototype and pseudomonas aerogenosa more specific for corneal ulcers), which break down the connective-tissue molecule into relatively small fragments and which can cleave the molecule at the extremities as well as anywhere along its length.

2. The *animal collagenases* which were identified five years later (GROSS & LAPIÈRE, 1962; LAPIÈRE & GROSS, 1963). They always act on the same place and break down the molecule into a larger (75%) and a smaller (25%) fragment (GROSS & NAGAI, 1965; RANG et al., 1966; DRAKE et al., 1966). This single cleavage reduces the viscosity to 40% and does not affect the helicoidal structure. This is indeed characteristic of all animal collagenases. The difference in the enzymatic action between the animal and the bacterial collagenases lies at the basis of the various effects of collagenase inhibitors and activators.

Solutions of cystein, ethylene-diamino-tetra-acetate (E.D.T.A.) and serum inhibit nearly all collagenases (NORDWIG, 1971).

The *sub-stratum* affected by this enzyme is the *collagen*. The cornea consists of 90% collagen. This collagen molecule (M.W. 300 000) has a helicoidal structure of three peptide chains (M.W. 100 000), each of which contains some 1000 amino-acids. Two of these chains are identical, and the third differs slightly in structure (collagen type $\alpha 1\ \alpha 1\ \alpha 2$) (PUZ et al., 1963; DAVISON & BERMAN, 1973).

In solution, the collagen molecule consists of long rods 3000 Å in length and 15 Å in width, with an intrinsic viscosity and a marked negative optical rotation. At a temperature of 37° C and pH of 7, the molecule polymerises into insoluble fibrillae. Denaturation by pH or temperature changes result in a break-down of the helicoidal structure and a reduction of the intrinsic viscosity (RAMACHANDRAN, 1967).

Trypsin, chymotrypsin and pepsin can dissolve these molecules over a long period, by dissolving them very slowly from the polar extremities on or by detaching them at the level of the intermolecular bonds, but they in no way alter the helicoidal structure of the collagen molecule.

COLLAGENASE IN VARIOUS HUMAN TISSUES

Since GROSS & LAPIÈRE (1962, 1963) were able to isolate collagenases under physiological conditions during the metamorphosis of Anura, in particular, from the epithelial cells and to a lesser degree from the mesenchyme; collagenases have been identified in normal human tissues, such as the skin, kidneys, intestinal tissue and bone, as well as in pathological tissues, such as these from gingivitis, dermatomyositis and polymyositis, skin wounds, neurinomata, epithelial tumours of the intestinal tract, cervix uteri or prostate, rheumatoid arthritis and cholesteatomata. Granulocytes can also produce collagenase (FRANÇOIS & CAMBIE, 1972).

It is characteristic that these tissue homogenates or extracts present no collagenase activity, as after freezing and again thawing no enzyme activity could be demonstrated. The enzyme can, however, be clearly demonstrated in cell cultures. This indicates that collagenases are produced only by living cells and are not accumulated in the cells or tissues, except perhaps in amounts not detectable up to the present (GROSS & LAPIÈRE, 1962, 1963).

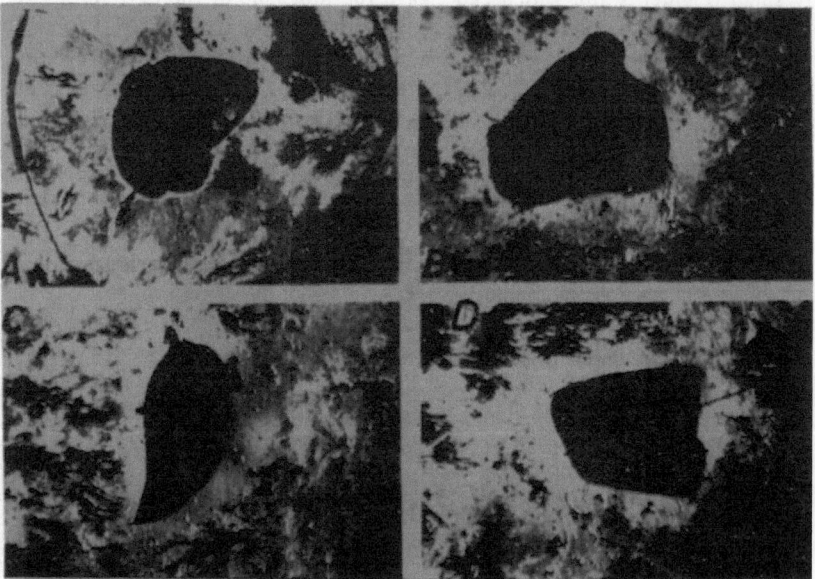

Fig. 1. Collagen substratum to control the lysing effect of the chemically burned corneas. During the first seven days no lysis (A), but after 10 (B), 12 (C) and 14 (D) days there is lysis.

Up to the present, experiments have indicated that the animal collagenases cleave the collagen molecules of different types and of different species always at the same place (DAVISON & BERMAN, 1973). It is not known whether that place is determined by well-defined amino-acid sequences or by a specific configuration, but the place appears to have been well preserved in the phylogenetic development from the agnatha to the primates. These observations confirm the phylogenetic stability already known of the collagen molecule.

COLLAGENASE IN ANIMAL CORNEAS

SLANSKY et al. (1968) were the first to demonstrate in the normal homogenised corneal epithelium of the cattle, collagenase which was inhibited by E.D.T.A. On the other hand, no author was able to demonstrate collagenase activity in normal corneas of rabbits (BROWN & WELLER, 1970). However, when the corneas of the animals were burned with NaOH, it was

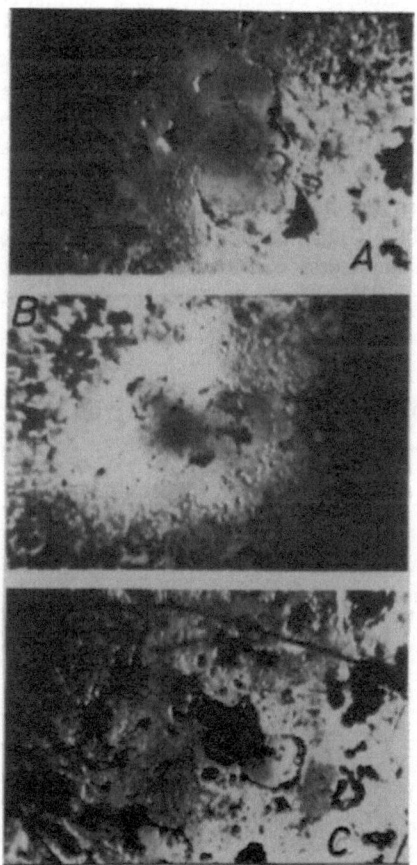

Fig. 2. Collagen substratum with grafts of corneal stroma (A and B) and epithelium (C) 12 days after a chemical burning. Obvious lysis in A and B, none in C.

possible to identify collagenase, after a latency period of at least seven days, at the level of the edges of the central ulcer (Fig. 1 and 2). This collagenase diminished progressively in concentration toward the periphery (BROWN et al., 1969; FRANÇOIS & CAMBIE, 1975). It was concluded therefrom that there existed a correlation between the liquefaction of the corneal stroma and the concentration of collagenase produced by the altered epithelium (SLANSKY, 1968; SLANSKY et al., 1969) and by the corneal granulation tissue (BROWN, 1971).

If now a corneal extract of collagenase is obtained from this lesion and injected into a normal, non denatured cornea, no perforation is obtained. When this extract is injected into a freshly burned cornea, a perforation is obtained within two days (Fig. 3). This indicates that, as long as the collagen fibres retain their normal mucopolysaccharide sheaths, collagenase is inactive (FRANÇOIS & CAMBIE, 1975).

COLLAGENASE IN THE HUMAN CORNEA

No collagenases could be demonstrated in a normal cornea, nor in parenchymal dystrophies, healed keratitides or scar tissue. Collagenase can, however, be demonstrated in keratitides with epithelial lesions, such as infectious or chemical keratitis, keratitis rosacea, ocular pemphigoid, keratitis e lagophthalmo, keratitis in rheumatoid arthritis, the Stevens-Johnson syndrome and scleroderma (SLANSKY & DOHLMAN, 1970).

Collagenase can be produced only by lesions of the corneal epithelium. In other words, as long as there exists no epithelial erosion, no collagenase production will be possible. Consequently, only unhealed ulcers can benefit from collagenase inhibitors.

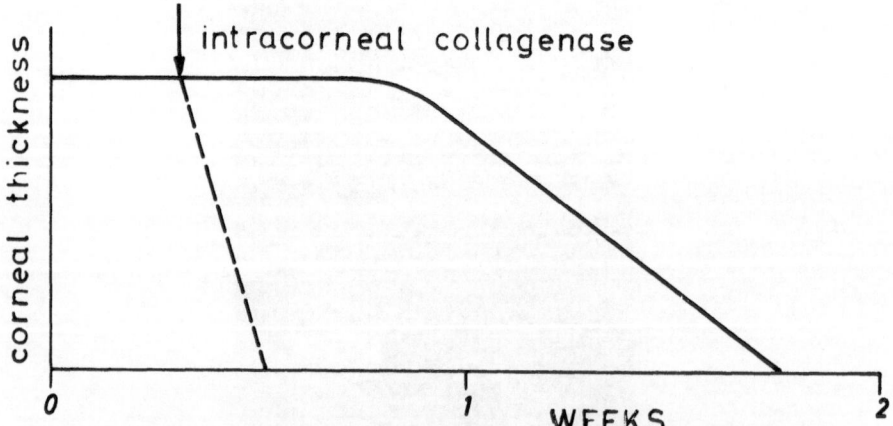

Fig. 3. Diagram of the normal evolution of the corneal liquefaction after chemical burning. The lysis starts after the 7th days and the cornea perforates between the 10th and the 15th day. The intracorneal injection of collagenase very rapidly produces a perforation of the previously burned cornea (more or less 1 day). Thickness of the cornea in ordinate, time in weeks in abscissa.

10

E.D.T.A., cystein and serum neutralise the proteolytic action of collagenase (NORDWIG, 1971). E.D.T.A. (ITOI et al., 1969), cystein (BROWN & WELLER, 1970), acetyl-cystein (EVANS et al., 1972), cystin (FRANÇOIS & CAMBIE, 1972), penicillamine (FRANÇOIS et al., 1972, 1973) (aspecific inhibitors) and serum (PUCHKOVSKAYA & NEPOMIASHCHAYA, 1969) (specific inhibitor) are able to inhibit corneal collagenase (Fig. 4).

With the aspecific collagenase inhibitors, it is a question of chelation of the Ca ions (BROWN & WELLER, 1970), which is necessary for the action of collagenase. Na-E.D.T.A. should then also be much more efficient than Ca-E.D.T.A. (BROWN & WELLER, 1970).

It seemed to us that as cystein, which is a poor chelator for Ca, gave a better inhibition than Na-E.D.T.A., which is a very good chelator for Ca, the Ca ions played merely a secondary role. When it appeared that penicillamine, which is a good chelator for Zn and a poor chelator for Ca, gave good results in the case of collagenase inhibition, we then postulated zinc as metal for the metallo-enzyme collagenase (FRANÇOIS et al., 1972, 1973), and this was later confirmed by the incorporation of radioactive Zn in the collagenase molecule, whereby a correlation was found between the quantities of Zn absorbed and the collagenase activity (BERMAN & MANABE, 1973).

The *chelation of Zn ions* is consequently a first form of *indirect collagenase inhibition.* Clinically, cystein, cystin and penicillamine appear to give the best results, probably because of their specificity for the Zn chelation, by virtue of which they leave untouched the Ca ions needed for other vital processes.

A second form of collagenase inhibition is a rather physiological defence against the overproduction of collagenase. Since it became known that a considerable improvement of corneal infectious or chemical ulcers occurred after the local and subconjunctival administration of fresh blood, it has been found that serum can inhibit certain collagenases (EISEN et al., 1970; WELLER et al., 1971). In this serum there are two proteins α1-AT (α1 antitrypsin) and α2-M (α2 macroglobulin) (EISEN et al., 1970), which are responsible for this and also inhibit the corneal collagenases (BERMAN et al., 1973, 1975). Moreover, in patients with corneal ulcers, these two serum antiproteases increase in the tears, whereas they remain unchanged in normal corneae or inflamed conjunctivae (BERMAN et al., 1973, 1975).

OUR VIEW ON THE CORNEAL LYSIS INDUCED BY COLLAGENASE

In the experiments carried out by us (chemical burns of rabbits' corneas with 1% Na OH), there occurs, after the immediate death of the affected cells, also a denaturation of the mucopolysaccharide ground substance.

At least seven days after such chemical burns collagenolysis occurs, and this even in the absence of epithelium, which can be mechanically removed. Consequently, the epithelium is of little or no importance in the production of collagenase.

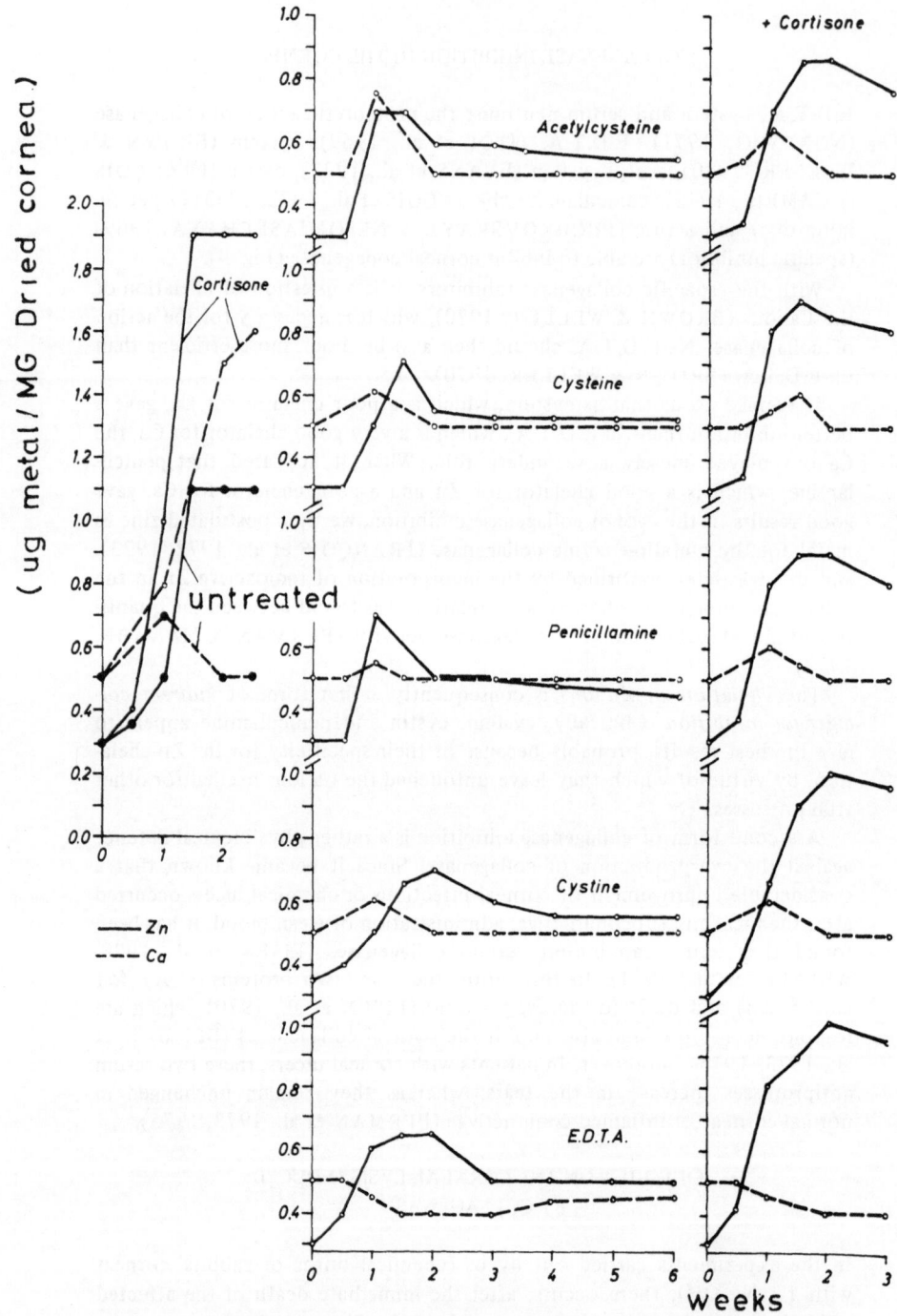

Fig. 4. Mean values of the metal content in the cornea measured by atomic absorption. On the left the values of the non-treated and corticoid (prednisolone acetate) treated corneas. In the middle the values of corneas treated by different chelators. On the right the values of the corneas treated by different chelators in association with corticoids (prednisolone-acetate).

12

Histologically we see that after a severe chemical burn, the keratocytes are destroyed, whereas after a slight chemical burn, the keratocytes can survive the injury. Therefore, the more active the cell remains, the lesser the collagenase production, and the greater the destruction of the cell, the greater the collagenase production. The keratocytes are, consequently, also of no or little importance in the production of collagenase.

When we review the literature, we see that all the publications concentrate on these two cells, namely epithelial cells and keratocytes. FRANÇOIS et al. (1973) were the first to stress the correlation between the granulocyte infiltration and the collagenase production. It is evident that the leucocytes introduced the collagenases which are responsible for the lysis and neither the epithelial cells nor the keratocytes. The administration of cortisone increases the granulocyte infiltration and accelerates the liquefaction of the cornea, whereas the administration of penicillamine reduces and even prevents the granulocyte infiltration (Fig. 5). There is consequently a clear correlation between the lysis and the infiltration of granulocytes, which we were able to demonstrate histologically. By means of the scanning and transmission electron microscope, we found that the lysis occurs in particular at the level of the wall of the granulocytes, where the lysosomal structures clearly increase during the lysis process (FRANÇOIS & CAMBIE, 1975) (Fig. 6). Epithelium and connective-tissue collagenases play an unimportant part and this in contrast with the active collagenase secretion of the granulocytes (VAES, 1969).

A second important point to which no attention has been paid, is that collagenase extracted from a lysing cornea never liquefies an intact cornea, whereas it does so when the mucopolysaccharide sheath around the stroma fibrillae is destroyed (1% NaOH). The mucopolysaccharides consequently play a much greater part than has up to now been attributed to them in counteracting connective tissue liquefaction.

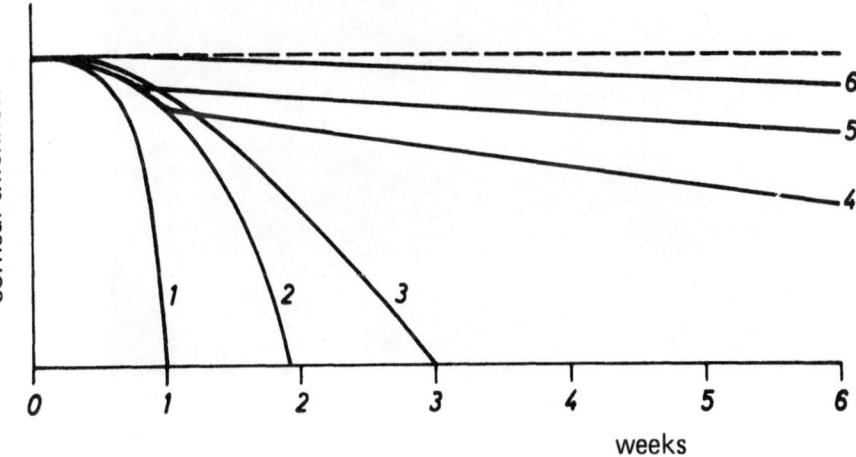

Fig. 5. Diagram of the corneal liquefaction: (2) normal evolution, (1) after administration of corticoids, (3) after administration of Cleland's reagens, (6) after administration of penicillamine from the beginning, (5) after the 3rd day and (4) after the 1st week.

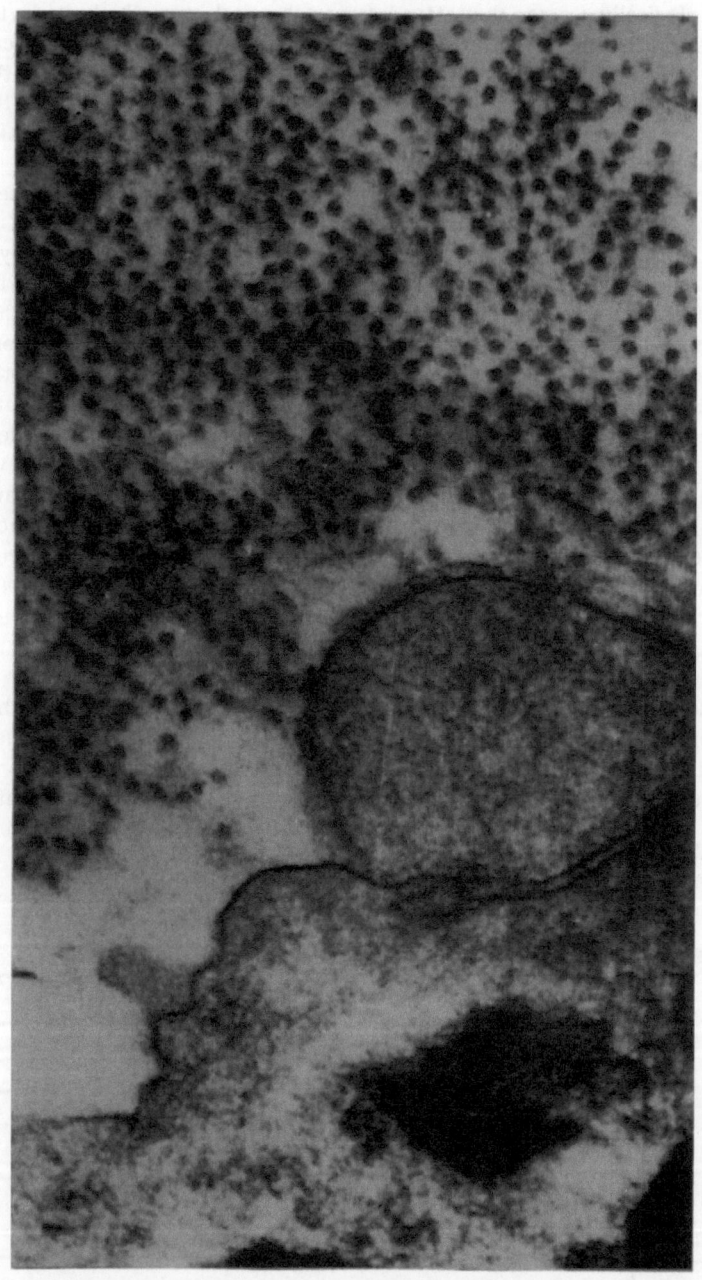

Fig. 6. Electronmicroscope. Aspect 10 days after the chemical burning of the cornea. The lysis is obviously situated around the white blood cells.

14

Another important clinical experience is that, in the case of good neo-vascularisation of the cornea, the ulcer either perforates less frequently or, after perforation, simply closes again. This indicates the presence of an important antiprotease factor in the serum.

In the case of corneal ulcers, we must consequently administer locally not only an indirect (chelator) collagenase inhibitor, but also a direct collagenase inhibitor (serum, fresh blood or the specific antiprotease). The harmful effect of the corticosteroids in the case of corneal ulcers lies consequently only in the fact that they promote the granulocyte invasion and increase the collagenase acitivity.

SUMMARY

The granulocytes are the most important producers of collagenase in the ulcered cornea. Epithelium cells and keratocytes play no part in the production of the collagenase during the process of perforation.

Zinc chelators play a part in the inhibition of the metalloenzyme collagenase. Moreover, penicillamine and cystin counteract the leucocyte migration in the damaged cornea, which gives them, besides their chelating, also an anti-inflammatory action.

The antiproteases (α1-antitrypsin and α2-macroglobulin) inhibit the corneal as well as the leucocyte collagenases. In the case of corneal ulcers they favour the healing of an ulcer by their increased concentration in the tears.

Penicillamine appears, up to now, to be the best indirect collagenase inhibitor and has, besides the Zn chelation, also an important anti-inflammatory action.

REFERENCES

BERMAN, M.B., BARBER, J.C., TALAMO, R.C. & LANGLEY, C.E. Corneal ulceration and the serum antiproteases. I. α_1-Antitripsin. *Invest. Ophthal.*, 12, 759-770, 1973.

BERMAN, M.B., GORDON, J., GARCIA, L.A. & GRACE, J. Corneal ulceration and the serum antiproteases. II. Complexes of corneal collagenases and α_2-macroglobulins. *Exp. Eye Res.*, 20, 231-244, (1975).

BERMAN, M.B., KERZA-KWIATECKI, A.P. & DAVISON, P.F. Characterisation of human corneal collagenase. *Exp. Eye Res.*, 11, 255, (1973).

BERMAN, M.B. & MANABE, R. Corneal collagenases: evidence for zinc metalloenzymes. *Annals of Ophthal.*, 5, 1193-1209, (1973).

BROWN, S.I. Collagenase and corneal ulcers. *Invest. Ophthal.*, 10, 203-209, (1971).

BROWN, S.I. & WELLER, C.A. Cell origin of collagenase in normal and wounded corneas. *Arch. Ophthal.*, 83, 74-77, (1970).

BROWN, S.I. & WELLER, C.A. Collagenase inhibitors in the prevention of ulcers of alkali-burned cornea. *Arch. Ophthal.*, 83, 352-353, (1970).

BROWN, S.I., WELLER, C.A. & WASSERMAN, H.G. Collagenolytic acitivity of alkali-burned corneas. *Arch. Ophthal.*, 81, 370-373, (1969).

DAVISON, P.F. & BERMAN, M. Corneal collagenase: specific cleavage of types $(\alpha 1)_2$ α_2 and $(\alpha 1)_3$ collagens. *Connective Tissue Res.*, 2, 57-64, (1973).

DRAKE, M.P., DAVISON, P.F., BUMP, S. & SCHMITT, F.O. Action of proteolytic enzymes on tropocollagen and insoluble collagen. *Biochemistry*, 5, 301-307, (1966).

EISEN, A.Z., BAUER, E.A. & JEFFREY, J.J. Animal and human collagenases. *J. Invest. Dermatol.*, 55, 359. (1970).

15

EVANS, R.M., MC CRARY III. J.A. & CHRISTENSEN, G. Mucomyst (acetylcysteine) in the treatment of corneal alkali burns. *Ann. Ophthal.*, 4, *320-328*, (1972).

FRANÇOIS, J. & CAMBIE, E. Collagenase and the collagenase inhibitors in torpid ulcers of the cornea. *Ophthalmic Res.*, 3, *145-159*, (1972).

FRANÇOIS, J. & CAMBIE, E. Unpublished data, (1975).

FRANÇOIS, J., CAMBIE, E., FEHER, J. & VAN DEN EECKHAUT, E. Penicillamine in the treatment of alkali-burned corneas. *Ophth. Res.*, 4, *223-236*, (1972/73).

FRANÇOIS, J., CAMBIE, E., FEHER, J. & VAN DEN EECKHOUT, E. Collagenase inhibitors (Penicillamine). *Ann. Ophthal.*, 5, *391-408*, (1973).

GALLOP, P.M., SUFTER, S. & MEILMAN, I. Studies on collagen. I. The partial purification, assay and mode of activation of bacterial collagenases. *J. Biol. Chem.*, 227, *891*, (1957).

GROSS, J. & LAPIERE, C.M. Collagenolytic activity in amphibian tissue: a tissue culture assay. *Proc. Nat. Acad. Sci., Wash.*, 48, *1014-1022*, (1962).

GROSS, J. & NAGAI, Y. Specific degradation of the collagen molecule by tadpole collagenolytic enzyme. *Proc. Nat. Acad. Sci., Wash.*, 54, *1197-1204*, (1965).

ITOI, M., GNÄDINGER, M.C., SLANSKY, H.H. & DOHLMAN, C.H. Prévention d'ulceres du stroma de la cornée grâce à l'utilisation d'un sel de calcium d'E.D.T.A. *Arch. Ophtal.*, 29, *389-392*, (1969).

KANG, A.H., NAGAI, Y., PIEZ, K.A. & GROSS, J. Studies on the structure of collagen utilizing a collagenolytic enzyme from tadpoles. *Biochemistry*, 5, *509-515*, (1966).

LAPIERE, C.M. & GROSS, J. Animal collagenases and collagen metabolism. Ed. Soganaes. Mechanisms of hard tissue destruction. *Amer. Ass. Adv. Sci., Washington D.C.*, 75, *663-694*, (1963).

MANDL, I. Collagenase. Gordon and Breach, Science Publishers. New York, (1972).

NORDWIG, A. Collagenolytic enzymes. In: Advances in enzymology. Ed. F. Nord. Interscience Publishers, New-York, vol. 34, 155-205, (1971).

PUCHKOVSKAYA, N.A. & NEPOMIESHCHAYA, V.M. Basic tactics in the treatment of severe ocular burns. *Oftalmol. Zh.*, 24, *486*, (1969).

PUZ, K.A., EIGNER, E.A. & LEWIS, M.S. The chromatographic separation and aminoacid composition of the subunits of several collagens. *Biochemistry*, 2, *58*, (1963).

RAMACHANDRAN, G.S. Chemistry of collagen vol. I. Academic Press, London, (1967).

SLANCKY, H.H. Collagenolytic activity in corneal epithelium. Ass. Res. Ophthal., Nat. Meeting, Chicago, Oct. (1968).

SLANSKY, H.H. & DOHLMAN, C.H. Collagenase and the cornea. *Survey of Ophthal.*, 14, *402-416*. (1970).

SLANSKY, H.H., FREEMAN, M.I. & ITOI, M. Collagenolytic activity in bovine corneal epithelium. *Arch. Ophthal.*, 80, *496-498*, (1968).

SLANSKY, H.H., GNÄDINGER, M.C., ITOI, M. & DOHLMAN, C.H. Collagenase in corneal ulcerations. *Arch. Ophthal.*, 82, *108-111*, (1969).

VAES, G. Lysosomes and the cellular physiology of bone resorption. *Frontiers in Biology*, 14A, *217-243*, (1969).

WELLER, C.H., BROWN, S.I. & IWANIJ, W. Characterization and inhibition of corneal collagenase. *Invest. Ophthal.*. 10, *496*, (1971).

Key Words: Collagenase (corneal); Collagenase-inhibitors; Cornea.

Author's address
J. François
Graaf de Smet de Naeyerplein 15
Ghent
Belgium

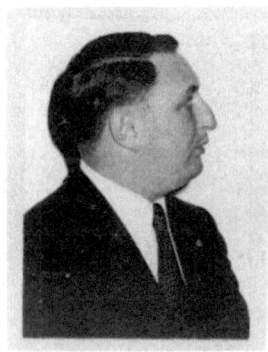

TECHNICAL ADVANCES IN CORNEAL TRANSPLANTATION

J. DRAEGER

(Bremen, Germany)

Very early, even before having solved the biological problems of corneal grafting, attempts were made to improve the cutting technique by means of motorized instruments. The aim was to make use of the smoother movement of a rotating trephine, to avoid the discontinuity of manual trephination, causing irregular wound edges. The surgeon's fingertips not only had to guide the trephine, but also to cut by rotating it. VON HIPPEL was the first to try a motorized trephine (Fig. 1).

VON HIPPEL considered the continuous motion of the blade superior to the discontinuous manual cutting technique.

LÖHLEIN (Fig. 2) tried to improve this instrument by use of an electric motor.

Quite a number of similar instruments was designed later on; however, none of them has found its way into clinical use. This was especially due to

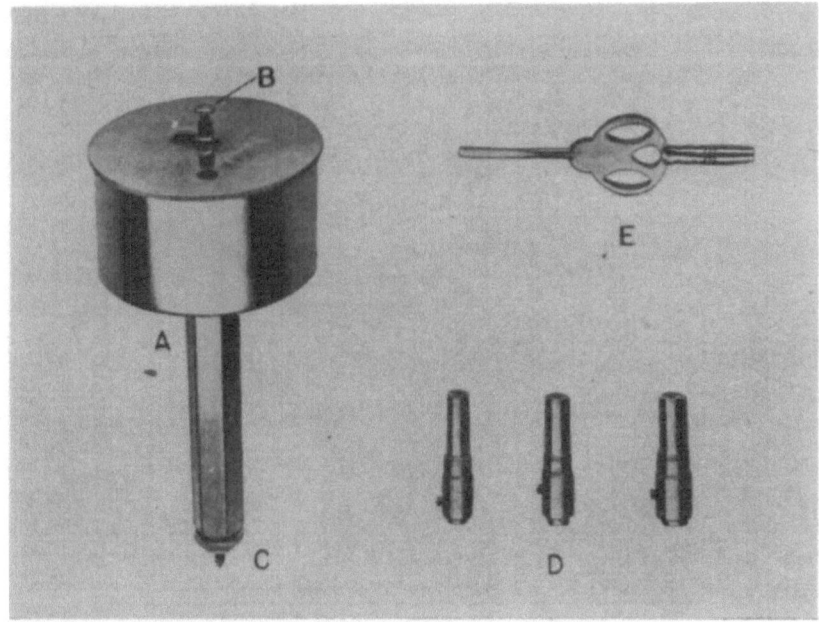

Fig. 1. Clock spring driven trephine by V. HIPPEL.

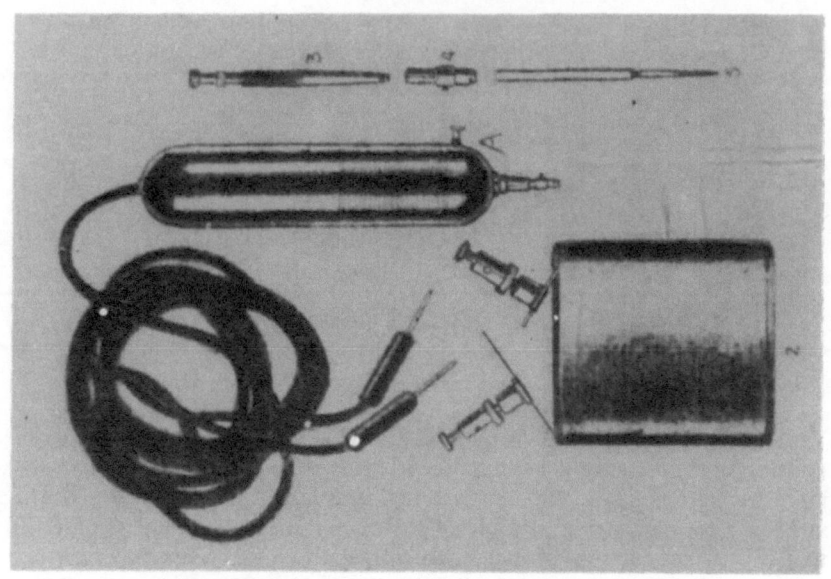

Fig. 2. Electric motor driven trephine by LÖHLEIN.

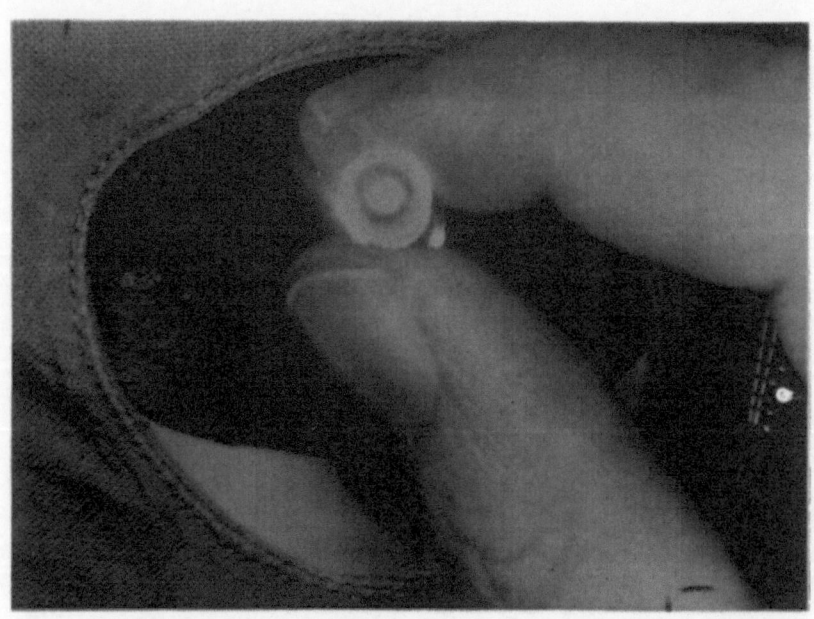

Fig. 3. Poor observation of surgical field using manual trephine.

the big diameter of all these instruments: Under the microscope the surgeon was not able to overlook the actual field of surgery (Fig. 3).

Under vertical observation trephine and fingertips cover the direct view, under oblique observation the foot of the trephine hides the opposite side of the blade. Therefore, an instrument was needed, which enables the surgeon's hand to perform precise incisions and on the other hand to have perfect optical control of the surgical field (Fig. 4).

The very low instrument approaches the eye from the side; handle and gear are outside the microscopical field (Fig. 5). So under vertical observation the corneal surface inside the trephine can be controlled (Fig. 6).

Appropriate illumination is helpful using these new instruments: Oblique illumination produces a cast shadow, which allows a good control of the depth of the anterior chamber. On the other hand, coaxial light illuminates the interior of the trephine allowing a perfect control of the button. The new microscope can easily be switched to the appropriate angle.

Besides better optical control a very low cutting pressure was the unexpected advantage of the new system. Experimental studies were performed to prove the correlation between cutting speed and pressure transmitted to the tissue. Experimental incisions were made on 108 pig's eyes and 18 enucleated human eyes. The eyes were mounted to the scale of an electronic precision balance (Fig. 7).

The action of the blade was observed through a standard surgical zoom microscope, magnification 10-15 times. All incisions had to be made under vertical direction, the light pointer deflection and the time elapsed were recorded. As the shape of an incision is also dependent on the intraocular pressure this was controlled by a handapplanation tonometer and a manometric gauge.

Incisions were performed in 3 pressure ranges: Below 10 mm Hg, between 10-20 mm Hg, and above 30 mm Hg. An unexpectedly close correlation between the cutting speed of the blade and the cutting pressure was

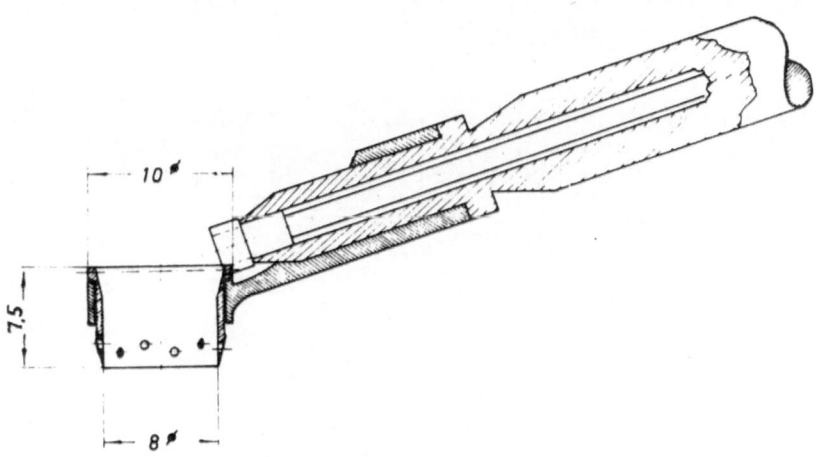

Fig. 4. Rotary trephine, cross section.

found: Increasing the cutting speed 10 times means decreasing the cutting pressure to a tenth! This inverse proportion was found in all 3 pressure ranges! This is clinically especially important in soft eyes where not too much cutting pressure can be used. Motorized instruments allow precise incisions under even less favourable conditions. The little motor turns up to 18000 RPM, and due to the gear ratio 275 revolutions are achieved. This means

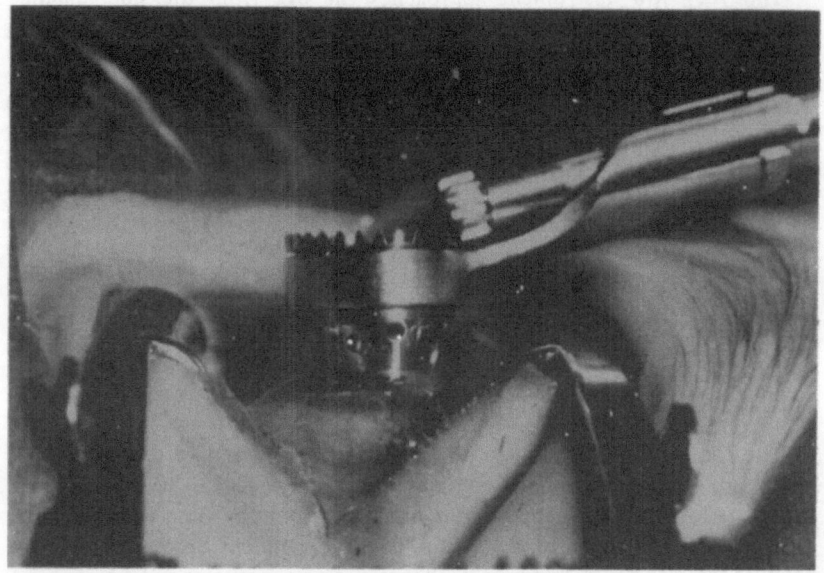

Fig. 5. Rotary trephine, side view.

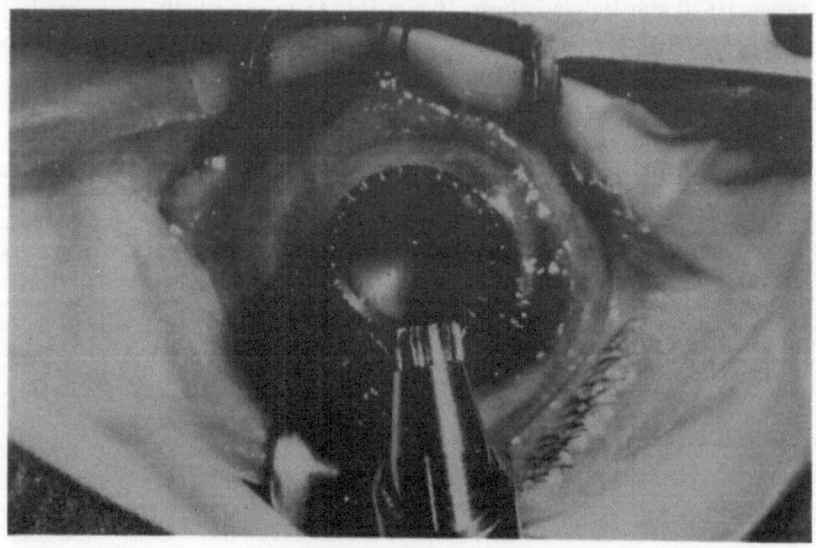

Fig. 6. Rotary trephine observed through microscope.

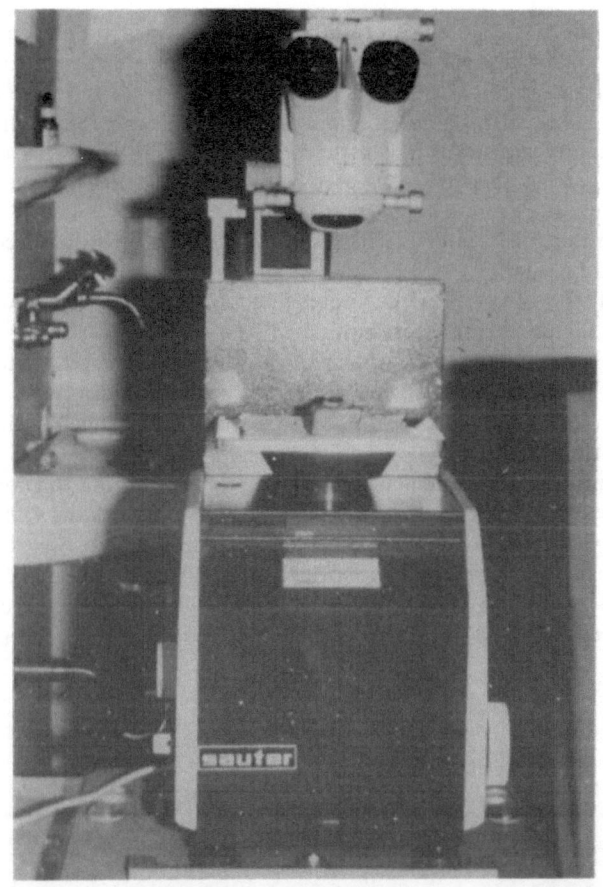

Fig. 7. Balance and microscope.

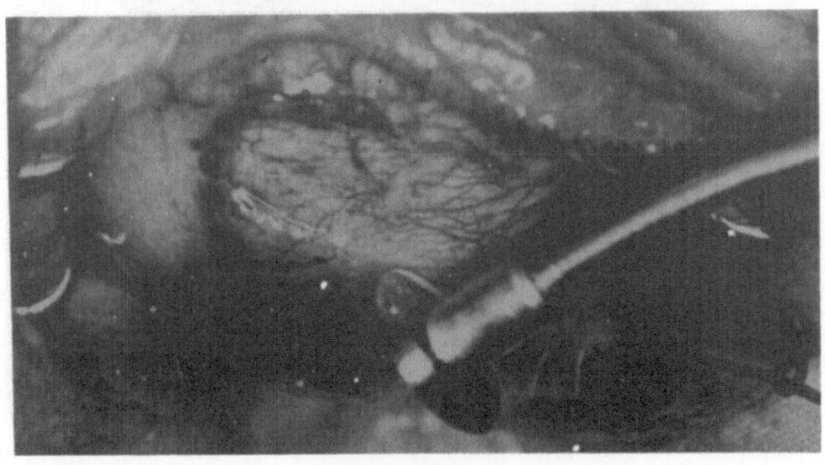

Fig. 8. Rotary knife.

0.1 m/sec speed of the blade or 600 cm/min, which is more than 10 times the speed of any manual instrument. Needing 42 p using a manual trephine only 3 p transferred to the eye by a rotary trephine of the same diameter using the same cutting time of about 20 sec are needed. These differences are even more marked using a little rotary knife (Fig. 8), which needs less than 1 p cutting pressure compared with 37.7 p applied by the sharpest razor blade.

Due to the adhesion at the flanks of the blade an opposite force reduces the pressure needed.

A small rotary keratome facilitates punctate incisions, also needing only a tenth of the usual cutting pressure.

Speed and torque can be changed by using different gears and also by changing the voltage on the panel of the microsurgical unit.

The surgeon can start and stop the action of the instruments without the least vibration.

When performing a lamellar graft the dissection in both the donor's and the recipient's eye is even more difficult than in a perforating graft. Several attempts were made to facilitate the lamellar dissection (Fig. 9).

Like a hair clipper oscillating motions of the blade are used to dissect the tissue. No doubt the cutting pressure is also decreased, but the discontinuous movement does not allow completely smooth wound edges. Besides

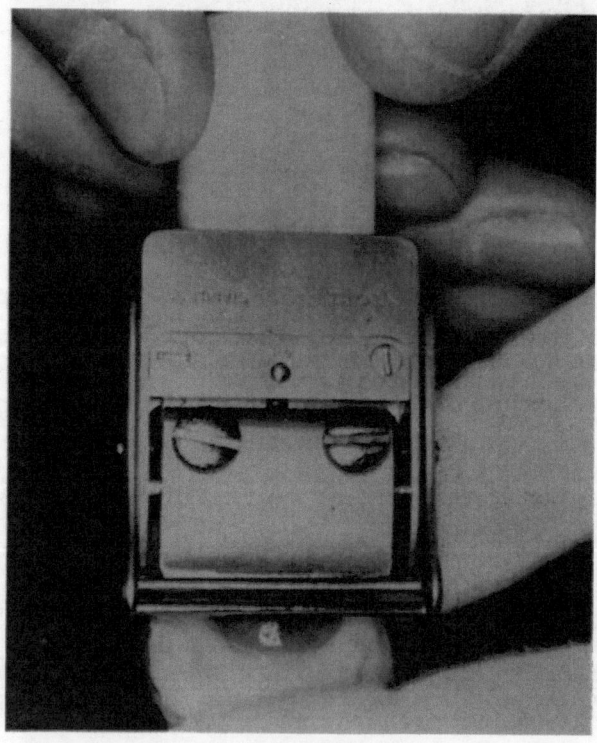

Fig. 9. Castroviejo lamellar keratome.

this, depth and direction of the incision are not precisely controlled as the instrument has to be guided manually.

Another problem has to be overcome in lamellar grafting: The lateral wound edges of the button also have to be marked. This means a second procedure, using a trephine with internal guide to mark the circumference of the button as well as the thickness of the lamella to be dissected. By

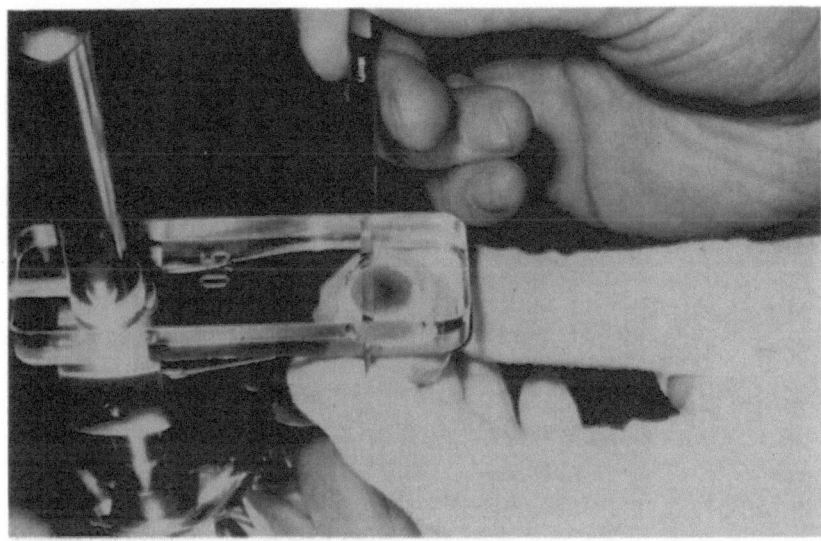

Fig. 10. HALLERMANN's device for lamellar dissection from donor's eye.

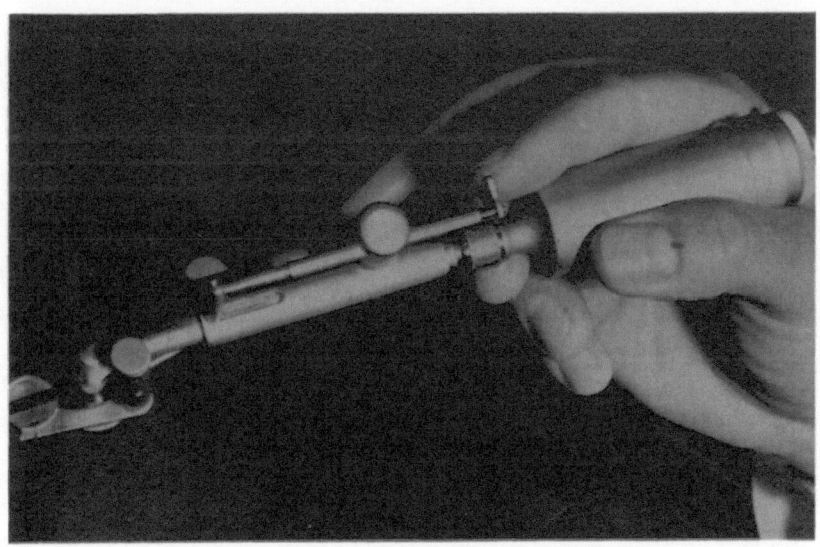

Fig. 11. Automatic lamellar keratome.

manual dissection it is very difficult to obtain a lamella of equal thickness with smooth surface.

Using HALLERMANN's device (Fig. 10) at least at the donor's eye a better quality can be achieved.

It is obvious that this technique cannot be used in the recipient's eye.

Therefore, our aim was to design a simple instrument, which could be used on both the donor's and the recipient's eye assuring a lamella of exactly the same thickness and diameter (Fig. 11).

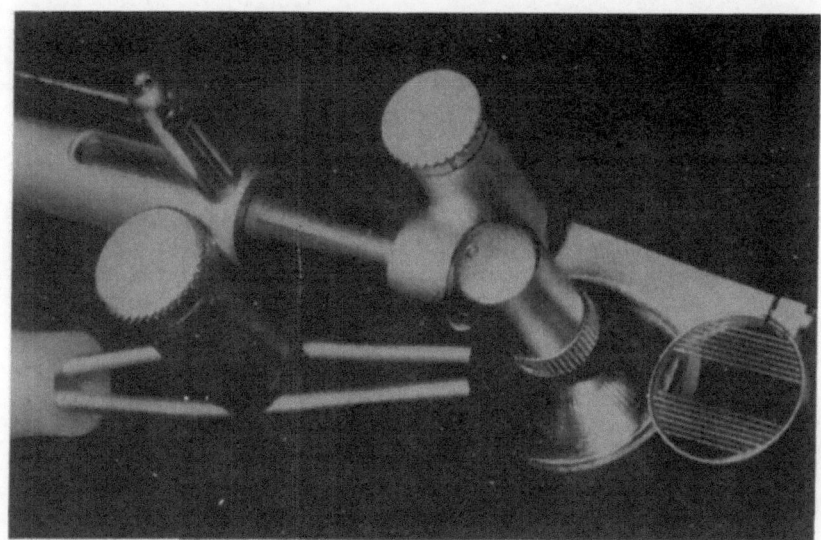

Fig. 12. Rotary blade, 2 micrometer controls.

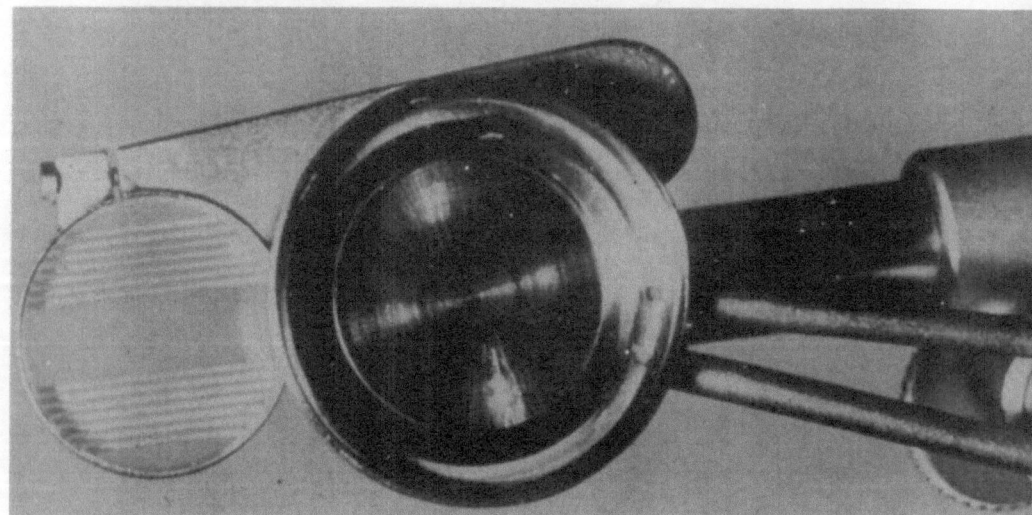

Fig. 13. Rotary blade, suction ring.

Using the same rotary principle as mentioned earlier, a little instrument was designed, the blade of which is rotating continuously. The position of the blade is determined by means of a suction ring, which keeps the instrument to the limbus; the vacuum is applied from the microsurgical unit. Two micrometers allow adjustment of the thickness and the diameter of the lamella (Fig. 12).

To reduce the capillary adhesion at the flanks of the blade, irrigation is provided onto the blade's edge. Because of the small dimensions the instrument can be used both on the donor's as well as on the recipient's eye. Therefore, thickness and diameter of the two dissected lamellas are exactly equal. Without any further step the graft can be directly used. The smooth surface of the wound edges guarantee optimal optical conditions. When healing – scar formation is reduced to a minimum.

Summarizing five years of experience with motorized cutting instruments in corneal grafting we hope that our new method means an improvement in the performance of these difficult and delicate procedures.

REFERENCES

DRAEGER, J. Neue Schneidetechnik in der Mikrochirurgie. *Klin. Mbl. Augenheilk.* 159, *293-303*, (1971).

DRAEGER, J. Ein neuer Motortrepan für die Keratoplastik. *Ber. dtsch. Ophthal. Ges.* 71, *318-322*, (1972).

DRAEGER J. & HACKELBUSCH, R. Experimentelle Untersuchungen und klinische Erfahrungen mit neuen Rotor-Instrumenten. *Ophthalmologica* 164, *273-283*, (1972).

DRAEGER, J. Ein Halbautomatisches elektrisches Keratom für die lamelläre Keratoplastik. *Klin. Mbl. Augenheilk.*, im Druck.

Author's address:
Zentralkrankenhaus
Augenklinik
St. Jürgen-Strasse
Bremen
Germany

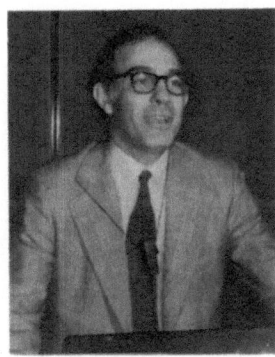

RECURRENT CORNEAL EROSION

A.J. BRON & N.A.P. BROWN*

(Oxford and London, England)

Recurrent corneal erosion is a disorder of epithelial adherence. It is common and familiar and in the majority of patients it is the first sign of corneal disease in that individual. In many it is secondary to trauma, in a few it is secondary to existing corneal disease. Inheritance of recurrent erosion has in the past been regarded as rare, but we may in time have to revise that opinion. In the last five years a cluster of biomicroscopic features in the cornea have been found in the recurrent erosion syndrome and are thought to be of causative significance.

INCIDENCE AND PRECIPITATION

It is difficult to find data on the incidence of recurrent erosion following trauma. GUYARD & PERDRIEL (1961) saw no recurrences in 40 abrasions. JACKSON (1961) saw one recurring in 150. The condition is evidently not a common event after trauma and it is natural that some effort has been made to establish a predisposing factor, such as the mode of injury. In a recent study (BROWN & BRON, 1975 in press) of 80 patients with recurrent erosion, 83% of those related to trauma were secondary to injury with organic material (finger nails being responsible for over half, the rest represented by claws, twigs, paper or card); 17% were due to a metallic object, foreign body, or in one case contact lens wear. However, it is significant that recurrent erosion was unrelated to trauma in 40%.

FORM OF EROSION

The existence of the non-traumatic group of recurrent erosion, which is well accepted, again suggests that affected individuals might be predisposed to a loosening of their corneal epithelium, either as a spontaneous event, or in response to trivial or specific trauma. CHANDLER (1945) noted two forms of clinical erosion; a macroform characterised by a severe attack with frank epithelial loss, and a microform characterised by less severe discomfort, though more frequent attacks, and the presence of clusters of epithelial dots, without frank loss of epithelium. He noted that the microform was more common in the spontaneous group of recurrent erosion patients. We

* Mr Brown is from the Institute of Ophthalmology, London.

have confirmed these findings in two studies (BRON & BROWN 1971, BROWN & BRON 1975). In the most recent, 56% of recurrent erosion patients showed the microform, 13% the macroform, and 31% showed a mixed picture with one or other form in different attacks. The pure microform was almost twice as common in the spontaneous group of recurrent erosion (i.e. 42% of patients in the traumatic group, 78% in the spontaneous group.)

TABLE I

80 patients presenting with recurrent erosion (BROWN & BRON 1975(b))

Age: Range 24 – 73 years.   Mean age 42 years.
Sex: M/F 1:0.9

Traumatic: 60%
Non-traumatic: 40%

Microform erosion 56%
Macroform erosion 13%
Mixed forms   31%

	Percentage of cases with microform
Traumatic Group	42%
Non-traumatic group	78%

Patients with fingerprints, blebs, nets or maps	59%
(66% of these cases bilateral)	
Patients with microcystic changes	59%
Patients with neither change	11%
Eyes with fingerprints, blebs, nets or maps	49%
Control eyes with fingerprints, blebs, nets, maps	
or cysts (See text)	5%

This difference in clinical behaviour might imply a difference of mechanism between the two groups, no doubt with some overlap between the two.

AETIOLOGICAL FACTORS

Until recently the aetiological basis for recurrent erosion syndrome, other than trauma, was unknown. Even to invoke trauma as a cause was unsatisfactory since this did not explain the low frequency of recurrent erosions considering the high incidence of traumatic erosions themselves. The most promising lead derived from a few reports of dominantly inherited recurrent erosion (FRANCESCHETTI 1928), which at least implied that recurrent erosion could be due to an inherited defect in epithelial adherence. Similar arguments applied to reports of recurrent erosion in relatives of patients with lattice corneal dystrophy (HERMANN 1946). Other disorders in which recurrent erosive events were well known included the classical inherited corneal dystrophies (REIS BUCKLER's, macular, lattice and to some extent granular dystrophy), (BRON & TRIPATHI 1971) Here, as in metaherpetic keratitis (KAUFMAN 1964) and bullous keratopathy, the erosive attacks were related to well-defined clinical and histopathological entities affecting the epithelium and/or Bowman's layer of the stroma, so that it was less

28

difficult to accept that epithelial adherence might become disturbed in these conditions. In recurrent erosion syndrome there appeared to be no antecedent corneal disease.

Within the last decade it has become clear that the majority of recurrent erosion cases occur in predisposed subjects and it is possible that this predisposition is inherited. The first indication was from a paper by KAUFMAN & CLOWER (1966) in which an association was found between recurrent erosion and fingerprint lines of the cornea, in addition to other changes at the level of Bowman's layer. VOGT (1930) had himself identified such lines in relation to recurrent erosion, though their significance had not been stressed. The term fingerprint lines was coined by GUERRY who described them in detail in 1950. Epithelial dots or microcysts were recognised as a part of the disorder in the active or healed state before KAUFMAN & CLOWER's study and were discussed by CHANDLER (1945).

In 1971 BRON & BROWN described 40 patients, of whom the youngest was 39, who showed unusual changes in their superficial corneae including epithelial microcysts, fingerprint lines and curious bleb and net-like patterns in the sub-epithelial region. 39% of the patients had symptoms of recurrent erosion. The changes were bilateral in 73% which suggested that this was a dystrophic or degenerative disorder predisposing to recurrent erosion.

TABLE II

40 patients presenting with a superficial corneal disorder (Bleb, net and fingerprint pattern) (BRON & BROWN 1971)

Age: Range 39 – 81 years.   Mean age 57 years.
Sex: M/F 1:1.5

Bilateral: 73%
Recurrent erosion: 39%

TROBE & LAIBSON (1972), in a study of 35 patients of similar age and sex distribution, added another clinical feature to the disorder. They noted a high incidence of recurrent erosion (60%) in association with epithelial dots (or cysts), fingerprint lines and map-like changes. The grey intra-epithelial maps had been observed by GUERRY (1965) as part of the epithelial microcystic disorder of COGAN (COGAN et al. 1964). TROBE & LAIBSON regard COGAN's microcystic disorder as part of the picture in their cases of recurrent erosion. LAIBSON & KRACHMER (1974) have since described the familial occurrence of these changes. The original patients described by COGAN et al. (1974) with microcystic disorder had been relatively asymptomatic, complaining of blurring or minor irritative symptoms.

A new picture of recurrent erosion syndrome has thus emerged, in which it is conceived that the erosive attacks occur in a background of a distinctive superficial corneal disorder (S.C.D.). These changes may be described briefly.

The fingerprint lines are arranged in a concentric whorl-like pattern. They are fine, refractile and best seen by retro-illumination. They raise up the epithelium in their neighbourhood so that tear thinning is seen over them. Other lines may be seen of similar appearance on retro-illumination but of differing configuration, forming rings, or arranged in a crazed pattern. These forms are uncommon, but a more common form is a demarcation line which separates off an area of fingerprints or blebs from clear areas (BROWN & BRON 1976).

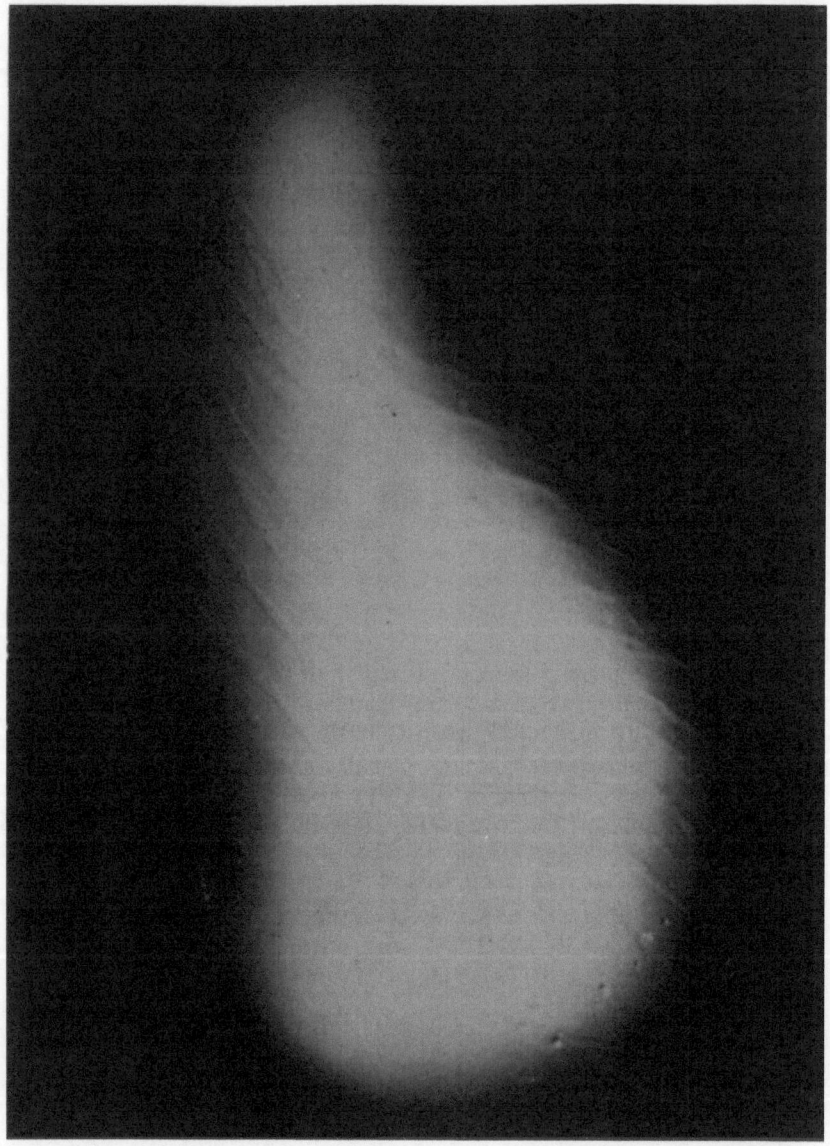

Fig. 1. Fingerprint lines of the cornea. Retroillumination photograph.

The bleb pattern is an appearance like that of pebbled glass, seen best by retro-illumination against the red reflex. It is rarely visible in focal illumination. Large areas of the cornea may be affected by the change. At times a more sparse but geometric arrangement is present in which the blebs are organised in a polygonal network corresponding to the anterior corneal mosaic. This net pattern may also be created by an arrangement of parallel bars or lines (BRON & BROWN 1971).

Fig. 2. (a) Bleb pattern. Retroillumination photograph. (b) Net pattern. Retroillumination photograph.

The map pattern consists of a patchy disturbance of the corneal epithelium with irregular geographical margins. Here and there there are clear zones whose borders may be more regular.

The characteristic epithelial cysts associated with the map pattern are the opaque putty grey microcysts originally described by COGAN et al. (1964) as part of their microcystic disorder, and later shown by GUERRY (1965) to be related to the map pattern. They may reach a size of over one millimeter in diameter and usually do not take fluorescein stain. Other epithelial cysts seen in recurrent erosion syndrome are more irregular in shape, may

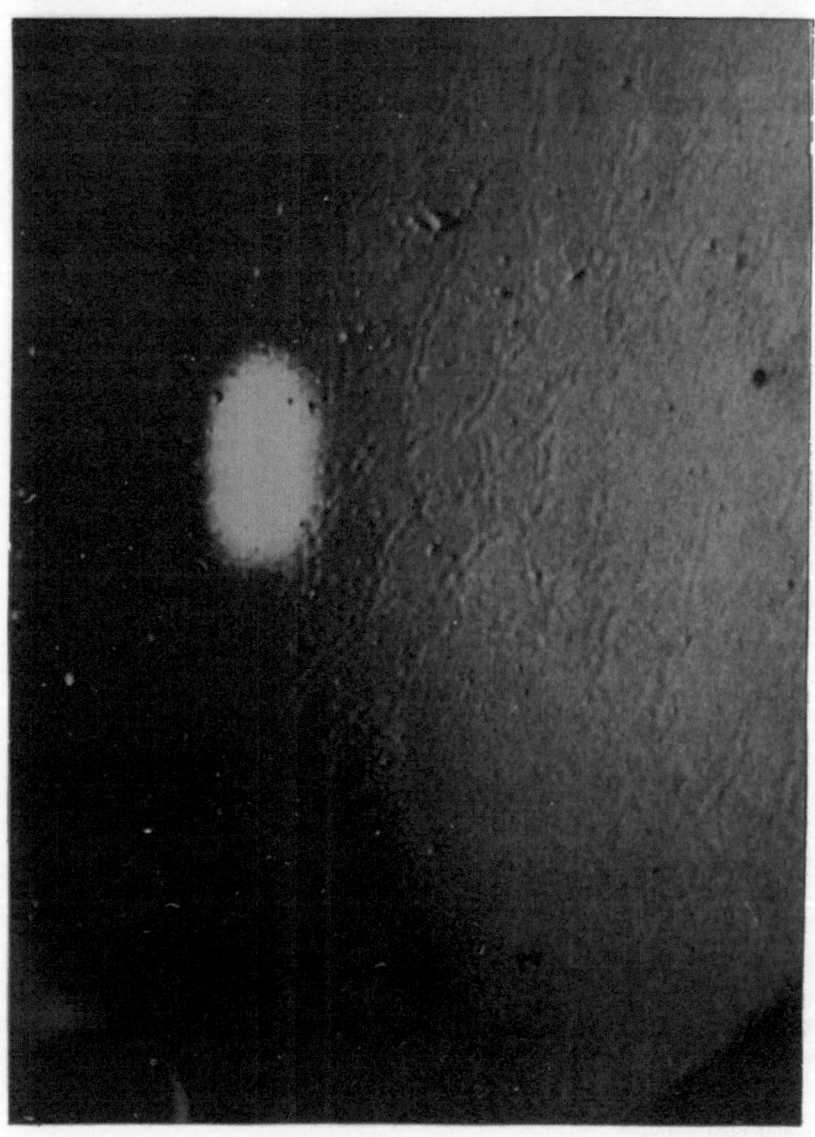

form conglomerate arrangements and often take up fluorescein stain. They sometimes appear in focal showers during an erosion attack.

The superficial corneal changes described above are more often bilateral than unilateral. In a given eye any one of the changes may be seen alone, or they may be found in varying combinations. The eye showing such changes may never have given rise to recurrent erosion symptoms. Indeed it may be the asymptomatic fellow eye in a patient with unilateral recurrent erosion.

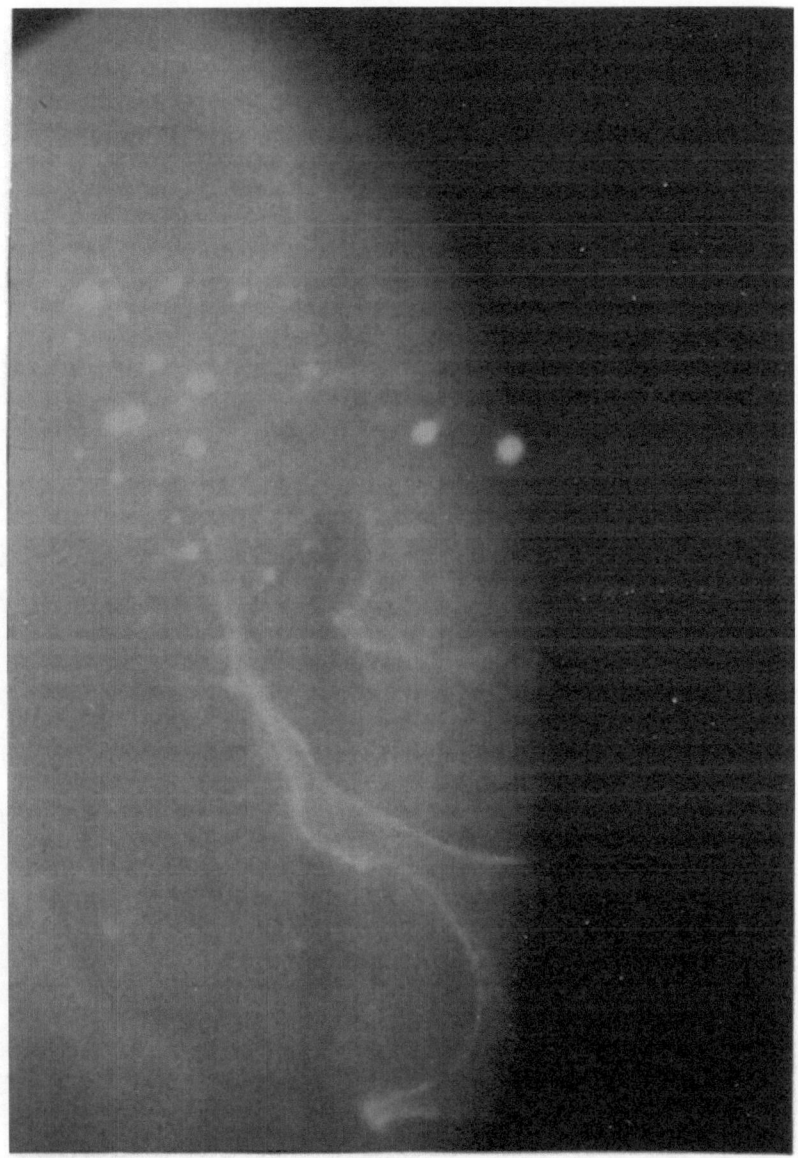

Fig. 3. Grey map-like changes in the corneal epithelium with numerous opaque micro-cysts of the Cogan type.

The relationship between these changes and recurrent erosion is brought out by a recent study (BROWN & BRON 1975(b)). A group of 100 control patients without symptoms of external eye disease were compared with 80 patients presenting with recurrent erosion. In the controls, 5% of the 200 eyes showed superficial corneal changes, including fingerprint lines (1.5%), blebs (2%), and microcysts (1.5%).

In the recurrent erosion group 49% of the 160 eyes were affected by

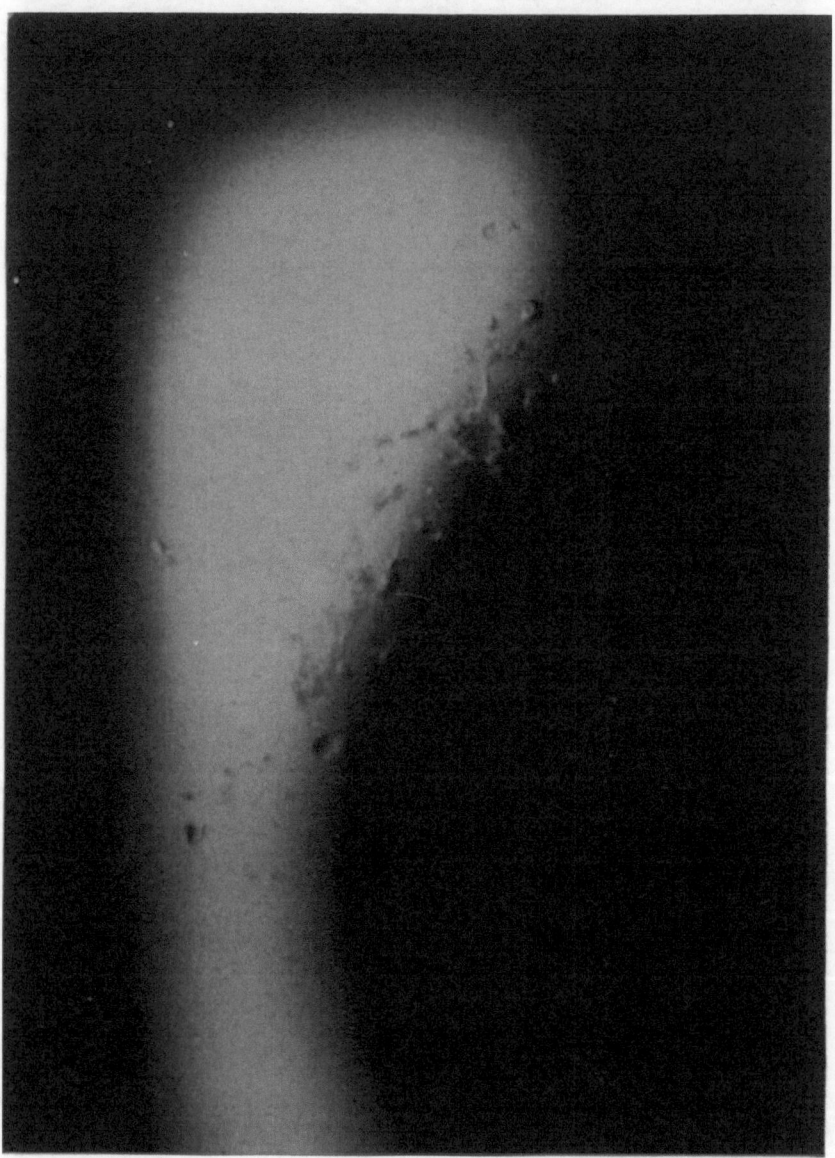

Fig. 4. Epithelial microcysts visible during a recurrent erosion attack. Note that the cysts are relatively empty and contain only a small proportion of cellular debris.

line, bleb (or net) and map changes. (The changes were bilateral in 66% of these, so that in fact 59% of patients showed such changes in at least one eye). In addition to this, 59% of the patients showed microcystic changes in at least one eye. (These changes were in the eye with the erosion only in 49% and in the unaffected eye in 24%.) In only 11% of all patients were there neither microcysts nor other superficial corneal changes in either eye.

MORPHOGENESIS OF CORNEAL LESIONS

There have been abundant reports of anomalous basement membrane-like material and of other connective tissue sheets both within and under the corneal epithelium in association with COGAN's microcystic disorder, both in the absence of clinical map-patterns (COGAN, DONALDSON, KUWA-BARA & MARSHALL 1964, and COGAN, KUWABARA, DONALDSON & COLLINS 1974) and in their presence (GUERRY 1975, WALTER & GEERAETS 1972, TRIPATHI & BRON 1973, RODRIGUES, FINE, LAIB-SON & ZIMMERMAN 1974, FOGLE, KENYON, STARK & GREEN 1975). BRODRICK, DARK & PEACE (1974) demonstrated the presence of a fibrillogranular material within intra- and sub-epithelial extensions in a patient with fingerprint lines. This material is assumed to be the product of disordered epithelial cells and lying sub-epithelially it may further disturb adhesion between epithelium and Bowman's membrane.

The extensive sheets of connective tissue material within the epithelium correspond to the grey maps seen biomicroscopically. The clear zones within the maps correspond to discontinuities in the intra-epithelial sheets. Our own observations (BRON & TRIPATHI 1973) and those of others (RODRIGUES, FINE, LAIBSON & ZIMMERMAN 1974) suggest that the typical opaque cysts of Cogan's microcystic disorder remain sequestered behind the anomalous basement membrane material for long periods, hindered in their movement to the surface by this barrier. This is thought to account for their large size and the persistence of cellular debris within them which is the reason for their opaque appearance. Those cysts which come to be next to fenestrations in, or on the edge of, such sheets, may obtain egress to the surface where they discharge their contents. At this point they may appear clear and take up stain.

MECHANISM OF RECURRENT EROSION

The relevance of basement membrane abnormalities to recurrent erosion has been clarified in recent years. KHOUDADOUST, SILVERSTEIN, KENYON & DOWLING (1968) showed experimentally the importance of basement membranes and of the hemidesmosomal attachment structures of the basal epithelium to epithelial adherence. A defective basement membrane was demonstrated in traumatic recurrent erosion by GOLDMAN, DOHLMAN & KRAVITZ (1969), and in spontaneous recurrent erosion by TRIPATHI & BRON (1972) who also noted an absence of hemidesmosomes in relation to affected basal cells. KENYON (1969) suggested that deficiencies in the formation of basement membrane complexes were responsible for the looseness of the epithelium in bullous keratopathy and more recently stressed that defective production of basement membrane, hemidesmosomes and attachment fibrils accounts for the erosive events encountered in REIS BUCKLERS' dystrophy, Cogan's microcystic dystrophy and non-traumatic recurrent erosion. (FOGLE, KENYON, STARK, & GREEN 1975).

LOWE has suggested that looseness of the corneal epithelium may be demonstrated in the healed cornea of recurrent erosion subjects by rotating a contact lens over the surface of the cornea to produce epithelial wrinkling (LOWE 1964 and 1970). This is apparently a harmless manoeuvre. What produces the acute attack is still not clear. The role of nocturnal epithelial oedema has been thoroughly studied by COGAN (1941) and is the basis for the current use of hyperosmotic topical agents at night. The role of lid contact and adhesion is uncertain but provides the rationale for the use of lubricants in the form of parolein and various oculents.

It has been the purpose of this paper to demonstrate that the majority of patients who present with recurrent erosion occur in a background of a distinctive underlying superficial corneal disorder (S.C.D.). It is essential to examine both corneae of affected patients with great care and to use retro-illumination with the pupil dilated. Knowledge of the predisposing condition is of great assistance in advising patients on the nature of their ocular problem.

SUMMARY

It is well recognised that only a small percentage of patients who develop corneal erosion go on to develop the recurrent erosion syndrome. However, recurrent erosion is a common and disabling disorder and recent studies suggest that the majority, particularly in the older age groups, are associated with specific antecedent disease of the superficial cornea. This presumably explains the fact that 40% of recurrent erosion cases are non-traumatic and that such 'spontaneous' cases are more likely to be bilateral. The superficial corneal dystrophies predisposing to recurrent corneal erosion are described in detail, together with their histopathological features. The management of recurrent corneal erosion is briefly discussed.

REFERENCES

BIETTI G.B. Contribution à la connaissance des dégénérescences cornéennes séniles. *Arch. Ophthal. (Paris)* 15: *37-42* (1965).
BRODRICK, J.D., DARK, A.J. & PEACE, W. Fingerprint dystrophy of the cornea. A histologic study. *Arch. Opthal.* 92: *483-489* (1974).
BRON, A.J. Anterior corneal mossaic. *Brit. J. Ophthal.* 52: *659-669* (1968).
BRON, A.J. & JONES, D.B. Net-like degeneration of Bowman's membrane. *Brit. J. Ophthal.* 53: *490-492* (1969).
BRON, A.J. & BROWN, N.A.P. Some superficial corneal disorders. *Trans. Ophthal. Soc. U.K.* 91: *13-29* (1971).
BRON, A.J. & TRIPATHI, R.C. Cogan's Epithelial Microcystic disorder. Presented at the autumn meeting of the A.E.R., Edinburgh (1973).
BROWN, N.A.P. Macrophotography of the anterior segment of the eye. *Brit. J. Ophthal.* 54: *697-701* (1970).
BROWN, N.A.P. Visibility of transparent objects in the eye by retroillumination. *Brit. J. Ophthal.* 55: *517-524* (1971).

BROWN, N.A.P. & BRON, A.J. Recurrent erosion of the cornea. *Amer. J. Ophthal.* (1975) (in press). (1975(b)) in preparation.
BROWN, N.A.P. & BRON, A.J. Superficial Corneal Lines. *Amer. J. Ophthal.* 81: *34-51* (1976).
BRÜCKNER, A. Kurze Mitteilungen. I. Entoptische Beobachtungen. II. Rezidivierende Erosion. *Ophthalmologica (Basel)* 120: *38-43* (1950).
CHANDLER, P.A. Recurrent erosion of cornea. *Amer. J. Ophthal.* 28: *355* (1945).
COGAN, D.G. Bullous Keratitis with particular reference to the pathology of experimental corneal vesiculation. *Arch. Ophthal.* 25: *941-968* (1941).
COGAN, D.G., DONALDSON, D. KUWABARA, T. & MARSHALL, D. Microcystic dystrophy of the corneal epithelium. *Trans. Amer. Ophthal. Soc.* 62: *213-225* (1964).
COGAN, D.G., KUWABARA, T., DONALDSON, D. & COLLINS, E. Microcystic dystrophy of the cornea. A partial explanation for its pathogenesis. *Arch. Ophthal.* 92: *470-474* (1974).
DARK, A., BRODRICK, J.D. & PEACE, G.W. IRCS Int. Comm. System (3) 24-2-1 (1973).
FLYNN, M.A & ESTERLY, D.B. Bilateral recurrent erosion of cornea. *Amer. J. Ophthal.* 62: *964-966* (1966).
FOGLE, J.A., KENYON, K.R. STARK, W.J. & GREEN, W.R. Defective epithelial adhesion in anterior corneal dystrophies. *Amer. J. Ophthal.* 79: *925-940* (1975).
FRANCESCHETTI, A. Hereditäre rezidivierendem Erosion der Hornhaut. *Z. Augenheilk.* 66: *309-316* (1928).
FRAUNFELDER, F.T., HANNA, C., CABLE, M. & HARDBERGER, R.E. Entrapment of ophthalmic ointment in the cornea. *Amer. J. Ophthal.* 76: *475-484* (1973).
GOLDMAN, J., DOHLAM, C. & KRAVITT, J. The basement membrane of the human cornea in recurrent epithelial erosion syndrome. *Trans. Amer. Acad. Ophthal. Otolaryng.* 73: *471-481* (1969).
GUERRY, D. Fingerprint lines in the cornea. *Amer. J. Ophthal.* 33: *724-726* (1950).
GUERRY, D. Observations on Cogan's microcystic dystrophy of the corneal epithelium. *Trans. Amer. Ophthal. Soc.* 63: *320-334* (1965).
GUYARD, M. & PERDRIEL, G. A propos du traitement des erosions récidivantes de la cornée. *Bul. Soc. Ophthal. Paris* 7-8: *579-582* (1961).
HANNA, C., FRAUNFELDER, F.T., CABLE, M. & HARDBERGER, R.E. The effect of ophthalmic ointments on corneal wound healing. *Amer. J. Ophthal.* 76: *193-200* (1973).
HERMANN, C. La dystrophie grillagée de la cornée. *Ophthalmologica* 112: *350* (1946).
JACKSON, H. Effect of eye-pads on healing of simple corneal abrasions. *Brit. Med. J.* 2: *713* (1960).
KAUFMAN, H.E. Epithelial erosion syndrome: metaherpetic keratitis. *Amer. J. Ophthal.* 57: *983-987* (1964).
KAUFMAN, H.E. & CLOWER, J.W. Irregularities of Bowman's membrane. *Amer. J. Ophthal.* 61: *227-230* (1966).
KENYON K.R. The synthesis of basement membrane by the corneal epithelium in bullous keratopathy. *Invest. Ophthal.* 8: *156-168* (1969).
KHOUDADOUST, A.A., SILVERSTEIN, A.M., KENYON, K.R. & DOWLING, J.E. Adhesion of regenerating corneal epithelium. The role of basement membrane. *Amer. J. Ophthal.* 65: *339-348* (1968).
KING, R.G. JR. & GEERAETS, R. Cogan Guerry microcystic corneal epithelial dystrophy: a clinical and electron microscopic study. *Med. Coll. Va. Quartly.* 8: *241-246* (1972).
LAIBSON, P.R. & KRACHMER, J.II. Familial occurrence of dot map fingerprint (microcystic) dystrophy of the cornea. ARVO Spring Meeting, p. 44. Sarasota, 1974.
LEVITT, J.M. Microcystic dystrophy of the corneal epithelium. *Amer. J. Ophthal.* 72: *381-382* (1971).
LOWE, R.F. Recurrent erosion of the cornea. *Amer. J. Ophthal.* 57: *397-400* (1964).
LOWE, R.F. Recurrent erosion of the cornea. *Brit. J. Ophthal.* 54: *805-809* (1970).

37

LUXENBERG, M.N. & GREEN, K. Reduction of corneal edema with topical hypertonic agents. *Amer. J. Ophthal.* 71: *847-953* (1971).

LUXENBERG, M.N., FRIEDLAND, B.R. & HOLDER, J.M. Superficial microcystic corneal dystrophy. *Arch. Ophthal.* 93: *107-110* (1975).

RODRIGUES, M.M., FINE, B.S., LAIBSON, P.R. & ZIMMERMAN, L.E. Disorders of the corneal epithelium. A clinicopathologic study of dot, geographic, and fingerprint patterns. *Arch. Ophthal.* 92: *475-482* (1974).

SZILY, A. VON, SR. Ueber Disjunction des Hornhautepithels. *Albrecht v. Graefe's Arch. Ophthal.* 51: *486-531* (1900).

THEODORE, F.M. The use of tension-lowering drugs and other aids in the management of recurrent erosions. *Eye, ENT Monthly* 43: *62(2)* (1964).

THYGESON, P. Observations on recurrent erosion of the cornea. *Amer. J. Ophthal.* 47; 48 (pt II): *48-52* (1959).

TRIPATHI, R.C. & BRON, A.J. Ultrastructural study of non-traumatic recurrent corneal erosion. *Brit. J. Ophthal.* 56: *73-85* (1972).

TRIPATHI, R.C. & BRON, A.J. Cystic disorders of the corneal epithelium. II Pathogenesis. *Brit. J. Ophthal.* 57: *376-390* (1973).

TROBE, J.D. & LAIBSON, P.R. Dystrophic changes in the anterior cornea. *Arch. Ophthal.* 87: *378-382* (1972).

VALLE, O. Hereditary recurring corneal erosions. A familial study with special reference to Fuch's dystrophy. *Acta Ophthal. (Kbh.)* 45: *829-836* (1967).

VOGT, A. Die rezidivierende Hornhauterosion. Lehrbuch und Atlas der Spaltlampenmicrokopie. Vol. I, p. 244, Springer, Berlin, 1930.

VOGT, A. Lehrbuch und Atlas der Spaltlampen-mikroscopie des Lebenden Auges. Berlin, Springer 1930, Vol. I, pp. 1-313.

WOLTER, J. & FRALICK, F. Microcystic dystrophy of corneal epithelium. *Arch. Ophthal.* 75: *380-383* (1966).

Authors' address:
University of Oxford
Nuffield Laboratory of Ophthalmology
Walton Street
Oxford OX2 6AW, England

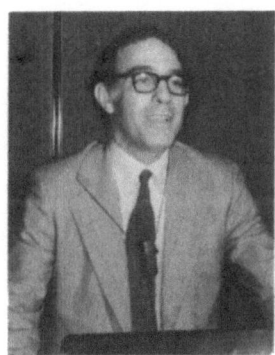

THE TREATMENT OF BACTERIAL INFECTIONS OF THE EYE

A.J. BRON

(Oxford, England)

ABSTRACT

The healthy eye is remarkably well protected from the common bacterial pathogens which are found around the lids and the conjunctival sac. The majority of serious intraoccular bacterial infections result either from a failure of these protective mechanisms or as a result of direct inoculation of microorganisms into the eye. The causes of intraocular infections such as corneal abscess and endophthalmitis are discussed.

An approach to the selection of antibacterial agents for the immediate and continuing treatment of such infections is presented including the routes of administration and the selection of supportive therapy, such as corticosteroids.

INTRODUCTION

The eye may be exposed to bacterial pathogens introduced into the conjunctival sac or reaching it via the blood stream. Exogenous or direct infection may arise as a result of surgical or accidental trauma, surface infection such as conjunctivitis in the normal or diseased eye, and the spread of organisms from neighbouring infections or reservoirs. Organisms may also be inoculated accidently when the eye comes into contact with contaminated materials such as drops and contact lenses. Endogeneous or metastatic bacterial infection is usually associated with septicaemia, secondary to an obvious septic focus. This may occur in a patient with a predisposing disorder such as alcoholism or immunodeficiency disorder (ARONSON et al, 1971).

To some extent the normal eye is protected from infection by the constituents of the tears. These include immunoglobulins, A, G, and E, lysozyme, which is no longer regarded as an important antibacterial substance, and the recently discovered non-lysozymal antibacterial factor. Transferrin, which is also found in the tears, may also have an antibacterial function by reason of its ability to reversably bind iron required by certain organisms. It has also been shown that certain commensal organisms found in the conjunctival sac are capable of secreting powerful anti-bacterial substances.

Studies by ALLANSMITH et al (1969) have shown that in normal subjects S. Aureus may be found on about 30% of the lids cultured, and that S. Albus was present on over 80% of lids. Even this organism may act as a pathogen on occasion. Organisms such as Pneumococci, Streptococcus pyogenes, Proteus, and E. coli were found in about 5% of subjects. NORN has shown that staphylococci may reside in the lash follicles (1970). It is clear

39

that the eyes are constantly exposed to pathogenic bacteria which none the less do not cause infection. In fact few organisms are capable of causing a direct infection in the absence of a breach in the epithelium. The Neisseria are capable of doing this, however.

TREATMENT OF BACTERIAL INFECTIONS OF THE EYE

Severe, potentially blinding, bacterial infection in the form of bacterial corneal ulceration and endopthalmitis represent an emergency demanding prompt and effective therapy. Effective therapy begins with the clinical diagnosis, which leads to microbiological confirmation and specific anti-microbial and supportive therapy.

The clinical diagnosis is suggested by the speed of development of the signs and symptoms which may clearly differentiate it from fungal disease. Viral infection, particularly Herpes simplex kerato-uveitis, may present a differential diagnostic problem. These possibilities must always be taken into consideration in the diagnostic work-up. Clinical features of severe bacterial infection include increasing pain, visual failure, lid swelling, discharge, and chemosis. The keratitis may take the form of a focal ulcer overlying a dense infiltrate or abscess with or without a hypopyon uveitis. The cardinal signs of endopthalmitis are the presence of cells in the vitreous and loss of the red reflex. This too may be accompanied by a hypopyon uveitis.

It is essential to identify the bacteria responsible for infection. For this, material must be taken directly from the site of infection. In keratitis, this must be obtained with a spatula from the ulcer itself. In endopthalmitis, an aqueous and sometimes vitreous tap must be performed. Smears are prepared for gram staining and material is innoculated into solid and liquid media. The media used is in part dependent on the amount of material available. Innoculation on to blood agar will permit the growth of the majority of ocular pathogens while use of thioglycolate permits growth of microaerophyllic and anaerobic organisms. Additional media may also be used (Figure 1). Brain-heart medium for fungal culture and viral transport medium will also be indicated on occasion.

The value of anterior chamber paracentesis in achieving a bacterial diagnosis has been shown in a number of instances (ALLANSMITH et al, 1970, TUCKER et al, 1971, D. JONES, 1974). A positive smear may be present alone or in combination with a positive culture. A positive smear may guide

---

MEDIA FOR CULTURE

BLOOD AGAR	The majority of ocular pathogens
THIOGLYCOLATE	Microaerophyllic and anaerobic
CHOCOLATE AGAR	Neisseria, Moraxella, Haemophilus
COOKED MEAT	Anaerobes
LOWENSTEIN	Mycobacteria

Fig. 1. Media for culture

the initial selection of antibiotic therapy and the subsequent cultural and sensitivity information allow a precise therapeutic regime to be formulated.

Chemotherapy

Route of administration of antibiotics

The route of administration of an antibiotic is no less important than the selection of the antibiotic itself. The chief routes are topical (including drops, ointments, corneal baths, and lavage) sub-conjunctival (and subtenons) and systemic (including intravenous, intramuscular and oral administration). In the normal eye there are significant barriers to penetration of antibiotics by the topical and systemic routes, while penetration from the sub-conjunctival route is by comparison excellent. However, the situation is greatly changed in the inflamed eye. Commonly in the treatment of severe bacterial infection, all routes are employed simultaneously, but it may be noted that in the presence of a small localised corneal abscess it may be sufficient to use only topical and sub-conjunctival therapy while in a metastatic endophthalmitis where the cornea may show little change in the early stages, the most effective therapy will be via sub-conjunctival and systemic routes. Bacterial corneal ulcer in the aphake should always be regarded as a potential cause of endophthalmitis and treated vigorously by all routes.

In the uninflamed eye, penetration from the conjunctival sac is impeded by the conjunctival and corneal epithelial barrier. In the presence of this barrier only drugs with a high lipid/water coefficient such as chloramphenicol and those sulphonamides which dissociate poorly will produce significant aqueous levels. Once this barrier is lost (which will occur with an abrasion, ulcer, or in the presence of epithelial oedema), then the lipid solubility of the drug ceases to be important and penetration into the cornea and aqueous depends on the concentration in the preparation used and molecular size. Highly water soluble drugs such as Neomycin, Streptomycin, and Penicillin, will than achieve better levels than poorly soluble drugs like Chloromycetin because they can be made up in high concentration.

BELLOWS & FARMER (1947) showed that when a rabbit eye was exposed to Streptomycin solution (50 mg. per ml.) in a corneal bath, the aqueous level was 12 μg. per ml. when the epithelium was intact and over 100 μg. per ml. when it was abraded after exposure. JONES (1973) advocates the use of fortified antibiotic drop preparations in the treatment of bacterial corneal ulcers.

The highest aqueous levels of antibiotic are achieved after sub-conjunctival and to a lesser extent subtenons injections. Subtenons injection is said to be less painful (GOLDEN 1974). The dose of antibiotic used depends on drug solubility, the volume which can be injected, and factors which are responsible for discomfort, such as irritative properties of the drug (e.g. Cephalothin) and probably pH and tonicity.

The early animal studies of SORSBY et al (1958) showed that with a drug that can be given in high concentration such as Neomycin, high antibiotic levels can be achieved in the aqueous and cornea, in the anterior and posterior tissues of the globe, and even in the vitreous, which normally presents a significant barrier to penetration (Fig. 2). Even after 48 hours therapeutic levels still remained in aqueous and vitreous. It will be seen from this figure that aqueous levels of antibiotic provide a satisfactory indication of levels in other parts of the eye excluding the vitreous.

One problem with the sub-conjunctival route of administration is the limited persistence of antibiotic in the ocular tissues. For instance, Gentamycin given in the lower concentrations may be absent from the aqueous in therapeutic concentration eight hours after injection (FURGUIELE, 1974) SORSBY et al (1958) has shown that concentration and persistence of antibiotic in the ocular tissues is enhanced by the inclusion of adrenaline in the sub-conjunctival preparation (e.g. 0.25 ml. of 1:1000 adrenaline in 1 ml. of solution). Thus in the rabbit the four hour aqueous Neomycin concentration was 290 μg. per ml. in the absence of adrenaline and 5000 μg. per ml. in the presence of adrenaline after a 500 μg. dose of Neomycin sulphate. The vitreous level at this time was 725 μg. per ml. and at the end of 48 hours the aqueous concentration was still 207 μg. per ml. (Fig. 3). Such an effect is important since it may ensure for many antibiotics that an adequate therapeutic concentration will exist at the site of infection for at least 24 hours. Daily sub-conjunctival injection is usually indicated in severe bacterial infections.

It has been noted that the ability of a drug to penetrate into the aqueous is often regarded as an indication of the drug's ability to reach other sites in the eye. Studies by BLOOME et al (1970) in uninflamed animal eyes have shown that the penetration of antibiotic into cornea, sclera and uvea exceeded that into the aqueous after parenteral (intramuscular and intravenous) administration of Penicillin G and Dihydrostreptomycin. Only levels in the vitreous and lens were lower than aqueous levels. The ability of antibiotics to enter the extra vascular compartments of the uninflamed eye from the plasma after systemic administration is limited by the blood-

Neomycin 500 mgs.		4 Hours	48 Hours
	CORNEA	330 μg/G	23 μg/G
	AQUEOUS	290 μg/ml	22 μg/ml
	VITREOUS	48 μg/ml	20 μg/ml
	ANT. TISS.	960 μg/G	11 μg/G
	POST. TISS.	900 μg/G	6 μg/G

Fig. 2. Penetration of Neomycin into the ocular tissues of the rabbit after subconjunctival injection (SORSBY & UNGAR 1958).

		4 Hours	48 Hours
Neomycin	CORNEA	195 μg/G	150 μg/G
500 mgs.	AQUEOUS	5000 μg/ml	207 μg/ml
with	VITREOUS	725 μg/ml	21 μg/ml
Adrenaline	ANT. TISS.	1500 μg/G	24 μg/G
	POST. TISS.	1750 μg/G	35 μg/G

Fig. 3. Inclusion of adrenaline solution in the subconjunctival injection improves the penetration of Neomycin (SORSBY & UNGAR 1958).

aqueous and blood-retinal barriers (LANGHAM 1951). In the presence of uveal inflammation the blood-aqueous barrier breaks down. This results in a greater approximation of the aqueous levels to those in the plasma. Certain antibiotics show relatively good penetration into the primary aqueous after systemic administration. These include ampicillin, chloramphenicol, dicloxacillin, lincomycin, the cephalosporins and sulphonamides (LEOPOLD 1971). Taking Cephaloridine as an example one may compare the penetration of this drug into the human eye after parenteral and sub-conjunctival injections. After a 30mg./kg. intramuscular dose of cephaloridine (RICHARDS et al, 1971) a primary aqueous level ranging from 0.4-3.7 μg. per ml. was found, while secondary aqueous levels up to 11 μg. per ml. were recorded. In another study (RECORDS 1969) after a 1 G. intravenous dose, secondary aqueous levels of up to 28.4 μg. per ml. were recorded after 1 hour. These values compare with an aqueous concentration of 100 μg. per ml. demonstrated in the human aqueous one hour after a dose of 125 mg. of Cephaloridine subconjunctivally. (FERNANDES et al, 1974) (Fig. 4).

Entry of antibiotic into the vitreous is influenced by lipoid solubility among other factors. High dose subconjunctival preparations may achieve prolonged therapeutic vitreous levels while low dose preparations may achieve negligible levels. In the inflamed eye it is likely that adequate thera-

CEPHALORIDINE DOSE	In Man ROUTE	AQUEOUS
30mg/kg	I.M.	1° 3.7μg/ml
		2° 11.0μg/ml
IG	I.V.	2° 28.4μg/ml
125mg	S.C.	1° 100.0μg/ml

Fig. 4. Penetration of Cephaloridine into primary and secondary aqueous after various routes of administration in man (see text).

ORGANISM	BACTERIAL ULCER	ENDOPHTHALMITIS
Staphylococcus	++	++
Pneumococcus	++	+
Streptococcus	+	+
Bacillus sp.	+	+
M. fortuitum	+	+
Pseudomonas	++	++
Moraxella	++	+
Enterobacter	+	++
Neisseria	+	
Serratia	+	+
Herellea	+	+

After Jones 1973 and 1974, and Leopold 1971

Fig. 5. Bacteria responsible for corneal ulcer and endophthalmitis.

peutic levels build up if high serum levels are maintained by parenteral therapy. This depends on the individual antibiotic. In studies in man by WILLIAMSON et al (1970) a vitreous level of sodium fusidate of 28.8 μg. per ml. was recorded in an enucleated eye corresponding to an aqueous fucidin level of 12.8 micrograms per ml. and a serum level of 84 μg. per ml. The patient had received 500 mg. of the drug eight hourly for three days.

Concern about the adequacy of antibiotic penetration into the vitreous has revived an interest in treating endopthalmitis with intravitreal injections (MAYLATH & LEOPOLD 1955). Peyman's group have demonstrated the persistence of therapeutic non-toxic levels of antibiotic in experimental animals for up to 96 hours after injection. They have reported the clinical use of a gentamycin (400 μg) and dexamethazone (360 μg) mixture made up in a 1 ml. solution, 0.1 ml. of which is injected into the vitreous, a similar volume being used to reform the anterior chamber after diagnostic paracentesis (PEYMAN, VASTINE, CROUCH & HERBST 1974).

Selection of antibiotic

In a proportion of patients the gram stain may indicate whether a gram positive or gram negative organism is responsible for the infection. In some this must await cultural identification and in others no bacterial diagnosis is made. A knowledge of the common organisms responsible for bacterial ulceration and endopthalmitis is of value in formulating a suitable antibiotic regime when information is lacking or is incomplete. D. JONES (1973, 1974) has collated data from several sources to show the organisms commonly responsible for corneal ulcer and endophthalmitis (Fig. 5). The bacteria commonly responsible for corneal ulceration are Staphylococcus, Strep. pneumoniae, Pseudomonas, and Moraxella. Less frequent pathogens have been Streptococcus pyogenes, E. coli, Aerobacter, Proteus, and Neisseria. More recently infection with Serratia marcescens, Mimae and Mycobacterium fortuitium have been recorded (LEOPOLD 1971). Staphylococcus aureus is the most common cause of post-cataract endophthalmitis, probably accounting for $\frac{2}{3}$ of cases (ALLEN & MANGIARACINE 1964) (BURNS 1959), (LEOPOLD 1952) (LOCATCHER-KHORAZO GUTIERREZ 1956). Streptococcus pyogenes and Streptococcus pneumoniae are of lesser importance among the gram positive organisms. B. Subtilis and Clostridium Welchii have been incriminated after trauma. Of the gram negative agents Pseudomonas and Enterobacter are the most important in the post cataract situation. Metastatic endophthalmitis is most frequently caused by Streptococcus and Pneumoccoccus. It is of interest that both Streptococcus viridans and Staphylococcus epidermidis, previously regarded as harmless saprophytes are now thought capable of causing severe ocular infection. S. Epidermidis may show a greater degree of antibiotic resistance than S. aureus.

Where the gram stains suggest a gram positive coccus as the causative organism, it is wise to regard the organism as a penicillinase-producing staphylococcus. Methicillin is a suitable penicillinase resistant penicillin which may be used sub-conjunctivally and systemically. A proportion of staphylococci are resistant to Methicillin and to certain alternative antistaphylococcal drugs, such as Erythromycin, Kanamycin, and Chloramphenicol, and to a lesser extent to Cephalothin and Lincomycin. In this situation, Vancomycin has been advocated by LEOPOLD (1971) for systemic therapy, though it must be recognised that this is a highly ototoxic and nephrotoxic drug. Gentamycin and Fucidin might well be suitable alternatives (Figure 6).

Where the gram stain suggests that a causative agent is a gram negative rod this must be assumed to be pseudomonas until proven otherwise. In this situation gentamycin is the drug of choice by all routes. Carbenicillin may be used in conjunction with this sub-conjunctivally and systemically. The synergistic effect of carbenicillin and gentamycin against P. aeruginosa has been demonstrated in certain circumstances and it is claimed that such a combined therapy may prevent the emergence of resistant strains during therapy. However, in a recent experimental study BOHIGAN et al, 1971 failed to demonstrate the synergistic effect when these drugs were used sub-conjunctivally against pseudomonas in rabbits.

Selection of the appropriate drugs for known organisms does not depend only on the in-vitro sensitivity of the organism to that drug. The response of the organism will depend partly on its sensitivity and partly on the concentration of the antibiotic achieved in the tissues at the site of infection. This will depend on the dose of the drug and the route by which it is given. This is brought out very clearly when the aqueous level of different antibiotics is compared after sub-conjunctival injections of standard doses. Figure 7 shows approximately peak aqueous levels of a number of antibiotics plotted against their sub-conjunctival dose. It is apparent and not unexpected that in general the higher the dose the higher the peak aqueous level. For instance, Lincomycin at a dose of 10 mg. gives an aqueous level of 10 μg./ml, Methicillin in a dose of 100 mg. gives an aqueous level of 166 μg per ml. It is of course clear that some drugs produce high aqueous levels after low dosage. Erythromycin in a 10 mg. dose gives an aqueous concentration of 50 μg./ml while Novobiocin in a 12.5 mg. dose gives an aqueous concentration of 90 μg per ml. It is an interesting exercise, though its practical validity may be questioned, to examine for individual organisms the ratio between aqueous level and the sensitivity of the organism to a particular drug. This produces an index which allows one to place each antibiotic in order of

Methicillin   — and other penicillinase
                                                  resistant penicillins
Erythromycin
Kanamycin
Chloramphenicol

Cephalothin
Lincomycin

Fucidin
Vancomycin
Gentamycin

Fig. 6. Systemic therapy against penicillinase-producing staphylococci.

its potential effectiveness against the organism in the *in-vivo* situation (Figure 8 and Figure 9). Although such charts cannot be used as a guide to management in individual cases, they do emphasize the importance of dosage and of maintained high tissue levels in effective therapy.

Where the gram stain does not yield an organism, then it is essential to devise a regime which will be effective against both gram positive and gram negative organisms. Gentamycin is the mainstay of such therapy since this drug is effective against pseudomonas and resistant staphylococci. Like

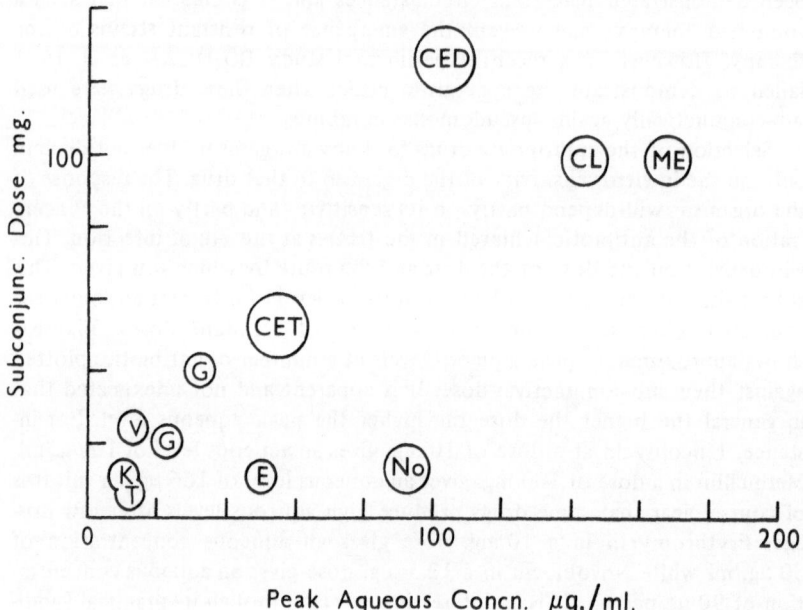

Fig. 7. Subconjunctival injection. The effect of dosage on peak aqueous levels achieved. (multiple sources.); CED = Cephaloridine; CET = Cephalothin; CL = Cloxacillin; E = Erythromycin; G = Gentamycin; K = Kanamycin; ME = Methicillin; No = Novobiocin; T = Tetracycline; V = Vancomycin.

PSEUDOMONAS SPECIES

Sub-Conjunctival Injection

DRUG	DOSE mg.	M.I.C. µg/ml	AQUEOUS LEVELS µg/ml	HRS.	A/M.I.C. Index
Colistin	10	0.12	56	3	467
Neomycin	500^	64	5,000	1	78
Streptomycin	500^	16-64	80	1	1 – 5
Gentamycin	40	1-8	32	1	1 – 4

Fig. 8. Listing of antibiotics effective against Pseudomonas in the order determined by sensitivity of the organism and penetration of the agent by the subconjunctival route. (Minimum Inhibitory Concentrations from GARROD & O'GRADY 1968; aqueous levels from multiple authors.) = with adrenaline.

46

other aminoglycosides it is weaker against streptococci than against other organisms. Combination with agents effective against gram positive organisms such as Methicillin provide a cover for this deficiency as well as an agent effective against resistant staphylococci. Both KANSKI (1974) and JONES (1974) employ these drugs in the form of a sub-conjunctival 'cocktail' (Fig. 10). KANSKI combines this therapy with systemic Fucidin 500 mg. 8 hourly. An alternative and effective sub-conjunctival preparation combines gentamycin with cephaloridine (Figure 11).

PROTEUS VULGARIS

Sub-conjunctival injection (Rabbit)

DRUG	DOSE mg	M.I.C. $\mu g/ml$	AQUEOUS LEVEL $\mu g/ml$	HRS.	A/M.I.C. Index
Neomycin	500´	4	5,000	4	1,250
Gentamycin	40	1-4	32	1	8 – 32
Ampicillin	100	64	1,000	1	16
Streptomycin	500´	8	80	2	10
Kanamycin	10	4	10	1	2.5

´= with adrenaline

Fig. 9. Listing of antibiotics effective against Proteus Vulgaris in the order determined by sensitivity of the organism and penetration of the agent by the subconjunctival route. (Minimum Inhibitory Concentration from GARROD & O'GRADY 1968; aqueous levels from multiple authors.)

SUBCONJUNCTIVAL COCKTAIL	G^+/G^- ORG.	
	DOSE	*VOL.*
Gentamycin	20 mg	0.5ml
Methicillin	150 mg	0.2ml
Mydricaine		0.3ml
		1.0ml

After Kanski 1974 b.

Fig. 10. Subconjunctival cocktail suitable against gram-positive and gram-negative organisms (Mydricaine is a mixture of adrenaline, atropine and procaine).

SUBCONJUNCTIVAL COCKTAIL	G^+/G^- ORG.
	DOSE
Gentamycin	20mg
Cephaloridine	125*–250mg

*See Fernandes et. al. 1974

Fig. 11. Alternative sub-conjunctival cocktail suitable against gram-positive and gram-negative organisms.

Adjunct to chemotherapy

The importance of adding adrenaline to the sub-conjunctival preparation to increase levels and persistence of antibiotic in the ocular tissues has been mentioned above. This should however be omitted in old and infirm patients with a cardiac disease. Probenecid 0.5 G. 8 hourly taken orally will significantly increase plasma penicillin levels by its action in blocking tubular excretion of penicillin drugs. Topical anticollagenese (disodium edetate) has been advocated in the treatment of pseudomonas infections of the cornea. However, it is likely that most such cases are so advanced at the time when diagnosis is made that it is already too late for such enzyme inhibitors to alter the course of the disease.

The studies of MAYLATH & LEOPOLD (1955) demonstrated a beneficial effect of cortico-steroids in conjunction with antibiotics on experimental intraocular infections in rabbits. ARONSON et al (1971) found that a combination of local cortico-steroids and antibiotics in the treatment of endophthalmitis produced better visual results than antibiotics alone. LEOPOLD advocates a delay of 24 to 48 hours prior to institution of corticosteroids in order to assess the initial response to antibiotics (LEOPOLD & APT 1960). FREEMAN & GAY (1969) were not able to demonstrate any benefit of including corticosteroids in the antibiotic therapy of post-cataract endophthalmitis. JONES (1974) points out that there are no strict guidelines for the selection of this adjunctive therapy. This must certainly be accepted. It is of interest that KANSKI (1974a) has used a combination of systemic prednisolone (10 mg. 4 times daily) and sub-conjunctival steroids (methyl prednisolone acetate (Depomedrone) 40 mg. initially, followed by Betamethazone (Betnesol 4 mg). in conjunction with sub-conjunctival and systemic antibiotics in the treatment of late endophthalmitis assocated with filtering blebs. No loss of acuity occurred in 16 out of 20 patients treated. In another series a further 20 patients with endophthalmitis following anterior segment surgery were treated with a similar regimen. For the overall series 85% of eyes were saved with some useful vision (counts fingers or better at 2 feet). 5% of eyes were enucleated or eviscerated and 10% were retained without useful vision. Comparing these results with five other series published between 1959 and 1971 (BURNS 1959, NEVEU & ELIOT 1959, THEODORE et al 1961, ALLEN & MANGIARACINE 1964 and HATTEN-HAUER & LIPSICH 1971), the figures were 25% saved with useful vision, 42% saved without useful vision. and 33% enucleated or eviscerated (60 patients in all). This appears to support the approach which KANSKI has adopted, though his studies lacked bacterial confirmation in the majority of instances. (KANSKI 1974 b).

As a guideline in the treatment of bacterial endophthalmitis with steroid I have relied on the degree of vitreous reaction present and the size of the hypopyon and anterior chamber coagulum. When these changes are marked then the risk of later sequelae in the form of synechiae pupillary membranes, and vitreous organization is high enough to justify steroid administration. My preference is for systemic administration. It would seem wise not to use systemic steroids in the presence of septicaemia.

SUMMARY

The effective treatment of bacterial corneal ulcers and endophthalmitis demand prompt action in obtaining smears and cultures for microbial diagnosis. When the organism is not known the initial therapy consists of providing broad antibiotic cover using multiple routes and doses capable of achieving high levels of antibiotic at the site of infection. With every drug selected the possibility of systemic or local toxicity should be kept in mind. Continuing therapy is modified according to the results of bacterial cultures and sensitivity findings, and an assessment of the patient's response to current therapy. Adjunctive measures may include, apart from cycloplegics, analgesics and heat, diamox for raised pressure and in selected instances of endophthalmitis, corticosteroids. At this stage the surgeon may be called upon to perform a conjunctival flap or corneal graft in treatment of a corneal perforation. In the post-infective stage management may involve corneal grafting, removal of pupillary membranes and cataract extraction.

REFERENCES

ALLEN, H.F. & MANGIARACINE, A.B. Bacterial endophthalmitis after cataract extraction: A study of 22 infections in 20,000 operations. *Arch. Ophthal.*, 72, *454* (1964).
ALLANSMITH, M.R., OSTLER. H.B. & BUTTERWORTH, M. Concomitance of bacteria in various areas of the eye. *Arch. Ophth.* 82, *37* (1969).
ALLANSMITH, M., SKAGGS, C. & KIMURA, S.J. Anterior chamber paracentesis. *Arch. Ophth.* 84, *745* (1970).
ARONSON, S.B., SUSSMAN, S.J., MOORE, T.E. JR., WILLIAMS, F.C. & GOODNER, E.K. Corticosteroid therapy in metastatic endophthalmitis. *Arch. Ophth.* 85, *61* (1971).
BELLOWS, J.G. & FARMER, C.J. Streptomycin in ophthalmology. *Amer. J. Ophth.* 30, *1215* (1947).
BLOOME, M.A., GOLDEN, B. & MCKEE, A.P. Antibiotic concentration in ocular tissues – penicillin G. and dihydrostreptomycin. *Arch. Opthal.* 83, *78* (1970).
BOHIGAN, G., OKUMOTO, M. & VALENTON, M. Experimental Pseudomonas Keratitis: treatment with and evaluation of carbenicillin and gentamycin in combination. *Arch. Ophthal.* 86, *432* (1971).
BURNS, R.P. Post-operative infection in an ophthalmic hospital. *Amer. J. Ophthal.* 48, *519* (1959).
FERNANDES, E., ZORAB, E.C., MARSHALL, M.J. & MILLS, P.M. Ocular use of Gentamycin and Cephaloridine, Pt. I. Intra-ocular penetration. *Canad. J. Ophthal.*, 9, *170* (1974).
FREEMAN, M.I. & GAY, A.J. Systemic steroid therapy in postcataract endopthalmitis. In: Current Concepts in Opthalmology, St. Louis, C.V. Mosby 163-177 (1969).
FURGUIELE, F.P. Discussion in Ocular Inflammatory Disease Golden, B., Ed. Illinois, Charles Thomas 182 (1974).
GARROD, L.P. & O'GRADY, F. Antibiotic and Chemotherapy 2nd Ed. London, E & S Livingstone (1968).
GOLDEN, B. Discussion in Ocular Inflammatory Disease. Golden, B., Ed. Illinois, Charles C. Thomas 161-179 (1974).
HATTENHAUER, J.M. & LIPSICH, M.P. Late endophthalmitis after filtration surgery. *Amer. J. Ophthal.* 72, *1097* (1971).
JONES, D.B. Early diagnosis and therapy of bacterial corneal ulcers in External Ocular Diseases. Diagnosis and Current Therapy. International Ophthalmology Clinics 13 No. 4, Laibson, P.R. & Trobe. J.D. Eds. Boston, Little, Brown & Co. 1-37 (1973).

JONES, D.B. The early diagnosis and management of bacterial endophthalmitis in Ocular Inflammatory Disease. Golden, B., Ed. Illinois, Charles C. Thomas 161-179 (1974).

KANSKI, J.J. Treatment of late endophthalmitis associated with filtering blebs. *Arch. Ophthal.* 91, *339* (1974) a.

KANSKI, J.J. The prevention and management of post-operative bacterial endophthalmitis. *Trans. Ophthal. Soc. U.K.* 94, *19* (1974) b.

LANGHAM, M.E. Factors affecting the penetration of antibiotics into the aqueous humour. *Brit. J. Ophthal.* 35, *614* (1951).

LEOPOLD, I.H. Surgery of ocular trauma. *Arch. Ophthal.* 48, *738* (1952).

LEOPOLD, I.H. Management of Intra-ocular infection. Doyne Memorial Lecture. *Trans. Ophth. Soc. U.K.* 91, *577* (1971).

LEOPOLD, I.H. & APT. L. Postoperative intraocular infections. *Amer. J. Ophthal.* 50, *1225* (1960).

LOCATCHER-KHORAZO, D. & GUTIERREZ, E. Eye infections following cataract extraction with special reference to the role of Staphylococcus aureus. *Am. J. Ophthal.* 41, *981* (1956).

MAYLATH, F.R. & LEOPOLD, I.H. Study of experimental intraocular infection. I. The recoverability of organisms inoculated into ocular tissue and fluids. II. The infleunce of antibiotics alone and combined on intraocular growth of these organisms. *Amer. J. Ophthal.* 40, *36* (1955).

NEVEU, M. & ELLIOT, A.J. Prophylaxis and treatment of endophthalmitis. *Amer. J. Ophthal.* 48, *368* (1959).

NORN, M.S. Localisation of bacteria on single eyelashes *Acta. Ophth.* 48, *237* (1970).

PEYMAN, G.A.,VASTINE, D.W., CROUCH, E.R., HERBST, R.W. JR. Clinical use of intravitreal antibiotics to treat bacterial endophthalmitis. *Trans. Am. Acad. Ophthalmol. Otolaryngol.* 78, *862* (1974).

RECORDS, R.E. Intraocular penetration of cephaloridine. *Arch. Ophthal.* 81, *331* (1969).

RICHARDS, A.B., BRON, A.J., RICE, N.S.C., FELLS, P., MARSHALL, M.J., & JONES, B.R. Intraocular penetration of cephaloridine. *Brit. J. Ophthal.* 36, *531* (1972).

SORSBY, A. & UNGAR, J. Neomycin in ophthalmology. *Ann. Roy. Coll. Surg. Eng.* 22, *107* (1958).

THEODORE, F.H., LITTMAN, M.L. & ALMEDA, E. The diagnosis and management of fungus endophthalmitis following cataract extraction. Arch. *Ophthal.* 66, *163* (1961).

TUCKER, D.M., MEIER, W.C. & FORSTER, R.K. Experimental osilation of intraocular bacteria via anterior chamber and vitreous aspiration. A.R.V.O. Meeting, Sarasota, April 1971 (Cited by D. JONES 1974).

WILLIAMSON, J. *et al.* Estimation of sodium fusidate levels in human serum, aqueous humor and vitreous body. *Brit. J. Ophthal.* 54, *126* (1970).

Author's address:
University of Oxford
Nuffield Laboratory of Ophthalmology
Walton Street
Oxford
England

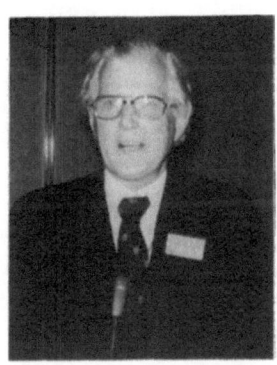

SOME ASPECTS IN THE MANAGEMENT OF ORBITAL DISEASE

FRANK W. NEWELL, M.D.

(Chicago, Illinois)

ABSTRACT

Computerized axial tomography provides a new dimension in the diagnosis of orbital disorders. It renders obsolete orbital phlebography, injection of contrast material in the orbit, and radionuclide orbital scanning. A history that excludes previous thyroid disease or systemic malignancies is important in the diagnosis of proptosis. Retraction of the upper eyelid and lag of the upper eyelid involving the globe in downward gaze are important. Choroidal folds are not diagnostically significant.

The year 1973 constituted a high point in the diagnosis and management of orbital disorders. The Second International Symposium on orbital disturbances was held in Amsterdam May 28-29, 1973. The proceedings of that symposium appeared as volume 14 in 'Modern Problems in Ophthalmology' in 1975 (STREIFF, 1975). This Symposium was followed by the Fifth Congress of the International Society for Ultrasonic Diagnosis in Ophthalmology, the proceedings of which also appeared in 1975 in 'Ultrasonography in Ophthalmology' (FRANÇOIS & GOES, 1975). In 1973, HENDERSON published his exhaustive monograph on orbital tumors.

In 1972, G.N. HOUNSFIELD first described computerized transverse axial scanning in which he used a photomultiplier tube to measure the intensity of the emergent x-ray beam. The impulses were recorded on a magnetic disk and processed by a computer, thus providing the most significant contribution to neurologic and orbital diagnosis since the introduction of cerebral angiography by Egas Moniz and pneumoencephalography by Walter Dandy. Transverse computerized axial tomography promises to provide to orbital diagnosis what photocoagulation, fluorescein angiography, and scleral buckling procedures provide in diagnosing retinal disorders.

This technique permits the physician for the first time, to see the shape and structure of lesions in the brain and orbit, and to locate them accurately in space, using a noninvasive technique with no discomfort or significant risk to the patient. Current scanning instruments direct a narrow beam of x-rays through the tissue and the intensity of the emergent beam is measured by a scintillation counter. The beam is rotated until the device has passed through 180 degrees. After the first scan, an iodine-containing contrast material is injected intravenously and as this circulates, greater contrast is provided to be compared to the first pass. Tissue density ranges from 0

51

for water to 500 for bone and the absorbtion characteristics vary both with the tissue density and the atomic number of the tissue molecules. As iodine has an atomic number of 52 and calcium an atomic number of 22, the first instrument required a water bath surrounding the tissue to be studied and its usefulness was limited to the head. Newer instruments do not require a water bath and are suitable for whole body tomography.

Suggestive of the instrument's value was a study of brain scans from the Mayo Clinic in which 25% of patients thought to have multiple sclerosis were found to have intracranial tumors or parenchymal lesions; 21% of the patients with suspected brain infarcts had similar findings as did 20% with seizure disorders, 17% with focal cerebral dysfunctions, and 8% with headaches.

Despite the contribution of computerized tomography, conventional roentgenography is essential in the diagnosis of many orbital abnormalities. The standard frontal projection permits a composite view of the bones forming the orbit. When both orbits are photographed in the same field, their dimensions and density can be compared. Water's technique is necessary for detailed study of the roof of the orbit; separate oblique views are required for examination of the inner and outer walls. The Caldwell position is used for demonstration of the superior orbital (sphenoidal) fissure; visualization of the inferior orbital fissure (sphenomaxillary) is necessary to demonstrate orbital floor fractures.

Computerized axial tomography has certainly rendered obsolete a number of special methods used to demonstrate particular defects. Cerebro angiography to demonstrate the ophthalmic artery and its branches in the orbit appears necessary solely in those disorders caused by an aneurysm and other vascular abnormalities. Orbital phlebography by means of catheterization of the angular vein at the medial canthus of the frontal vein on the forehead, to demonstrate displacement of the ophthalmic vein, is no longer necessary. Laminography also seems to have limited value. Injection of radiopaque material into the orbit to demonstrate its escape into adjacent nasal sinuses, or to outline structures within the orbit, seems to have a limited application. Radionuclide orbital scanning also seems to have no further use.

Ultrasonography, using either A or B scan is useful in the diagnosis of orbital disorders. However, the geometry of the orbit is such that these scans must be recognized as solely auxillary.

Most reports concerning orbital disorders deal with specific abnormalities. The factors underlying the clinician's approach are seldom emphasized: 1. intraocular or extraocular disease; 2. neoplasm, inflammation, or systemic disease; 3. origin from contiguous sinus or brain, or metastatic; and 4. actual proptosis or its simulation by a local abnormality of the orbital bones or contents.

I am impressed that much of the difficulty in diagnosing and managing orbital disease arises because of an incomplete history, inadequate physical examination, or failure to use the appropriate diagnostic test. Proptoses, with the exception of those caused by aneurysms and acute orbital inflammations, do not constitute a medical emergency. It is thus possible to obtain an appropriate history, physical examination, and diagnostic studies systematically.

The age of the patient is important. Abnormalities in the size and shape of the orbit and its contents are more likely to be evident in children than in adults. Simple steps such as refraction and measurement of the intraocular pressure will exclude monocular myopia or congenital glaucoma with enlargement of the globe, which have been mistaken for proptosis.

Previous treatment for hyperthyroidism or systemic malignancy is indicative of either thyroid ophthalmopathy or a tumor metastatic to the orbit. Previous enucleation alerts the examiner to the possibility of localized recurrence, as does surgery for removal of meningioma, in any region in which the dura mater is adjacent to the orbit. A history of sudden onset with rapid progression is suggestive of either an aneurysm or an acute inflammation.

Intermittent proptosis suggests an orbital varix or a lesion that can discharge through a paranasal sinus. Pain is most often associated with an inflammation of the orbital contents. Bruits and sounds in the head suggest an aneurysm.

General physical examination should be directed to signs that may be associated with orbital disease, such as café au lait spots or other evidence of phakomatosis or signs and symptoms of hyperthyroidism. A neoplasm in a structure adjacent to the orbit, particularly in the nasal pharynx or accessory nasal sinuses, requires direct observation.

The severity and direction of the proptosis should be studied. In a compensated proptosis, the eyelids will cover the globe, with little danger of exposure keratitis. Masses in the muscle cone cause symmetric proptosis and a relatively small tumor may cause displacement. Masses outside of the muscle cone must be larger to displace the globe; the proptosis is then asymmetric. Tumors located in the anterior portion of the orbit may be palpated through the eyelids. Often, a lateral canthotomy or a conjunctival incision in the lower outer canthus will permit palpation of tissues deep in the orbit.

Marked congestion of the orbital vessels suggests an inflammatory process within the orbit, a thyroid abnormality with rapid progression of the proptosis, or a carotid cavernous sinus fistula.

Retraction of the upper eyelid and eyelid lag with downward gaze are of particular importance in the diagnosis of thyroid ophthalmopathy, provided there has not been a previous orbital fracture. Limitation of vertical movements of the eye associated with ocular muscle contracture is almost certainly a sign of thyroid disease. Increase in intraocular pressure with upward gaze is an unreliable sign and occurs with orbital tumors other than thyroid ophthalmopathy, although this is the abnormality with which it is most commonly associated. Increased amplitude of pulsation with tonography suggests a carotid cavernous sinus aneurysm. Choroidal striae and related signs are of scant value because they also occur with a variety of other disorders.

Blood studies should be carried out to exclude syphilis, leukemias that may affect the orbit, and other causes of chronic granulomas. Mucormycosis should be considered when there is diabetes mellitus with acidosis.

The thyroid gland plays a particularly important role in the diagnosis of orbital abnormalities. The hypothalmic releasing factor (TRF) causes release of pituitary thyrotropic hormone (TSH), which controls the trapping rate of circulating iodine by the thyroid gland and causes the release of two hormones, thyroxine (T_4) and triiodothyronine (T_3), from the thyroid globulin of the thyroid gland. These hormones are bound mainly to the serum protein in the blood and only a minute amount circulates in the free, physiologically active form.

Recently, the tests for thyroid function have been reevaluated. The basal metabolic rate is no longer available at many institutions. The protein-bound iodine test – though economic, reproducable, and automated – is nonspecific and the results are invalidated by the use of iodine in health foods, contrast media in radiology, and in patients using contraceptive pills. Currently, the total serum thyroxine is measured and then the free thyroxine index is measured. This test measures the availability of unsaturated thyroxine-binding sites, being directly proportional to the unbound or free thyroxine in the serum, and it presumably represents the metabolically active form of the hormone. This test should give results proportional to the actual metabolic status of the patient irrespective of the level of binding proteins in the serum. This test is useful in patients who have received iodine, who have severe liver disease, in patients who are pregnant or are taking contraceptive pills, and the like. The test should indicate definite hypothyroidism, hyperthyroidism, or euthyroidism (REFETOFF et al., 1974).

In patients with equivocal increase in the free thyroxine index, particularly in those with proptosis or suspected Graves' disease, a serum triiodothyronine test or a triiodothyronine suppression test is indicated (BRITTON et al., 1975).

The triiodothyronine suppression test is commonly used in the diagnosis of thyroid ophthalmopathy; initially the uptake of the thyroid gland is determined by using radioactive technetium and scintillation techniques. The patient then receives a full replacement dose of triiodothyronine (Cytomel) for one week; scanning of the thyroid gland is then repeated. A normal thyroid gland is suppressed by the Cytomel and shows a decreased uptake of radioactive technetium. In thyroid ophthalmopathy, both the hyperthyroid gland and the thyroid gland continue to take up the radioactive isotope as before. The test is particularly valuable when Graves' disease occurs in the absence of acute hyperthyroidism.

Thyroglobulin hemagglutination antibodies are present in a high titer with thyroiditis. Patients with chronic lymphocytic (Hashimoto's) thyroiditis have highest titers. A high level of antibodies is also present in patients with Graves' disease, exophthalmos, and primary thyroid disease (possibly a thyroiditis).

Measurement of circulating thyroid microsomal hemagglutination antibodies is more sensitive. Of adult patients with Hashimoto's thyroiditis, 90% to 95% have positive tests as contrasted with only 50% to 60% who have positive thyroglobulin agglutination antibodies. Of patients with Graves' disease, some 80% have positive microsomal hemagglutination antibodies as contrasted with 20% to 30% who have positive thyroglobulin tests.

The long-acting thyroid stimulator is an immune globulin, present in the blood in about one half of the patients with active Graves' disease. It is also found in the blood of patients who, in the absence of thyrotoxicosis, have other manifestations of Grave's syndrome such as ophthalmopathy with or without dermopathy. It is commonly present in patients with exophthalmos, although it does not appear to be the primary cause of the disorder.

The test is difficult, time-consuming, and cumbersome. It requires a determination of the release of labelled thyroid hormone from the thyroid gland of mice. It is particularly valuable in the differential diagnosis of unilateral exophthalmos; a persistently high or an increasing long-acting thyroid stimulator may correlate with progression of exophthalmos. The test, however, should be used in only selected instances.

A group at the University of Chicago has long been interested in choroidal folds. These folds have been characteristic, although an extremely uncommon sign of expanding orbital tumors. In recent years, however, this has been recognized as both a common sign and one not associated soley with orbital tumors. These tumors were first described histologically in 1915 by BIRCH-HIRSCHFELD & SIEGFRIED. In a review of patients seen at the University of Chicago in 1972, we found 15 instances of choroidal folds: eight caused by orbital tumors and seven associated with Graves' disease, postoperative hypotony, hypermetropia, papilledema, disciform macular disease, and uveitis.

Choroidal folds consist of parallel folds involving the posterior pole that on ophthalmoscopy appear to be composed of alternating bright and dark streaks. The peaks of the streaks are bright while the valleys are dark. On fluorescein injection, there is hyperfluorescence of the peaks and no fluorescein leakage. The folds may be horizontal or vertical and may involve the temporal or nasal side of the disk.

When folds persist for a long time they become broader and whiter and may become pigmented. The pigmentation may be diffuse or may be linear and bead-like, appearing along the slope of a fold. These folds may become associated with areas of deep pigmentation.

Choroidal folds may be easily missed unless one seeks them. They may often be seen on fluorescein angiography, when they have not been appreciated on light ophthalmoscopy. They are easily seen with retroillumination by directing an ophthalmoscopic light directly adjacent to the lesion and observing the fields in the light passing behind the lesion.

Retinal folds may give rise to a more or less similar pattern on light ophthalmoscopy, although the reinal folds are often associated with increased tortuosity of blood vessels; additionally, the fluorescein pattern is normal. Conspicuous choroidal vessels may be confused with choroidal folds or angioid streaks.

Histologically, Bruch's membrane appears to be closely attached to the choroid and fewer choroidal vessels seem to be in the region of a fold. All experimental attempts to produce the lesion have failed.

REFERENCES

BIRCH-HIRSCHFELD, A. & SIEGFRIED, C. Zur Kenntnis der Veraenderungen des Bulbus durch Druck eines Orbitaltumors. *Arch. f. Ophth.* 90: *404* (1915).

BRITTON, K.E., QUINN, V., BROWN, B.L. & EKINS, R.P. A strategy for thyroid function tests. *B.M.J.* 3: *350-352* (1975).

HENDERSON, J.W. Orbital Tumors. W.B. Saunders Company. Philadelphia, (1973).

HOUNSFIELD, G.N. A. The EMI Scanner system. The Congress of the British Institute of radiology, (1972).

FRANÇOIS. J. & GOES, F.: eds. Ultrasonography in Ophthalmology. S. Karger, Basel. (1975).

REFETOFF, S., DEGROOT, L.G., HAGEN, R. & O'NEILL, J. Thyroid function test – Internal memorandum to medical staff of the University of Chicago, Feb. 7, (1974).

STREIFF, E.B. Modern Problems in Ophthalmology, Vol. 14. Orbital Disorders, Eds: Bleeker. G.M., Garston, J.B., Kronenberg, B., Lyle, T.K., Karger, S., Basel . (1975).

Key words: Computerized axial tomography, Thyroid disease, Choroidal folds.

Author's address.
University of Chicago
Department of Ophthalmology
950 East 59th Street
CHICAGO, Illinois
USA

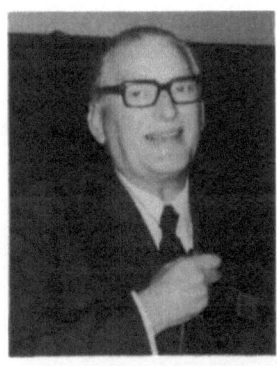

EXOPHTHALMOS BY ARTERIO-VENOUS COMMUNICATION AND THE CAVERNOUS SINUS

G.M. BLEEKER, H.J.F. PEETERS,
J.P.A. GILLISSEN & T.H. OEI

(Amsterdam)

Pulsating exophthalmos is not necessarily a consequence of arterio-venous communication in the cavernous sinus and a carotid-cavernous communication does not necessarily produce pulsating exophthalmos. This quotation of WALSH & HOYT (1969) is the subject of today. Of the 4 main causes of pulsating exophthalmos, the defects in the orbital roof and the orbital vascular tumours will be left out and we will confine ourselves today to the carotid-cavernous communications and the external carotid-orbital venous fistula.

As a classical representative of the traumatic carotid cavernous shunt a man is presented of 59 years old (Fig. 1). Four weeks after a motor-accident, complicated by a left orbital fracture, a pulsating bruit started in his left orbit. Ectasy of palpebral veins and conjunctival congestion were gradually completed to the classical signs of the carotid cavernous fistula:
a. Pains and buzzing in the head, pulsating exophthalmos.
b. Arterialisation of the orbital veins, motility disturbances, impaired vision and glaucoma.

The loss of vision may be consequent to direct lesion of the optic nerve by the trauma or to indirect lesion by disturbance of the vascular supply of the optic nerve. Disturbance of the retinal circulation is relatively infrequent. Glaucoma on the other hand is very common, because of elevated episcleral venous pressure.

Motility disturbances again can be a consequence of direct damage to nerves at the site of the fracture. Abnormal conditions and pressure within the cavernous sinus can be responsible for delayed diplopia as well as passive motility disturbance by congested orbital veins and oedema.

Angiography revealed the carotid-cavernous communication by clouding the venous orbital pathways immediately. In the course of time an efficient system of collaterals increases the arterial supply to such an extent that both internal carotid arteries have a share in the supply of blood to the fistula. This comes to our aid when ligation of the carotid artery is performed, because exactly these collaterals take over the blood supply as soon as the affluent carotid artery is occluded.

In our patient, the internal carotid was ligated between the fistula and the circle of Willis. This being well tolerated, the common carotid was clamped, a piece of muscle tissue was inserted into the arterial lumen and floated upward into the fistula by releasing the clamp. Finally, the common

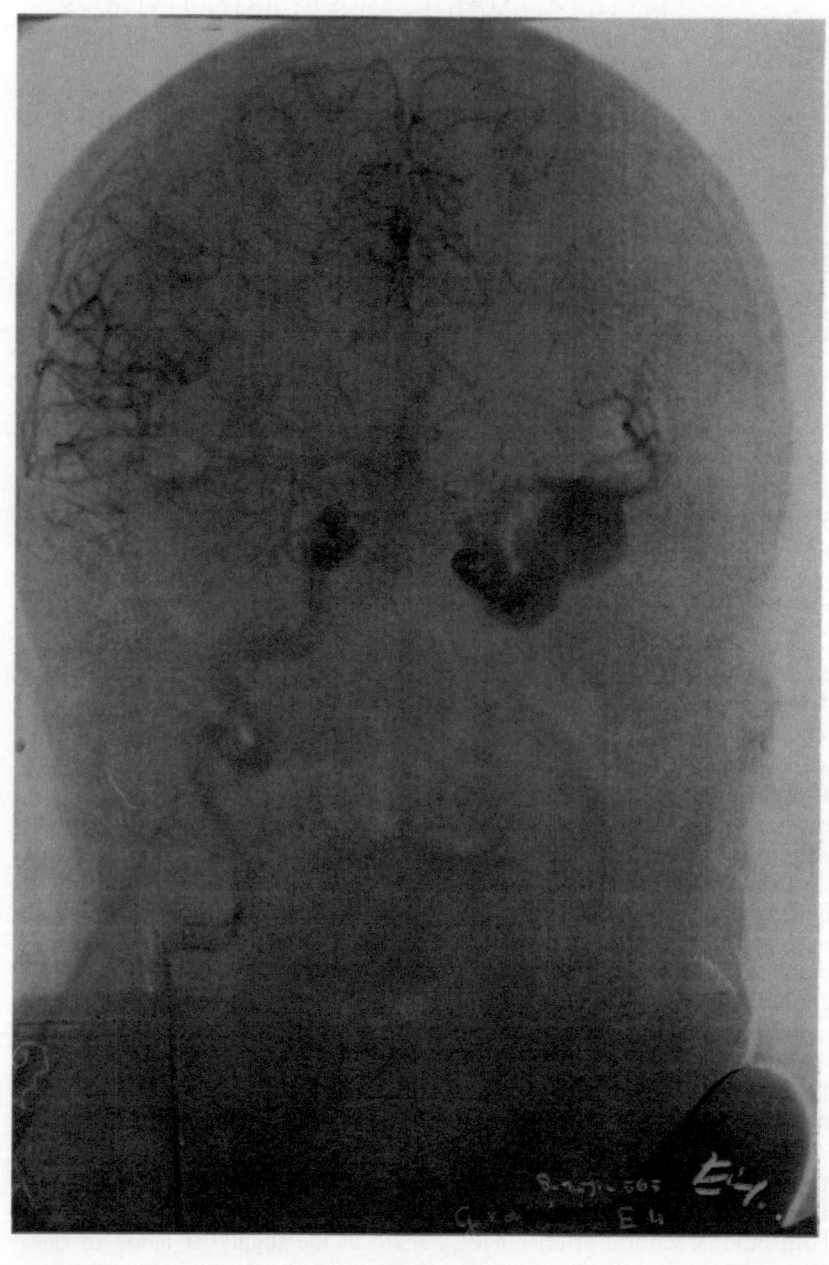

Fig. 1. Mr. v.d.W. 59 years of age. Classic traumatic carotid cavernous fistula on the left side. Severe damage to the homolateral orbital contents. Abundant communication with the right carotid artery.

carotid was ligated and the patient is doing well ever since.

If pulsating exophthalmos is manifest immediately after trauma, there must be a traumatic rupture of the artery or branches thereof.

One to several weeks interval after trauma suggests damage to the arterial wall, traumatic aneurysm, and late rupture or leakage.

In about one third of the cases there is no preceding trauma. These usually concern elder women. As an example, a woman of 77 years reported to have a gradually increasing strange feeling in the right ear and orbit (Fig. 2). She had 7 mm of exophthalmos with swollen eyelids and congested conjunctival veins. Vision was reduced and a choked disc was easily visible. The intraocular pressure on the right side was 30 mm Hg., and internal examination revealed hyperfunction of the thyroid gland. Any objective or subjective sign of buzzing was absent.

Phlebography provided more evidence for the existence of an intraorbital process. The orbital veins did not fill on the affected side. Carotid angiography revealed a carotid cavernous fistula and abnormal filling of the orbital vein. It was, however, a small fistula and because of the age of the patient agressive therapy was not advised. In the course of a year the situation is ameliorating very gradually.

A similar case concerned a woman of 59 years with headache in the right orbit for 7 years (Fig. 3). In May last year she had a slight head injury, in August exophthalmos developed on the right side in three days, in October diplopia became manifest and in December severe pain and glaucoma developed. There was no sign of a pulsating bruit. The stereoscopic X-rays of the skull were suggestive for the existence of a mucocele but carotid angio-

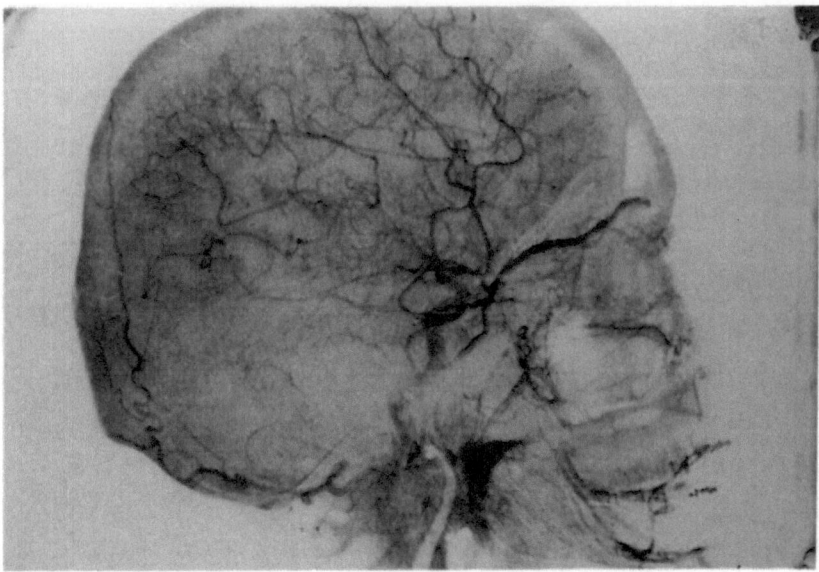

Fig. 2. Mrs v.d. V.-D. 77 years of age. Progressive exophthalmos on the right side. The patient proved to have a carotid-cavernous shunt without any sign of buzzing, probably by spontaneous rupture of an aneurysm.

graphy immediately revealed the true cause, being a small carotid cavernous fistula. Again this came as a surprise and therapy was refrained of. In the course of last year the signs and symptoms were vanishing spontaneously.

As an example of an external carotid fistula a girl of 18 years is presented with a record of four years buzzing in the right orbit. She had congested conjunctival vessels, but a normal fundus and vision (the left eye was convergent and amblyopic).

The stereoscopic X-rays of the skull revealed an enlargement of the right superior orbital fissure and the common carotid angiography promptly revealed a large carotid cavernous communication. However, selective injection of the internal carotid artery gave no sign of any communication with the cavernous sinus (Fig. 4). On the other hand, selective injection of the external carotid artery revealed a large communication of the internal maxillary artery with the plexus of the oval foramen and via the cavernous sinus with the superior ophthalmic vein (Fig. 5). This condition is relatively rare and means a fundamental difference with the fistula between the internal carotid artery and the cavernous sinus where, by trying to obstruct the fistula with artificial thrombi through the internal carotid, these thrombi may land in the cerebral tissue when the target, the fistula, is missed. Hence, the neurosurgeon always begins by ligating the carotid artery distal to the site of the fistula. Inserting artificial thrombi into the external carotid artery on the other hand is not dangerous. In case the thrombi might slip through the fistula, they will arrive somewhere in the venous plexus of the orbit or in the facial veins.

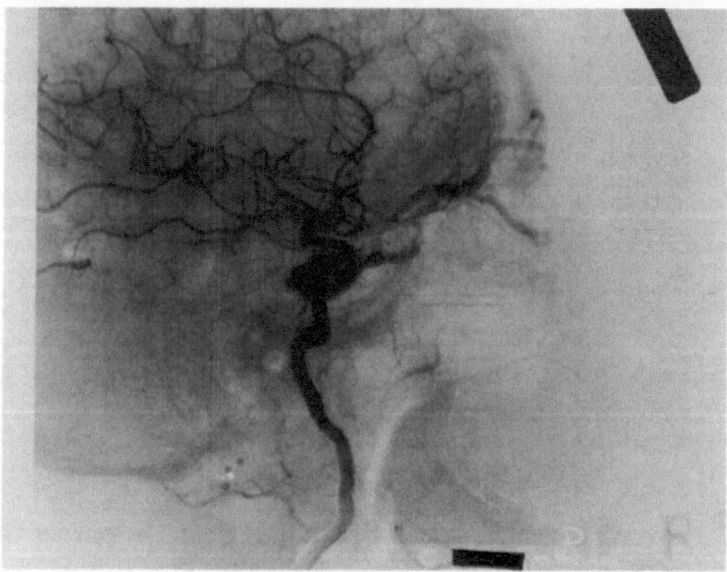

Fig. 3. Mrs O.K. 59 years of age. Example of spontaneous healing of carotid cavernous fistula (absence of pulsating bruit).

60

Correspondingly an effort was made to simplify the obstruction procedure of the fistula by using a Seldinger approach.* This method of Seldinger concerns a routine procedure to inject contrast medium into many of the main vessels of the body through long catheters inserted in the inguinal artery or vein. The external carotid artery was easily reached and the fistula

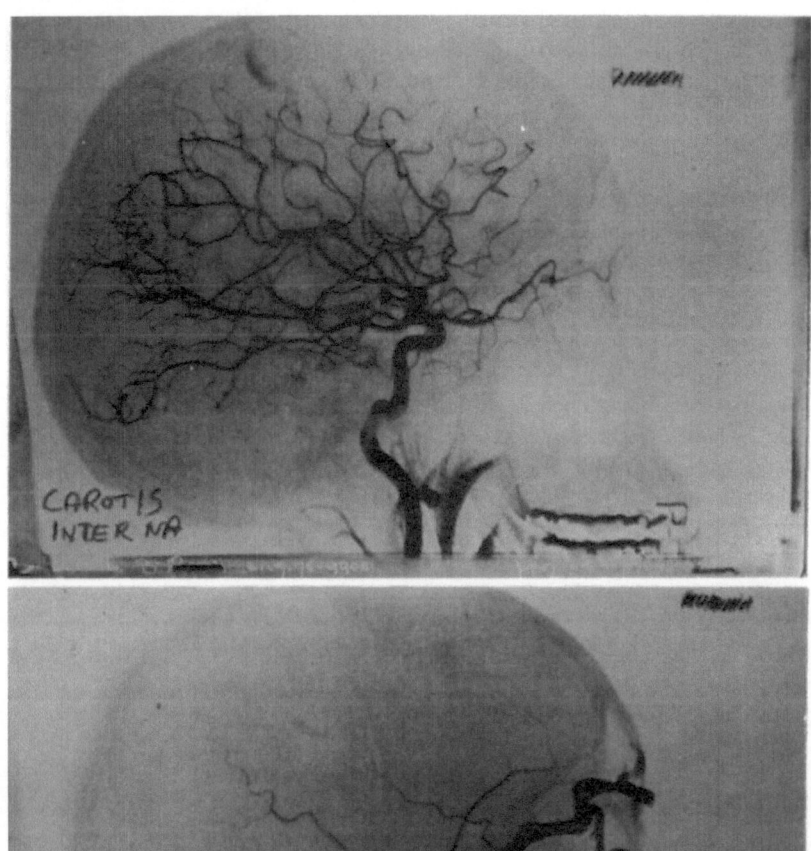

Fig. 4 and 5. Miss B.R. 18 years of age, with a record of four years of systolic buzzing on the right side. The internal carotid artery this time was not involved (Fig. 4), but the external carotid artery communicated with the cavernous sinus (Fig. 5).

* Prof. Dr. F.L.M. Peeters, neuroradiologist Wilhelmina Gasthuis Amsterdam.

was approached through the internal maxillary artery. Pieces of foam fibrine, with platinum markers, were injected but failed to enter into the shunt as if this was obstructed already. Without any hesitation all artificial thrombi floated outside the catheter in reverse direction into the lingual artery. Nevertheless, the buzzing had disappeared completely and after 5 months the girl was still in excellent condition. Apparently, the manipulation with the catheter had dislodged structures in the lumen of the shunting artery by which the fistula was obstructed definitively.

These examples may serve to demonstrate that pulsating exophthalmos and carotid cavernous fistula are not identical, but that many varieties and grades of arterio-venous shunt are influencing the clinical aspect and the treatment.

Seldinger catheterisation is a simple and effective method to direct thrombi to the fistula in certain instances.

REFERENCES

WALSH, F.B. & HOYT, W.E. Clinical Neuro-ophthalmology, Vol. II, p. 1714. The Williams & Wilkins Comp., Baltimore, (1969).

Authors' address:
Orbital Centre
Wilhelmina Gasthuis
Amsterdam, The Netherlands

PROPHYLAXIS IN RETINAL DETACHMENT

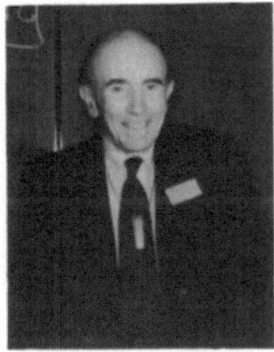

JAMES R. HUDSON

(London, England)

Prophylactic treatment of predisposing retinal lesions has been discussed in ophthalmic literature over many years, diathermy originally being the principal technique. The possibility of treatment with an instrument as easy to use as a direct ophthalmoscope was realized when the light coagulator was conceived by MEYER SCHWICKERATH and developed by him in conjunction with the Zeiss organization. It was consequent upon this important development that prophylactic treatment gained a firm hold upon the management of clinically recognizable retinal pathology, a position further strengthened by the re-introduction of cryotherapy by MCLEAN & LINCOFF in 1963. At the same time there was renewed interest in the distinction between benign and predisposing retinal conditions, a subject which remains controversial to the present day.

As with any new addition to our medical armamentarium, whether drug, diagnostic device or therapeutic instrument, enthusiasm in its use led to both favourable and unfavourable results appearing in the literature.

A simple example of a modality in which enthusiasm overcame clinical caution was in the treatment of macular holes. This led to a considerable difference of opinion as to what is and what is not a true macular hole. Increasing experience soon demonstrated that a high percentage of these are pseudo-holes, either due to the presence of a definite hole in another area of the retina, or to cystoid macular oedema, a condition now readily recognized by fluorescein angiography.

Other retinal lesions treated by light coagulation included areas of lattice degeneration, round holes, U-tears and the larger crescentic tears usually associated with lattice degeneration. The opercula of U-shaped and crescentic tears often exhibit vitreous traction and if this observation is confirmed surgery beyond simple light coagulation is certainly indicated. It was in this field of treatment that poor results were most frequently reported, not reflecting adversely upon the method but upon its application.

The re-discovery of cryotherapy in 1963 provided an undoubted alternative to diathermy and to it were ascribed other attributes giving it a potential advantage over light coagulation, for example the avoidance of vitreous changes. There has not, in my opinion, been any strong evidence that light coagulation, with the correct indications and properly applied, produces vitreous changes which will predispose to further retinal pathology to any greater extent than does cryotherapy. Evidence is stronger that the vitreous

63

pathology precedes the treatment, and that its sequelae will develop unless its proper recognition enables the surgeon to decide upon adequate measures as a primary procedure.

In general, therefore, some of the pioneers in the prophylactic treatment of retinal lesions by light coagulation are bound to have published results relatively unfavourable to its continued use, taking into account the degree of severity of the condition subjected to treatment.

It is my first purpose briefly to discuss the recent literature, in which a more conservative view is taken of the necessity for prophylactic treatment. As long ago as 1965, at the symposium in Houston dealing with the then new and controversial aspects of retinal detachment, SPIRA cited the dangers of the attitude prevalent in the preceding years, that the operative measures were easy, and demanded relatively little special experience. This led to the later recognition of complications – mild uveitis, hypotony, macular degeneration – and even more seriously to secondary retinal detachments with vitreous retraction and permanent visual loss. At that time SPIRA concluded that light coagulation was the only means of prophylactic treatment that was safe and effective. Should a detachment follow any form of preventive method, he considered that its management was much more difficult and he preferred to operate on a previously untreated eye.

More recently, further contributions to the literature have reiterated the importance of a conservative approach to prophylactic treatment. NEUMANN & HYAMS (1972) found that the continued observation of patients with asymptomatic retinal tears – albeit with considerable restriction upon their activities - was followed by no more complications than in cases that were treated.

The findings of DAVIS (1974) confirmed the earlier work of COLLYEAR & PISCHEL (1960), who found that in eyes with symptomatic fresh, horse-shoe breaks, between 30 and 50 per cent developed detachments if left untreated. DAVIS advised prophylactic cryotherapy for such cases. Observation is advised, however, in cases with free-floating opercula and with no evidence of vitreo-retinal adhesion.

He also holds the view that with modern techniques of detachment surgery the success rate will probably be as high as in cases treated prophylactically.

BYER (1974), dealing with a different sample of cases – asymptomatic breaks in first eyes -- has followed this series without treatment for 3-9 years. None of the breaks progressed to retinal detachment. He agrees, however, that treatment should be recommended in all cases with symptomatic breaks.

MORSE & SCHEIE (1974), on the other hand, advocate cryo-retinopexy when retinal breaks are identified. I would support this because firstly, I do not agree with DAVIS's view that the results of detachment surgery are as good as those of prophylactic treatment, and secondly, I consider that, particularly in fellow eyes, there is a significant risk of retinal detachment which can be minimised by prophylactic treatment.

The essential difference between the views expressed in these recent contributions and my own rests with the management of asymptomatic breaks. I support the use of treatment rather than observation because I think that the risk of intervention is less than that of a detachment developing in an untreated eye. This is obviously controversial when considering lesions in a first eye, but is less so in relation to fellow eyes, which achieve a degree of risk consequent upon first eye involvement, a risk variously estimated in the literature between 12 and 45 per cent.

My second purpose is to submit to you the indications which, in my opinion, should attract positive treatment. I am relying upon experience rather than statistics, and my preference for a philosophical approach is not any fear of contradiction, but my suspicion that figures tend to be indigestible when flung in quick succession upon the screen, often in a size beyond the discernment of anyone with less than telescopic vision.

These indications are:

1. Any retinal break, whether symptomatic or not, associated with evidence of vitreo-retinal traction, and especially if the upper half of the retina is involved.

2. Symptomatic breaks. These may present with an increase in muscae volitantes, with photopsiae, or with the symptoms of a vitreous haemorrhage. Our experience has been that over 60 per cent of cases with symptoms of a vitreous haemorrhage have fresh retinal breaks, the majority of them horse-shoe tears. Even occasional cases with evidence of relaxation of the vitreous traction (e.g. with floating opercula) are not immune to the development of detachments.

3. Predisposing lesions. Here I find Kanski's classification a useful one although, as I have already indicated, controversy persists when trying to classify benign and pre-disposing retinal pathology. Three remaining indications for treatment involve conditions which are relatively less frequent, but are nonetheless of paramount importance.

4. Retinal detachment in aphakia has a striking tendency to fellow-eye involvement, the risk being greater the shorter is the interval between cataract surgery and the onset of the detachment in the first eye.

Our retina unit has seen a sufficient number of cases with bilateral detachments following two cataract operations undertaken with a short intervening period for me to conclude that there should be an interval of at least three months between the two operations. If the first eye detaches during this period the fellow eye should undergo prophylactic treatment prior to cataract surgery.

5. The recognition of a giant retinal tear in one eye is a signal that the development of important retinal pathology in the fellow eye is, if not inevitable, highly probable. The second eye may become involved even in the absence of clinical evidence of a predisposition. I cannot over-emphasize the bilaterality of this condition, with an incidence of almost 50 per cent in non-traumatic cases, and an incidence of 84 per cent of fellow eye involvement in a detachment or with pre-detachment lesions. Our discouraging experience with giant retinal tears has made us wonder whether, in spite of any evident indication for the treatment of the fellow eye, it may not be justified by the poor prognosis.

6. A positive family history. This involves only 3 per cent of all cases (Cuendet), but our limited experience has been that the gravity of the detachment in these patients is greater and that the incidence of detachment

in fellow eyes is higher. The indication for prophylactic treatment is greater and it is my opinion that more radical rather than simpler techniques are the more reliable.

It is my third purpose to describe the methods of treatment of which we make use, bearing in mind always that the principle involved is that of producing the necessary protection with a minimum of surgical trauma, and with the least risk of initiating complications. All techniques involve the induction of choroido-retinal reaction and I need not comment further than to say that, of the methods currently available, cryotherapy and light coagulation are the most popular, with argon laser therapy and diathermy available as alternatives.

Prophylactic treatment can be undertaken:
1. Locally for single retinal breaks or limited areas of degenerative change.
2. Locally, for multiple areas of lattice degeneration with or without holes.

If there is any evidence of vitreous traction, or with larger tears, plombage should be associated with these two techniques.
3. By encircling cryotherapy or light coagulation, generally undertaken in two stages.
4. By a surgical encircling procedure in conjunction with such cryotherapy or light coagulation as may be necessary.

Over the past seven years we have selected certain cases for prophylactic treatment by a combination of cryotherapy and surgical encirclement with a silicone rubber rod or band. Eighteen of these were reported in 1973 (HUDSON, KANSKI & ELKINGTON) and at least a further seven have subsequently been treated. With evidence of moderate or severe vitreous traction, and when multiple equatorial holes or tears are involved, or when the first eye has undergone a series of unsuccessful surgical interventions, volume reduction in addition to the induction of local or circumferential choroido-retinal reaction should be considered. In our cases, complications have been minimal and in only one instance, when the encircling element was too tightly drawn up, was central vision adversely affected.

It is my conclusion from the clinical evidence which we have accumulated that, although over-enthusiasm in prophylactic treatment has undoubtedly led to new and sometimes grave problems, this is due in the majority of instances to lack of experience.

An over-conservative approach carries the risk of a higher incidence of retinal detachment and may involve patients in unnecessary 'ocular invalidism'.

Author's address:
36 Wimpole Street
London, W 1M 7AE
England

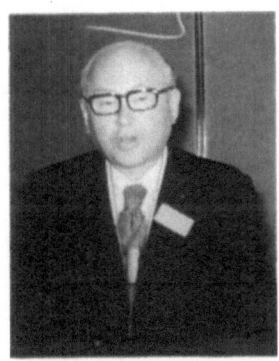

PHOTOCOAGULATION IN RETINAL DETACHMENT SURGERY

GERD MEYER-SCHWICKERATH

(Essen, Germany)

Gonin's principle, the sealing of retinal holes, is the most important step in the surgical treatment of retinal detachment. In former days when detachment surgery was mainly performed with surface- and penetrating diathermy, only a few variations of the operative procedure were known. Since eyeball-shortening, indenting and volume-reducing operations have been introduced we have a great variety of different techniques. This gives us a new opportunity to reflect upon Gonin's principle which rationally rests basically upon the two steps underlying all types of detachment surgery:
1. The retina has to be brought back into firm contact with the underlying pigment epithelium and choroid, at least in the area of the holes; and
2. the contact must be maintained whilst an inflammatory reaction causes the formation of a scar which involves both, retina and choroid and by this seals the retinal holes.

From the surgical point of view we can distinguish, therefore, between two steps:
1. Interventions for the re-application of the retina; (we call this 'active re-attachment operations').
2. Procedures for the permanent sealing of retinal defects.

The first step is *indispensable* for the operation of the second. Furthermore, the introduction of active re-attachment operations has made it possible to use photocoagulation for sealing off retinal defects.

I. INTERVENTION FOR THE RE-APPLICATION OF THE RETINA

The principles of this type of operations go back to the year 1903 when LEOPOLD MÜLLER in Vienna published his first cases of full thickness scleral resection called the 'Bulbusverkürzung'. Thirty years later by the publications of LINDNER this risky operation became somewhat more popular. The introduction of lamellar sclera-resection, which obviously was published simultaneously by LINDNER, DELLAPORTA, FRIEMANN-MARCHESANI, SHAPLAND & PAUFIQUE resulted in the fact that active re-attachment operations were accepted world-wide.

Only shortly thereafter the episcleral plombing operation of CUSTODIS and the encircling procedures of SCHEPENS & ARRUGA were added to the re-attachment operations.

It is interesting to note that WEVE (1949, 1950) whom we owe

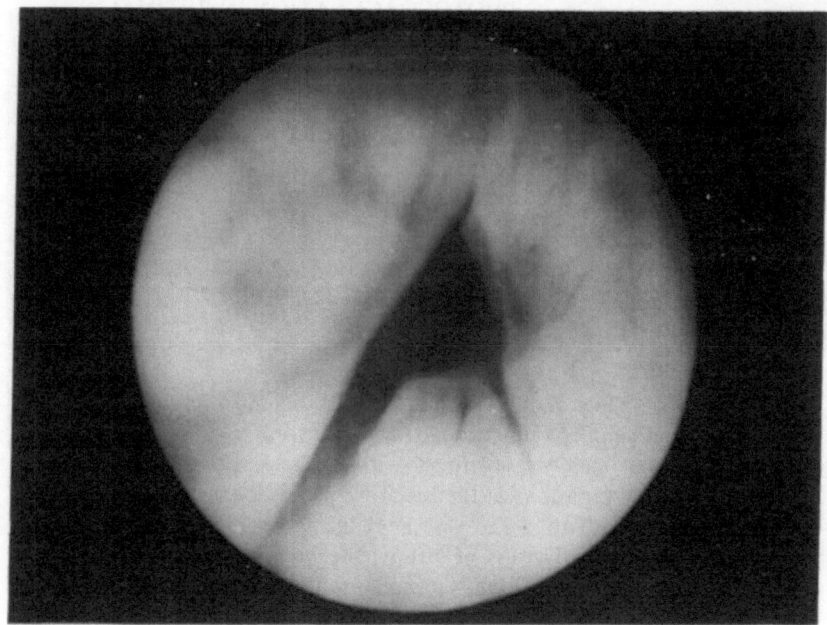

Fig. 1. Horse-shoe tear on a scleral infolding surrounded by photocoagulation.

the propagation of the use of diathermy in detachment operations noted, at the end of the Fourties, that diathermy does not only seal off retinal holes but that it has a considerable volume reducing and indenting effect on the sclera. The decrease of this effect about one week after diathermy application gave him the idea of the first scleral plastic operation in detachment surgery, the so-called *reefing*. Many good results of pure diathermy operations are certainly due to the volume-reducing effect of diathermy on the sclera.

Table 1 gives an estimated effect of the different re-attachment operations on the eyeball with regard to volume reduction, identation and shortening of the globe. The reduction of volume seems to be the most important and constant effect. Indentation, however, as well as the shortening, which

Table 1. The different effects of re-attachment operation to the size of the globe.

Redetachment Operations

	Volume red.	indenting	shortening
Diathermy	+	+	(+)
Tot. scl. Resect.	+ +	(+)	+ + +
Lam scl. Resect.	+ +	+ +	+ + +
Tot. scl. infolding	+ + +	+ + +	+ + +
Plombage	+ +	+ + +	+
Encircling	+ + +	+ + +	−

means myopia-diminishing effect, is quite different from one intervention to another. In encircling procedures the shortening effect is reversed!

With regard to the individual case and situation it is now important which type of re-attachment operation is to be chosen. The following factors play an important role in the choice of the re-attachment operation: The amount of subretinal fluid, the refraction of the eye, the thickness of the sclera, the presence or absence of traction by the vitreous and previous operations.

I cannot go into detail here, but I would like to give one example: In cases of high grade myopia we prefer a lamellar scleral resection or full thickness scleral infolding in the temporal circumference. We know that this eyeball shortening procedure, which reduces the myopia, has a good influence on the detached retina in such cases. If, however, in such a case the amount of subretinal fluid is such that with a scleral infolding over half the circumference a re-attachment of the retina is not possible, we might combine scleral infolding with an encircling procedure. *Different volume-reducing operations can be combined!*

Most 'active re-attachment operations' have been described by our school in detail.

II. PROCEDURE FOR THE SEALING OF RETINAL HOLES

There is a general tendency to use those procedures which produce little trauma to the ocular tissue and, more important, which can easily be applied.

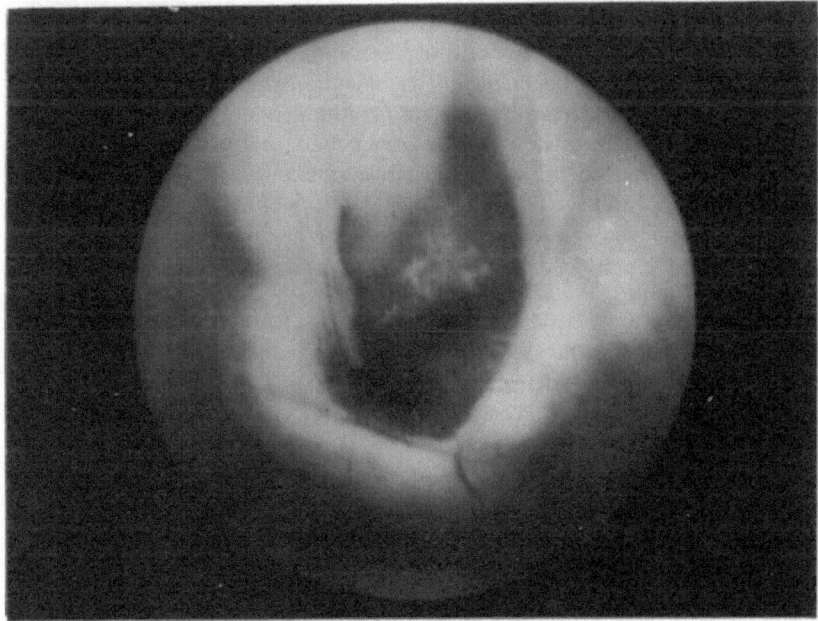

Fig. 2. Large horse-shoe tear on the buckle of a pocket- (episcleral) operation surrounded by photocoagulations.

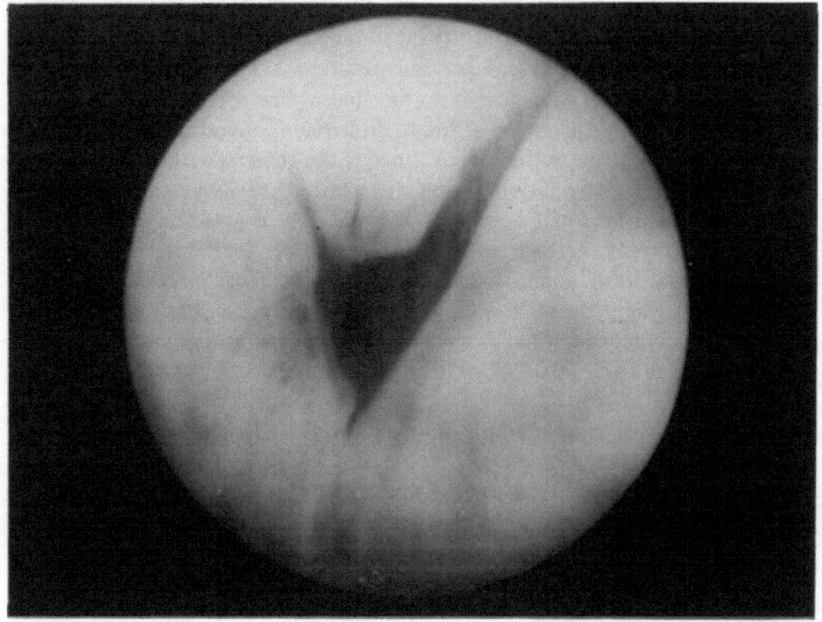

Fig. 3. V-shaped hole on the summit of an intrascleral pocket-operation surrounded by photocoagulation.

Diathermy-coagulation

Diathermy-coagulation is still one of the simplest and safest methods to produce a chorio-retinal adhesion. The objection that diathermy damages the sclera is unimportant as long as it is used moderately and as the sclera is infolded and the coagulated area is embedded. In cases of very flat and circumscribed detachments we use intrascleral-diathermy in form of a trap-doorprocedure. If this trapdoor is filled with lyophilized sclera or dura mater we have already a scleral pocket operation en miniature.

Cryo-coagulation

Cryo-coagulation has the great advantage that there is little damage to the sclera. It has the disadvantage that the application on the sclera, retina and choroid becomes almost invisible within a few seconds. Experience, of course, can overcome these difficulties.

Cryo-coagulation does not lead to shrinkage of the sclera as does diathermy. This can be regarded as an advantage. In cases, however, where some volume-reducing effect is desired, this is rather a disadvantage.

In spite of the fact that in some detachment centres cryo-coagulation has been picked up with great enthusiasm there are others with a tendency to to turn back to diathermy and photocoagulation. The inventor of cryo-coagulation, Professor BIETTI, in a recent paper comes to the same conclusion, himself.

The main purpose of this paper is to explain the advantages of photocoagulation in detachment surgery. We feel that in all cases in which photocoagulation can be performed it has all the advantages of diathermy *and* cryocoagulation without having their disadvantages. Because of this reason we have used photocoagulation progressively since more than 20 years in combination with operative procedures. Nowadays, 90% of all our detachment cases are finished with a photocoagulation procedure either at the end of the operation or a few days later. We do not coagulate retinal holes, tears or defects only, but also equatorial- (lattice-) degenerations. We like to combine areas with such changes with a chain of photocoagulation.

If an indentation or buckling operation has been performed it is important to realize that photocoagulation has to be applied to an area which is highly hypermetropic. This error in refraction has to be corrected either with a contact lens or by inserting a plus lens into the beam between the mirror of the photocoagulator and the patient's eye. The new photocoagulator of Zeiss (1975) contains a convergent-system up to 12 dptr. in order to facilitate photocoagulation of hypermetropic areas (Fig. 6).

The performance of photocoagulation at the end of the operation or a few days later has two more advantages compared with cryo-coagulation or diathermy application:

1. The coagulation is performed when the retina has settled. This means that failures of localization are avoided. The coagulation can be placed very

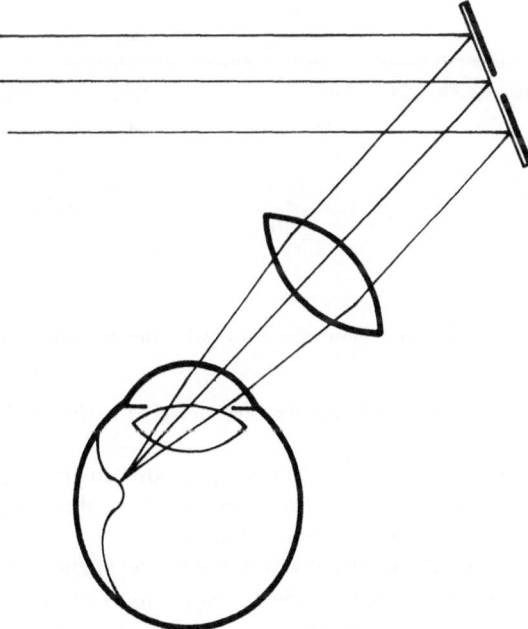

Fig. 4. Situation of introducing a plus lens (+14) in pathway of light between the mirror of the photocoagulator and the patient's eye by the surgeon. The new instrument (1975) has a convergent system incorporated.

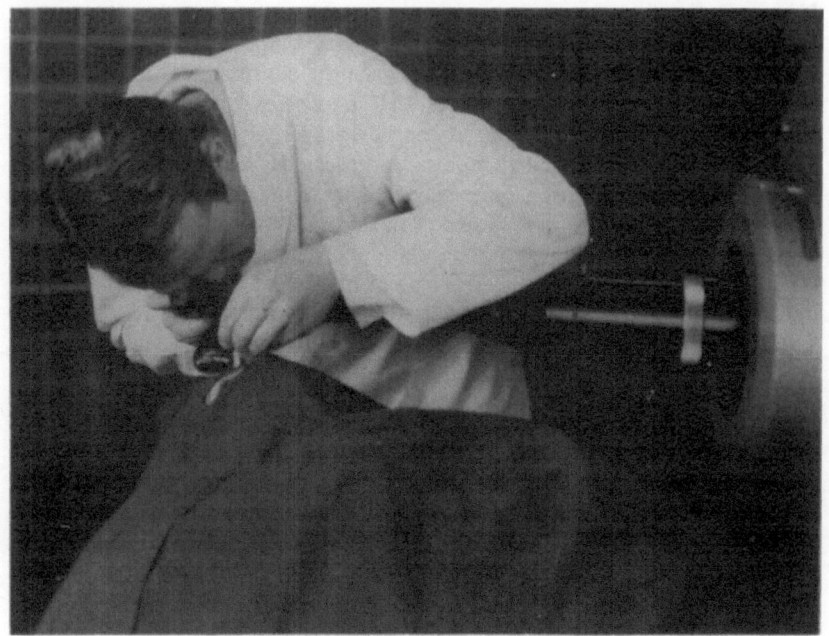

Fig. 5. Old Zeiss Photocoagulator and plus lens for coagulations on buckle.

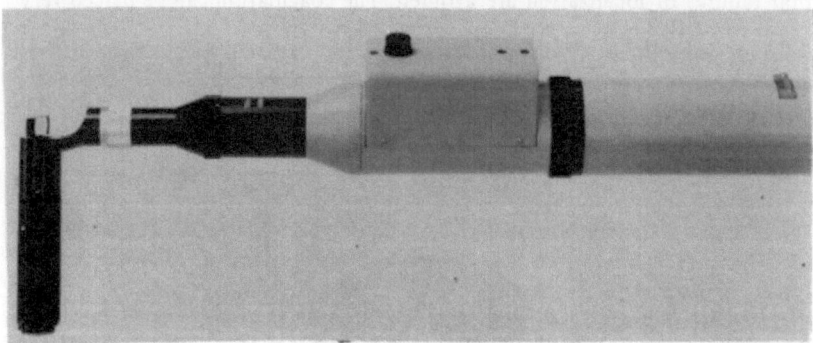

Fig. 6. New (1975) Zeiss Xenon-Photocoagulator with the possibility of convergent beam.

exactly and the destruction of unnecessary areas of retina and choroid is avoided.

2. In case the retina does *not* settle the coagulation can *not* be performed. Thus, unnecessary and uneffective destruction of choroid and pigment epithelium is avoided which otherwise would take place.

This latter is the most important advantage of the application of photocoagulation in detachment surgery, which will be appreciated by every surgeon who has to do many re-operations.

Photocoagulation is also very effective in cases of re-operations. In these cases it is unnecessary to re-coagulate areas which have previously been treated with diathermy or cryo-coagulation.

In his book: 'Le Décollement De La Rétine' A. URRETS-ZAVALIA (JR.) mentions several objections against photocoagulation in detachment surgery in discussing the paper of L. GIRARD. After 20 years of experience with this combined method I can accept none of his objections:

1. Cryo- or diathermycoagulation can be applied *simply*. This is certainly true but no argument against photocoagulation. The latter is certainly more difficult to apply but still has all the mentioned advantages.

2. The *size of the pupil* can be taken under control.

3. Opacities of the ocular media are extremely rare in well controlled cases and

4. Residual detachment in the area of the hole should lead to late post-operative photocoagulation.

5. Changes of refraction in the area of the hole can easily be corrected by the introduction of lenses or with the new Zeiss Photocoagulator.

6. 'Late' coagulation a few days after the operation is no problem for the surgeon if he has sufficient experience.

7. Postoperative changes such as chemosis of the conjunctiva or the lids do not interfere with the treatment.

8. The intervention is not more painful than before the operation, on the contrary.

9. The patient does not mind a 'second' intervention if he is prepared to it.

We usually tell the patient that the intervention (mostly in local retrobulbar anaesthesia) is necessary to prevent a recurrency.

We have never had difficulties in postoperative photocoagulation: I believe that this is mainly a question of experience.

III. PROPHYLACTIC TREATMENT OF RETINAL DETACHMENT

Prophylaxis is the treatment of retinal detachment before it has actually occurred. We recommend to perform prophylactic treatment with the conventional xenon-photocoagulator or with the argon-laser-coagulator in those cases in which one eye has a detachment and the second eye has holes or equatorial degenerations without detachment. The same rule is adapted for cases with a positive family history of retinal detachment.

For more than five years we have compared xenon-coagulation, laser-photocoagulation and cryo-coagulation for the purpose of prophylactic treatment. Our conclusion is that photo- and laser-coagulation is not always the easiest procedure but by all means the least traumatic and most accurate one. I cannot go into details and discuss all the problems of the risk of prophylactic treatment. The issue of the symposium of the German Ophthalmological Society (H. FANTA & W. JAEGER, 1970) contains many papers on this subject.

Retinoschisis

Our approach in cases of retinoschisis has not changed for the past 10 years. Since then we have treated the outer layer in retinoschisis with photocoagulation with the result that almost 80% of the cases settle completely. Further surgical intervention seems to be necessary only in cases in which retinoschisis is combined with retinal detachment. Then, of course, the rules of detachment operations come into action.

SUMMARY

The surgical treatment of retinal detachment has undergone a considerable change within the last 25 years. The introduction of volumereducing, globe-shortening and scleral-indenting operations has brought up a variety of new operations and has improved the results.

The introduction of active re-attachment operations has, at the same time, resulted in the fact that photocoagulation can be introduced as brake-closing procedure in surgical cases.

In contrast to diathermy-coagulation and to cryo-coagulation, photocoagulation has the advantage that it can be applied *only* in cases in which the retina is in close contact to the pigment epithelium and the choroid.

We have no doubt that the combined two-step operation technique with re-attachment in the first step and brake-closing procedure in the second step has brought about better results in detachment surgery. It is certainly not the easiest way of treatment but it is more accurate and less traumatic than any other brake-closing procedure. For this reason we feel that photocoagulation has a constant and growing place in the operative treatment of retinal detachment.

REFERENCES

ARRUGA, H. Technical variations in retinal detachment surgery. *Soc. Oft. Hisp.-Am.* 18: *55* (1958): *Zentralbl. Ophth. (Abstract)*, 74: *307* (1958).

BIETTI, G.B. Vergleichende Bewertung der Diathermie und der Cryo-applikation bei der Behandlung der Netzhautablösung. *Klin. Mobl. Augenhk.* 152, *181-194* (1968).

CUSTODIS, E. Observations on diathermy treatment of retinal detachment and new therapeutic approaches. 57th Meeting Deutsche, ophth. Gesellsch., p. 227, Sept. (1951).

DELLAPORTA, A. Experimental shortening of the eye through scleral folding (lamellar scleral resection). Ophth. Soc. Vienna, 9. Oct. (1950), *Graefes Arch. Ophthal.*, 152: *28* (1951).

DELLAPORTA, A. Shortening of the eye through scleral folding (lamellar scleral resection). *Klin. Monatsbl. Augenh.*, 119: *135* (1951).

FANTA, H. & W. JAEGER Die Prophylaxe der Ablatio retinae. Bergmann, München (1970).

FRIEMANN,W. Experiences in the treatment of retinal detachment through shortening of the eye, 56th Meeting Deutsche ophth. Gesellsch. p. 204, Sept. (1950).

GIRARD, L.J. & A.R. MC. PHERSON Bourrelet Scléral: Plissement total et circulaire avec cordonnet en coautchouc Silionique Associé. a la Photocoagulation. *Bull. Soc. franc. Ophthal* 74, *190-210* (1961).

GIRARD, L.J. & A.R. MC PHERSON Scleral Buckling. *Arch. Ophthal.* 67, *409-420* (1962).

LINDNER, K. Shortening of the eye by scleral folding (lamellar) scleral resection. Ophth. Soc. Vienna Meeting, 25. Nov. 1946; Wien, Klin. Woch., p. 206, 1949, *Zentralbl. Ophth.* (Abstract), 52: *190* (1950).

LINDNER, K. Attempts to cure retinal detachments with poor prognosis. *Ztschr. Augenh.*, 81: *277* (1933).

PAUFIQUE, L. & R. HUGONNIER Treatment of retinal detachment with scleral resection: Personal technique; indications and results, *Bull. Soc. Ophth. France*, 64: *435* (1951).

SCHEPENS, C.L. The scleral buckling procedures: Surgical techniques and management, I-IV. *A.M.A. Arch. Ophth.*, 58: *797* (1957); 60: *84* (1958); 60: *1003* (1958); 62: *445* (1959).

SHAPLAND, C.D. Scleral resection-lamellar. *Proc. Roy. Soc. Med.*, 44: *420* (1951).

URRETS-ZAVALIA, A. Le lécollement de la Rétine. Manou, Paris (1968).

WEVE, H. Shortening of the eye by reefing the sclera. *Opthalmologica*, 118: *660* (1949).

WEVE, H. Shortening of the sclerotic (reefing) in analogy with the furlings of sails. XVI Intern. Cong. Ophth. London, Vol. 2, p. 1179, (1950).

Author's address:
Universitäts-Augenklinik
Hufelandstrasse 55
Essen
Germany

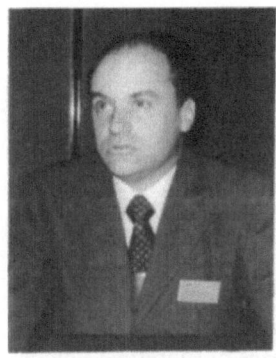

SURGICAL TREATMENT OF EQUATORIAL GIANT TEARS

A. WESSING

(Tubingen, West Germany*)

The difficulties in the surgical management of retinal detachment due to equatorial giant tears are well known. Extensive surgical techniques reaching from operations on hanging patients (SCHEPENS & FREEMAN 1967) intravitreal injection of liquid silicone (CIBIS 1965), the use of human centrifuges (NEAULT & MARTENS 1966, TEN DOESSCHATE 1968, RENELT & MEYER-SCHWICKERATH 1972) all the way to total vitrectomy combined with injection of air or gas (MACHEMER, AABERG & NORTON 1969, MCLEAN & NORTON 1974) demonstrate how far the therapeutic attempts may go.

At the same time these sophisticated methods clearly show the limits of such procedures. In an effort to find a simpler surgical method which can be applied for the majority of selected cases and which lead to comparable therapeutic success we arrived at a modified cerclage technique. This paper provides a description of the technique. Results, indications and contraindications of this method are discussed.

SURGICAL TECHNIQUE

TABLE 1

Surgical technique

---

1. Deviated encircling silicone rod corresponding to the location and extension of the tear and largely avoiding compression of vortex veins.
2. Drainage of subretinal fluid and of fluid vitreous with electrolysis.
3. Injection of Ringer's solution or hyaluronic acid (if needed).
4. Photocoagulation of the area of contact between retina and buckle.

The standard procedure is based on cerclage with a silicone rod of 2 mm diameter[1]. After careful localization of both the posterior edge and the lateral corners of the giant tear, the rod is sutured to the sclera in a

---

* In Anlehnung an: WESSING, A., SPITZNAS M. & A. PALOMAR, 'Management of retinal detachment due to giant tears', *Albrecht von Graefes Archiv für klinische und experimentelle Ophthalmologie* 192: 277-284 (1974).

[1] Leonhard Klein, Heidelberg, Germany

corresponding, slightly more posterior position. In many cases one or even two of the rectus muscles have to be temporarily removed, since it may be necessary to place the encircling element as far posteriorly as the region of the optic nerve or the macula. Toward the lateral extent of the tear the rod is brought forward to the equator (Fig. 1).

Thereafter, it runs at the equator and is closed at the opposite side of the eye. The posterior deviation of the cerclage in the area of the defect makes it possible to occlude tears of 180° or more without damaging the vortex veins on the other side of the eye.

In order to create stable and permanent conditions with definite contact of the re-attached retina at the edge of the buckle, subretinal fluid is drained by electrolysis puncture (Fig. 1). We feel that drainage of subretinal fluid is essential for two reasons. First, it allows a high indentation of the cerclage, which leads to a good contact between the edges of the tear and the cerclage buckle. Secondly, it is necessary for intravitreal injection. In cases where the retina is rolled over, hyaluronic acid[2] is injected under the flap using a long needle introduced through the pars plana (Fig. 1). Simultaneously, subretinal fluid and/or liquified vitreous are drained by electrolysis puncture, posterior to the buckle in the region of the tear (Fig. 1). With well controlled, step-wise injection and drainage it is often possible to unfold the retina completely or, at least, to bring it into good contact with the edge of the buckle.

Slight vitreous adhesions at the edge of the tear do not necessarily represent a contraindication for this technique. Only cases with massive vitreous strand formation and severe vitreous tractions are excluded.

The surgical procedure is concluded by photocoagulation. In cases where coagulation of the edge of the tear is not feasible, it is possible to coagulate the retina in contact with the buckle through the erect retinal flap (Fig. 2).

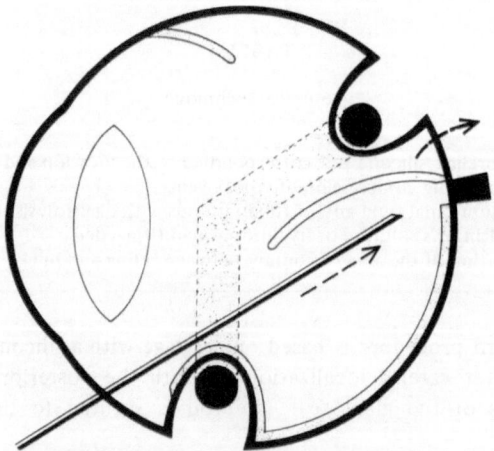

Fig. 1. Deviated cerclage technique in equatorial giant tears.

2   Healon-H, Biotrics Inc. 24 Beck Road, Arlington, Mass., U.S.A.

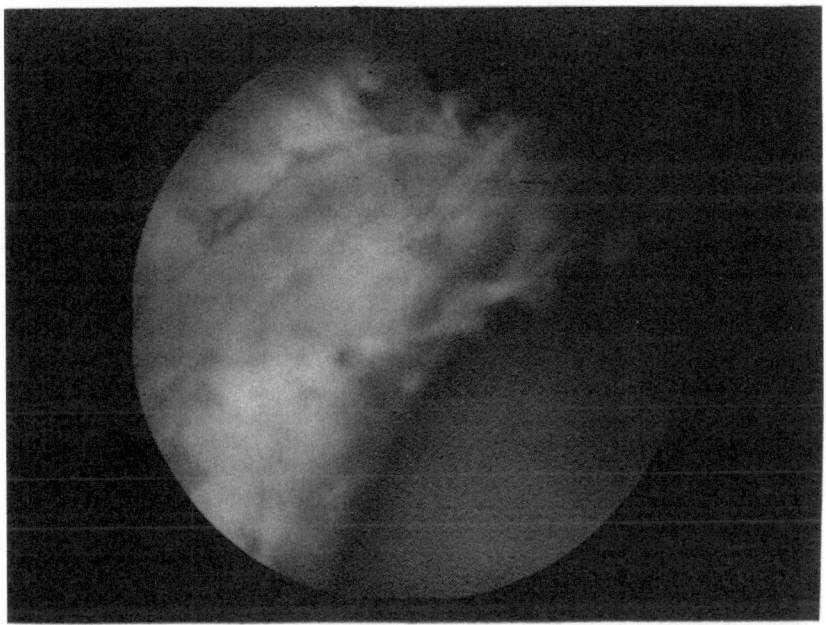

Fig. 2. Equatorial giant tear treated with deviated cerclage and photocoagulation.

If no reactions are obtained in this manner, it is often sufficient to coagulate the junction between attached retina and the buckle by directing the beam through the tear.

In these cases one should not hesitate to coagulate the exposed pigment epithelium and the underlying choroid until they shrink. The reactive exudation of fibrin is sufficient to create a solid contact between retina and buckle, which is maintained until scar formation is completed. At the corners of the tear the coagulations are extended up to the ora serrata. If this is not possible, a circular, i.e. 360° coagulation of the edge of the buckle is carried out. Photocoagulation may have to be performed in several sessions over a period of 1 to 2 weeks after surgery and must be continued until a firm occlusion of the defect has been achieved (Tab. 1).

In some important points our technique of operating retinal giant tears described here is different from other comparable procedures.

1. SIAM (1973) does not release subretinal fluid, which limits the method to relatively few cases with very favourable conditions. Giant tears with rolled-over retina cannot be treated.

2. In contrast to the oblique cerclage of PANNARALE the deviated cerclage gives less damage to the vortex veins and facilitates a watertight closure of the anterior corners of the giant tear.

3. The main and fundamental difference, however, is the use of photocoagulation. It is the great advantage of photocoagulation that the application can be done under optical controll and that the coagulation treatment can easily be repeated, if necessary.

79

RESULTS

The technique described was employed in eyes with partial or total retinal detachment due to equatorial giant tears of 90-240° (Tab. 2).

TABLE 2

Results in a total of 56 operated eyes

Retina	Immediately after surgery	Long term
Attached	48 (86%)	28 (50%)
Detached	8 (14%)	28 (50%)

A total of 56 eyes were operated, 8 of these twice or more. In 48 eyes the operation resulted in a re-attachment of the retina. Long term observations over a period of 2 months to 4 years, with a mean observation time of 6 months revealed permanent success in 28 eyes, i.e. 50%. Failures were all due to strand formation in the vitreous body or to M.V.R. Of the 28 cured eyes central vision remained unchanged or improved in 22 cases. In 6 instances it decreased due to 'macular puckering'.

FACTORS INFLUENCING THE RESULTS

There is a number of factors which may influence the results of surgery.

To our surprise, the degree of myopia did not seem to be important. The mean value of refraction was about the same in successful and unsuccessful cases (Table 3).

TABLE 3

Factors influencing the results: myopia

Retina	< −5.0 d	> −5.0 d	Average
Attached	13 (46%)	15 (54%)	−9.0 d
Detached	12 (43%)	16 (57%)	−8.5 d

The size of the tear, however, is of special importance. Surgical success rapidly decreased with increasing extention of the defect. This does not mean, that cases with tears of more than 180° are hopeless. The largest tear in a successfully treated eye was 240° (Table 4).

TABLE 4

Factors influencing the results: size of tear

Retina	100-150°	150−180°	> 180°	Average
Attached	16 (57%)	9 (32%)	3 (11%)	155°
Detached	11 (39%)	10 (36%)	7 (25%)	175°

Amazingly, rolling over or folding of the tear margin had no influence on the success of surgery. This demonstrates clearly the value of a combined injection-drainage technique (Table 5).

TABLE 5

Factors influencing the results: edges of tear

Retina	Rolled up	Straight
Attached	15	13
Detached	14	14

A very important factor was the extent of retinal detachment present. Surgical prognosis deteriorated with increasing extent of retinal detachment. Total detachment reduced the chances of success to a minimum. This fact has a corresponding finding in the pre-operative visual acuity. In the successfully treated eyes the mean pre-operative visual acuity was 0.15, whereas in the failures it was only 0.07 (Table 6).

TABLE 6

Factors influencing the results: extent of detachment

Retina	Total	Partial
Attached	4 (14%)	24 (86%)
Detached	20 (71%)	8 (29%)

Since the development of a total detachment of the retina is, at least in part, a question of time, a deterioration of the results has to be expected with an increasing time interval between the onset of the first subjective symptom and the date of surgery. The numbers in Table 7 confirm this tendency, which is also influenced by the slowly progressing secondary changes of the vitreous body (Table 7).

TABLE 7

Factors influencing the results: time interval between onset of symptoms and date of surgery

Retina	1 week	2–4 weeks	4 weeks
Attached	12 (43%)	14 (50%)	2 (7%)
Detached	7 (25%)	17 (61%)	4 (14%)

Additional ocular disorders such as subluxation of the lens, aphakia, glaucoma or buphthalmos, previous detachment prophylaxis and blunt or perforating injuries, all had an equally negative influence. This was especially true when trauma was the cause of the retinal detachment (Table 8). The presence of small additional holes does not seem to influence the results.

TABLE 8

Factors influencing the results:
additional ocular pathology

	Retina Attached	Detached
With additional pathology		
trauma	4 (14%)	9 (32%)
aphakia	2 (7%)	4 (14%)
glaucoma	1 (3.5%)	2 (7%)
prophylaxis	1 (3.5%)	2 (7%)
Total	8 (39%)	17 (61%)
Without additional pathology	20 (71%)	11 (29%)

The evaluation of pre-existing equatorial degenerations or other retinal detachment precursors is so uncertain in eyes with giant tears that they will not be further discussed here.

The state of the fellow eye does not give any useful prognostic hints. It should be mentioned, however, that in a remarkable number of cases the fellow eye showed peripheral retinal disease (Table 9).

TABLE 9

Factors influencing the results: state of the fellow eye

Retina	No changes	Equatorial degenerations	Ret. detachment or amaurosis
Attached	4 (14%)	14 (50%)	10 (36%)
Detached	9 (32%)	12 (43%)	7 (25%)

COMPARISON WITH RESULTS IN GIANT ORAL DISINSERTION

A comparison of these findings with the results of surgery in oral disinsertions seems to be worthwhile. As to be expected, the success rate was considerable higher, i.e. 88% primary success and 81% long-term success (Table 10).

TABLE 10

Results of surgery in 26 eyes with
giant oral disinsertion

Retina	Immediately after surgery	Long term
Attached	23 (88%)	21 (81%)
Detached	3 (12%)	5 (19%)

As in equatorial giant tears, a large extension of an oral disinsertion, total retinal detachment and additional ocular pathology had a negative influence on the surgical outcome (Table 11).

TABLE 11

Factors influencing the results in giant oral disinsertions

Retina	Size of defect, average	Extent of detachment		Additional pathology	
		total	partial	without	with
Attached	120°	7 (33%)	14 (67%)	12 (57%)	9 (43%)
Detached	140°	4 (80%)	1 (20%)	1 (20%)	4 (80%)

CONCLUSION

In conclusion, the following indications and contra-indications for surgery consisting of a modified cerclage technique, intravitreal injection of hyaluronic acid or Ringer's solution, if needed, and photocoagulation are proposed:

Indications	Relative indications	Contra-indications
1. Tears up to 200°	1. Tears between 200° and 240°	1. Tears larger than 240°
2. Partial detachment	2. Total detachment	2. Strand formation and retraction of vitreous
3. No major vitreous pathology	3. Aphakia	3. Severe preexisting ocular damage (e.g. trauma)
	4. Additional ocular pathology	

REFERENCES

CIBIS, P.A. Vitreoretinal pathology and surgery in retinal detachment. Mosby St. Louis (1965).

DOESSCHATE J. TEN. Reattachment of the retina by means of centrifugal force. *Mod. Probl. Ophthal.* 7: *325-326* (1968).

FREEMAN H.M., G.C. COUVILLION & G.L. SCHEPENS. Vitreous surgery. IV. Intraocular balloon. Clinical application. *Arch. Ophthal.* 83: *715-721* (1970).

MACHEMER R., T.M. AABERG & F.W.D. NORTON. Giant retinal tears. II. Experimental production and management with intravitreal air. *Amer. J. Ophthal.* 68: *1022-1029* (1969).

MACHEMER R. & F.W.D. NORTON. Vitrectomy, a pars plana approach. II. clinical experience. *Mod. Probl. Ophthal.* 10: *178-185* (1972).

MC LEAN E.B. & E.W.D. NORTON. Use of intraocular air and sulfur hexafluoride gas in the repair of selected retinal detachments. *Mod. Probl. Ophthal.* 12: *428-435* (1974).

NEAULT R.W. & T.G. MARTENS. Retinal detachment: use of human centrifuge in treatment. *Proc. Mayo. Clin.* 41: *145-149* (1966).

PANNARALE M.R. Techniques de traitement du décollement avec déchirures très postérieures. *Mod. Probl. Ophthal.* 4: *239-245* (1966).

RENELT P. & G. MEYER-SCHWICKERATH. Über die Beeinflussung von Netzhautrissen durch Zentrifugalkräfte. *Mod. Probl. Ophthal.* 10: *88-91* (1972).

SCHEPENS C.I. & H.M. FREEMAN. Current management of giant retinal breaks. *Trans. Amer. Acad. Ophthal. Otolarying* 71: *474-487* (1967).

SIAM A.L. Encircling silicone rod without drainage for retinal detachment with giant breaks. *Brit. J. Ophthal.* 57: *537-541* (1973).

Author's address:
Universitäts-Augenklinik
Abteilung und Lehrstuhl IV-Retinologie
Schleichstrasse 12
Tübingen
Germany

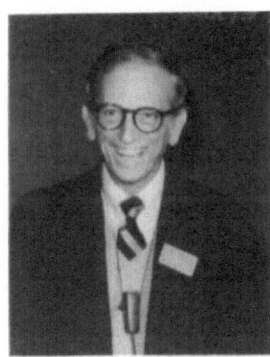

I. THE LIMITS OF CONSTRICTION FOR ENCIRCLING ELEMENTS

H. LINCOFF

SUMMARY

A constricting silicone band around the eye is a useful adjunct to the local scleral buckle procedure of Custodis. Subretinal fluid need not be drained. The required intrusion is predetermined and obtained by stretching the encircling element and utilizing its elastic return to drive intraocular fluid from the eye through internal channels over several hours.

The amount of constriction obtained without drainage of subretinal fluid is identical to what would be obtained by an equivalent shortening of the band in an eye in which subretinal fluid is drained. Studies on an animal model in 1967 suggested that a 20% shortening of the circumferential lenght was a maximum tolerable constriction. In the subsequent six years, 110 eyes among 800 retinal detachment patients were constricted between 10% and 20%. In 50 patients the operation was completed without drainage of subretinal fluid. The attachement rate in the undrained eyes was comparable to that in the drained eyes. Except for choroidal detachment, whose incidence is reduced by one-half, the rate of complications is not significantly altered by not draining.

II. PREFERENCE FOR RADIAL BUCKLING OVER CIRCUMFERENTIAL BUCKLING

H. LINCOFF

SUMMARY

More holes and in particular large horseshoe breaks, can be closed effectively with radially oriented buckles than can with buckles oriented circumferentially. Experience led us to a preference for this radial buckling in many instances as a solution to closing the retinal hole as the nondrainage technique for treating retinal detachment developed.

Circumferential buckles are frequently complicated by radial folds that leak beneath the posterior retina and radial buckles present no such complication. Radial buckling reaches its maximum usefulness in the treatment of large posterior horseshoe tears on the temporal side. The buckling of such tears poses the threat of distortion of the macula. When such a break is buckled circumferentially, a radial fold into the macula is a virtual certainty. On the other hand, no radial fold has occurred in our experience when the implant was oriented radially; we have on occasion extended a radial implant within two disk diameters of the macula with no consequent distortion.

Potential radial folds can be averted virtually without exception by relying on radial buckling. The buckle stretches the retinal break tightly across its surface and it fills a potential radial fold.

In many instances the combination of an encircling silicone band and radial silastic sponges is ideal (fig. 1).

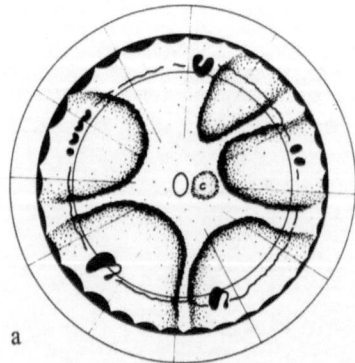
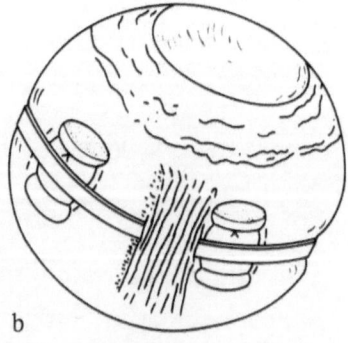

a   b

Fig. 1 Multiple holes connected by a line of circumferential traction in an aphakic eye were buckled with an encircling silicone band and radial sponges beneath the larger horseshoe breaks at 12.15, 5.15, and 7.30. *b* The inferior aspect of the eye demonstrating the encircling silicone band and two radial sponges at 5.15 and 7.30.

86

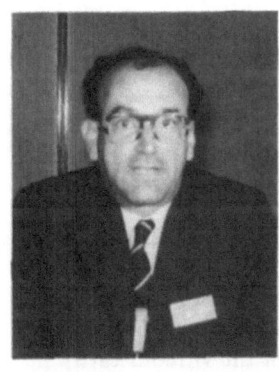

THE ANATOMY AND BIOMICROSCOPY OF THE VITREOUS BODY

GEORG EISNER

(Bern, Switzerland)

It may surprise that at a meeting on new developments in ophthalmology the anatomy and biomicroscopy of the vitreous should be dealt with. What new information is to be expected in that field, where methods of examination have remained unchanged for many years?

In fact, already in the last century many anatomical examinations of the vitreous were performed. Early investigators made out a peripheral portion concentrically laminated, and a central radiate portion (Fig. 15a) findings confirmed later by highly elaborate histological methods (SZENT-(GYÖRGYI) (Fig. 16a). However, doubts were expressed as to the validity of these observations since the methods employed did not exclude artefacts of preparation. With the increasing knowledge about the behaviour of gels they have become even more doubtful, as similar structures have been observed in artificial gels as well.

With the concept of the vitreous as being a gel and the structures recognizable therein a product of mere haphazard, interest in further investigations was lost for a long time. If clinical problems were discussed they usually delt with a heavily deteriorated vitreous, as in massive periretinal fibrosis or proliferative diabetic retinopathy.

New interest, however, has arisen, since the examination of the vitreous base in living eyes, made possible only recently with the introduction of indentation biomicroscopy (EISNER 1973) has revealed characteristic reactions of the vitreous depending on specific anatomical structures. As those reactions were not entirely compatible with vitreous concepts of that period, new anatomical examinations were undertaken.

In this paper I shall present some of the new findings and their clinical implications, trying to demonstrate that the examination even of normal or only slightly altered vitreous can yield valuable information to the clinician.

1. ANATOMY OF THE VITREOUS BODY

The closest approach to vitreous anatomy, as present in the living eye, is provided by the examination of unfixed autopsy eyes, where artefacts of fixation are excluded (EISNER 1971, 1973). The vitreous is exposed by removing the coats of the eye, including the retina (Fig. 1).

Slit-lamp illumination of such specimens produces the same optical phenomena as in biomicroscopic examination of the living eye (Fig. 3): optically denser structures are revealed through scattered light, inter-faces through reflection.

Three zones (Fig. 2) are to be distinguished in the vitreous:
— a preretinal zone
— an intermediary zone
— a retrolental zone.

The preretinal zone covers the vitreous wherever it is adjacent to the retina, ending thus at the ora serrata. The intermediary zone extends anteriorly towards the ciliary body resp. the free portion of the anterior hyaloid membrane. It contains several fine membranelles which originate in the region of the optic nerve head and proceed anteriorly through the vitreous cavity in an onion-peel arrangement. Outermost is the preretinal tract (Fig. 4 and Fig. 11c), separating the preretinal zone from the intermediary zone and inserting at the ora serrata. Next, two more tracts insert at fine bands of circular zonular fibres in the middle of the pars plana (median tract) and above the posterior third of the corona ciliaris (coronary tract). Innermost there is

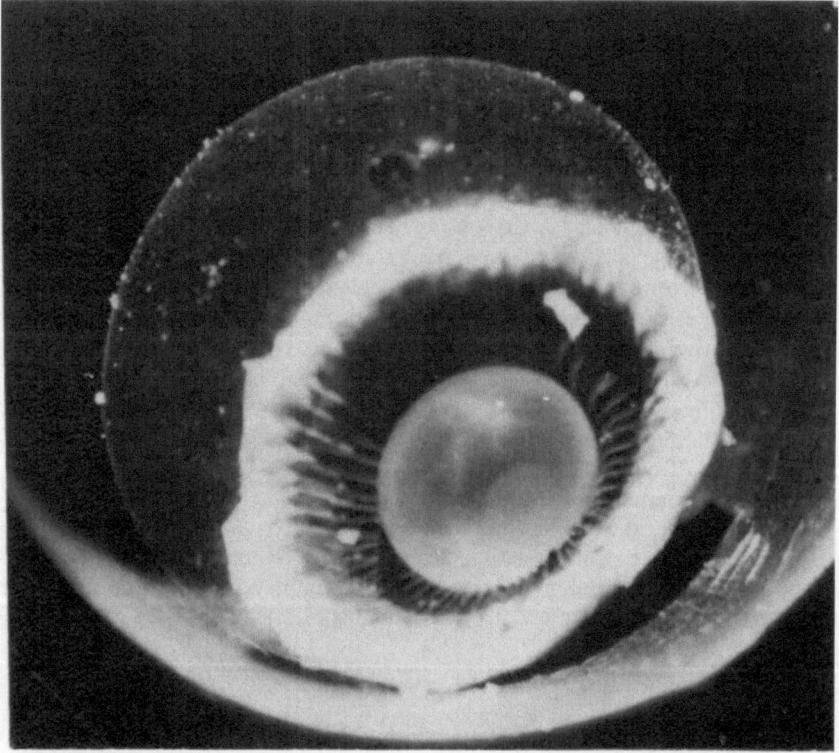

Fig. 1. Vitreous specimen of an unfixed autopsy eye (child). The anterior parts of the eye, the ciliary body and a small fringe of retinal tissue near the ora serrata have been left upon the vitreous whereas in the posterior part the retina is removed. In the upper center of the vitreous appears as a round defect, the prepapillary hole of the vitreous cortex.

the retrolental tract ('hyaloid tract'), separating the intermediary zone from the retrolental zone, inserting just behind the lens border. The retrolental zone is closed anteriorly by the patellar fossa. It contains no tracts but often remnants of Cloquet's channel and of the hyaloid artery.

In human eyes the preretinal zone is denser optically as well as mechanically, forming a cortex, as it were. The intermediary and the retrolental zones are transparent and semifluid. In animals (EISNER 1975) different vitreous patterns may be observed, e.g. a nuclear type with a dense retrolental zone and a semifluid preretinal and intermediary zone, in cats and dogs; or a homogeneous dense vitreous in cattle and sheep; or else a homogeneous semifluid vitreous in the horse and the rabbit.

The patterns described above are subject to alterations throughout growth and ageing (Fig. 3 and Fig. 5). In the premature infant we still find the hyaloid artery and Cloquet's channel. In the newborn they both have

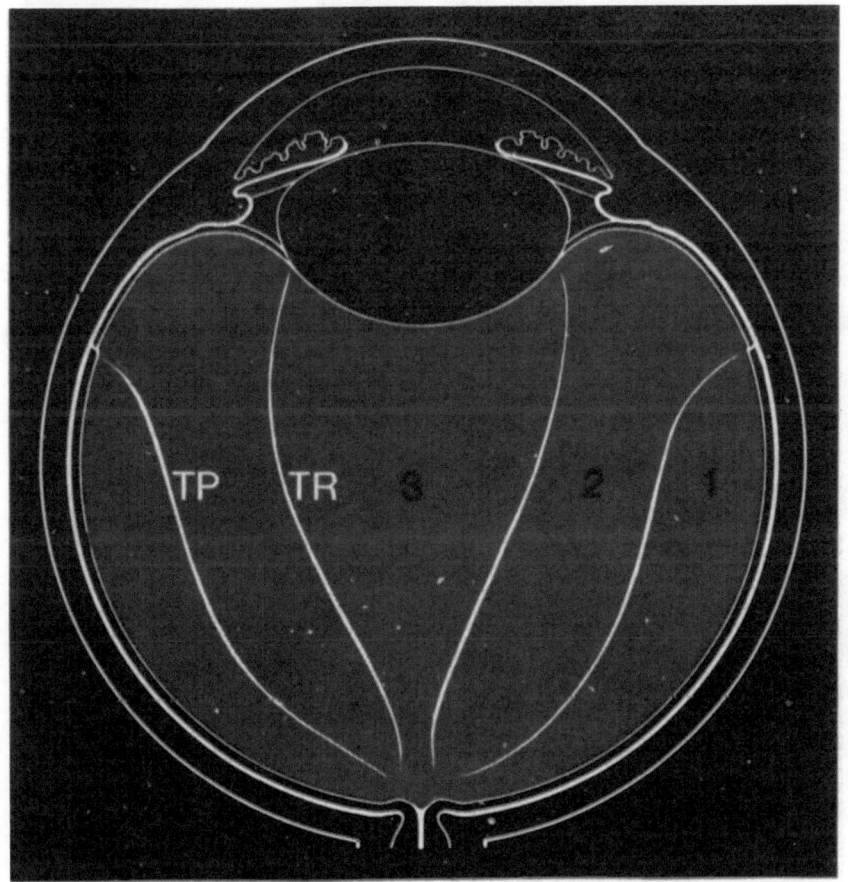

Fig. 2. Subdivision of the vitreous body into zones.
1. preretinal zone; 2. intermediary zone; 3. retrolental zone; TP preretinal tract; TH retrolental (hyaloid) tract.

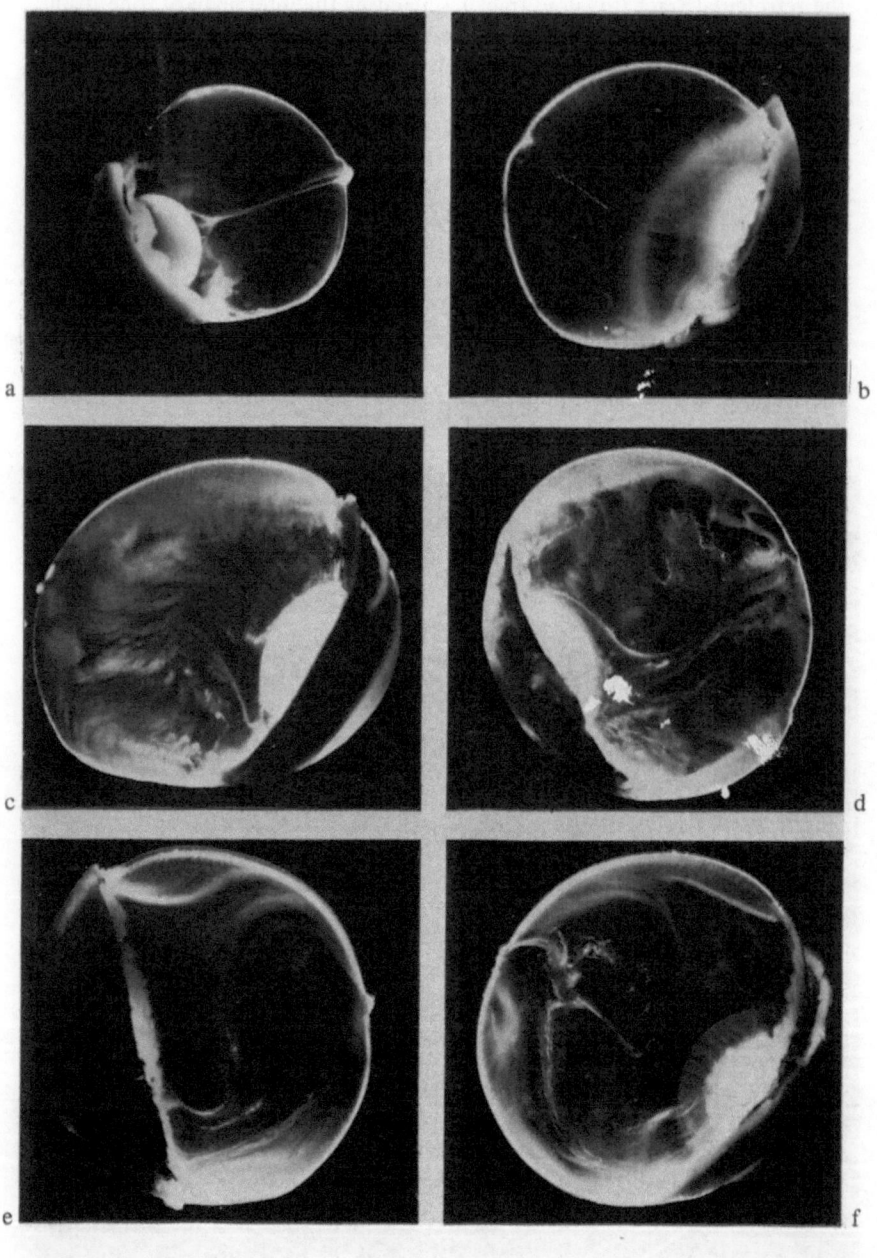

Fig. 3. Optical section through unfixed vitreous specimens. a) premature infant, 32nd week of pregnancy; b) child 7 months old; c) adolescent 14 years old; d) adult 31 years old; e) adult 70 years old; f) adult 80 years old.

almost completely disappeared and the vitreous space contains but secondary vitreous with a pattern of fine radial striation (Fig. 11a).

The differentiation into zones and the formation of vitreous tracts occur only later in the first few years of life, developing first in the anterior parts of the eye and gradually extending posteriorly in the course of a life time. Yet in adolescence already we find the first signs of involution, with the onset of the gradual destruction of the vitreous framework. The picture we observe in clinical practice represents therefore always a combination of simultaneous evolution and involution.

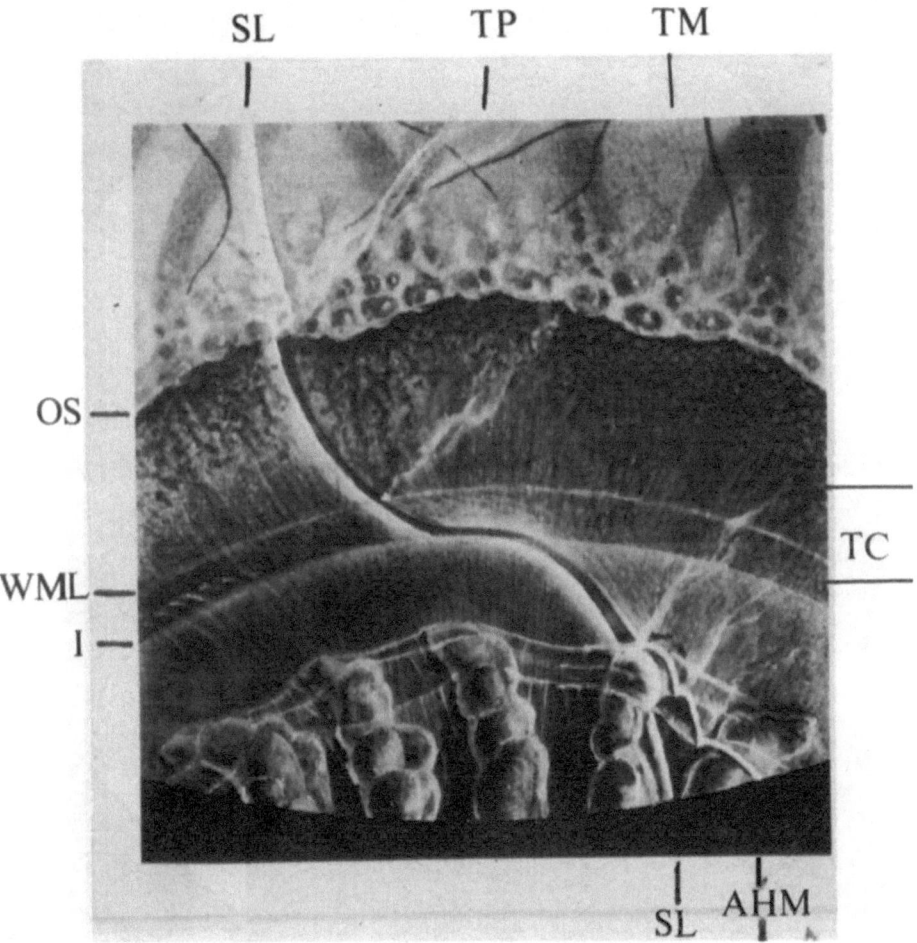

Fig. 4. Biomicroscopy of the insertion of the vitreous tracts in the peripheral fundus. SL Slitbeam; TP preretinal tract; TM median tract; TC coronary tract; AHM anterior hyaloid membrane; WML white midline of the pars plana; OS ora serrata; I summit of the indentation protuberance.

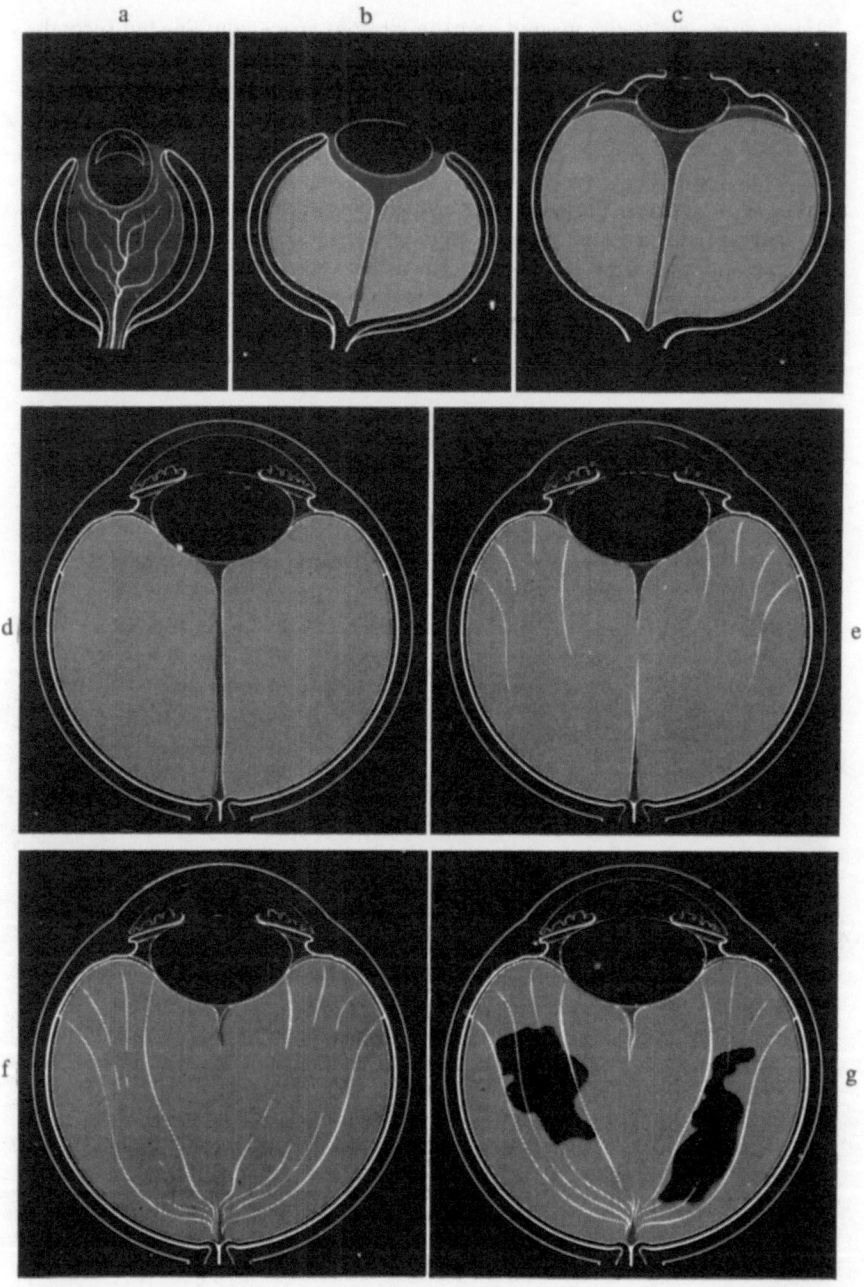

Fig. 5. Growth and ageing of the vitreous. a-c prenatal development (after Ida Mann): development and regression of the hyaloid system; d) newborn: Cloquet's channel still present; e) adolescent: development of vitreous tracts in the anterior portion of the vitreous; f) adult eye: vitreous tracts reaching the posterior segment; g) senile destruction with formation of liquified cavities.

The clinical significance of the vitreous space derives from the fact that it is a body cavity closely interrelated with the adjoining tissue. Pathological processes occuring within the innermost retinal layers affect the vitreous, just as vitreous diseases will affect the retina. In this context the visible vitreous structures described above are clinically relevant: owing to their mechanical properties they may on the one hand impede the passage of substances with larger molecule size and on the other hand transfer mechanical forces, i.e. traction towards their fixation points within the adjacent tissue.

TABLE I

POSTERIOR VITREOUS DETACHMENT	RHEGMATOGENEOUS DETACHMENT	ARRHEGMATOGENEOUS DETACHMENT
OCCURRENCE	Vitreous destruction and liquefaction	Concomitant sign of pathologic condition of adjoining tissues Vitreous shrinkage
MODE OF VOLUME TRANSFER	Through a hole in the posterior hyaloid membrane	Through an 'intact' posterior hyaloid membrane
MORPHOLOGICAL ASPECT		
General configuration	Typical	Atypical
Course of the tractus vitreales	Stretched towards the hole in the posterior hyaloid membrane	Normally curved, occasionally slightly deformed in direction of traction
Posterior hyaloid membrane	Loose, plicated	Taut, with occasional tractional folds
Holes in posterior hyaloid membrane	Cause of the detachment	If present, formed by secondary processes
Prefoveal and prepapillary holes	At typical position: initially vertical, later horizontal	Moved to atypical positions, deformed by traction
COURSE OF THE VITREOUS DETACHMENT	Rapid and sudden	Slow and steady
COMPLICATIONS		
Traction	Rapid and irregular	Slow and steady
Effect of traction on		
— vitreoretinal adhesions	Vitreous ripped off from the retina Tearing of the retina	Vitreous peeled off even at points of strong vitreoretinal adhesions
— posterior hyaloid membrane	Remains intact as a relatively thick membrane	Formation of retinal folds Is split into several lamellae
Type of induced retinal detachment	Rhegmatogeneous	Arrhegmatogeneous

2. PATHOLOGICAL CONDITIONS OF THE VITREOUS AFFECTING THE RETINA

As long as the vitreous is attached, mechanical stress produced by jactation movements of the central vitreous does not seem to affect the retina, the latter probably being protected by a buffering action of the cortex. If the vitreous is detached, however, tractional forces will affect the retina directly, which leads to the well-known complications of posterior vitreous detachment.

Since in vitreous detachment the total volume of the globe remains the same, part of it is bound to pass from the vitreous body into the newly formed retrovitreal space. The passage of fluid occurs in two different ways; accordingly, vitreous detachment may be subdivided into two types. (Tab. I).

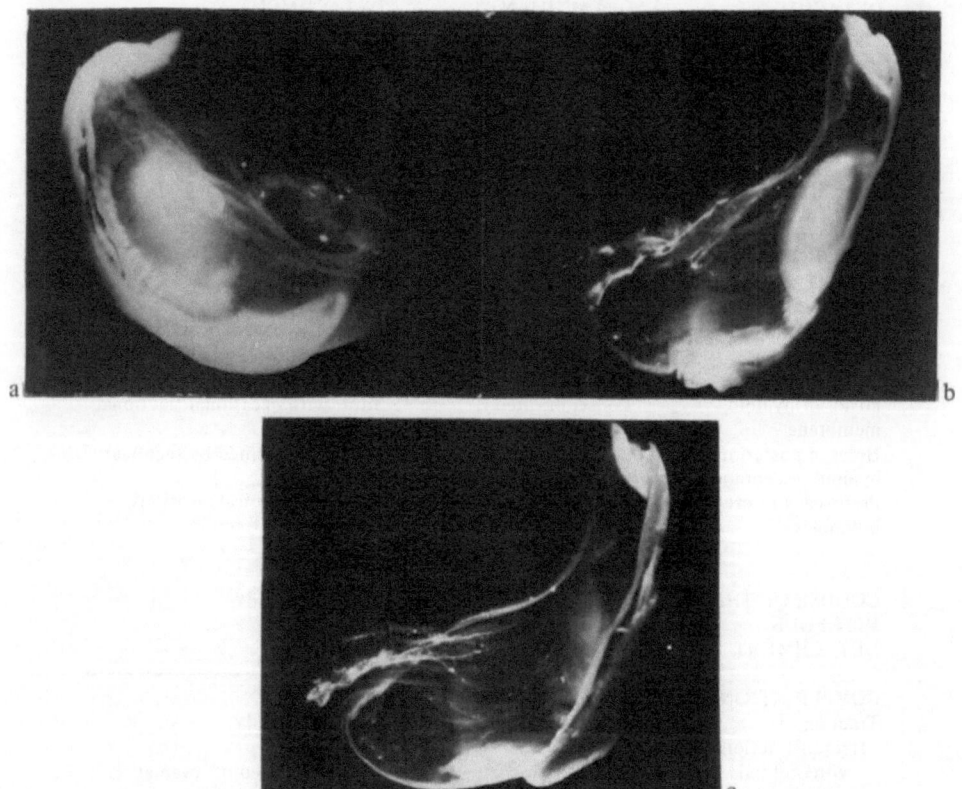

Fig. 6.   Rhegmatogeneous posterior vitreous detachment.
(unfixed vitreous specimen). a) diffuse illumination: the vitreous 'bag' has collapsed, the large prefoveal hole is well recognizable; b) optical section: just underneath the prolapsing vitreous the small prepapillary hole appears surrounded by an annular opacity; c) optical section through the prefoveal hole, showing prolapsing vitreous strands.

2.1. Rhegmatogeneous vitreous detachment

In rhegmatogeneous vitreous detachment there is always a *hole in the cortex* as an outlet for the liquified central vitreous (Fig. 6 and Fig. 7). The hole through which the passage occurs is usually the prefoveal hole at the posterior pole. In the living eye it is not easily detectable since it is too large to be seen in its entire circumference at one glance (Fig. 8). It is best seen in early stages of vitreous detachment, when still in a vertical position; later, with the completion of the detachment it assumes a horizontal position, where only its anterior margin can be made out well, the lateral and the posterior margins being blurred by the reflected retinal light. Rhegmatogeneous vitreous detachment always has a characteristic configuration (Fig. 6). The vitreous collapses like an empty bag. The posterior hyaloid drops from its insertion on the posterior border of the vitreous base, while the vitreous remaining within the 'bag' succombs into the inferior parts of the globe. Rhegmatogeneous vitreous detachment is due to senile resp. myopic vitreous destruction and is thus a part of normal senile involution. Its clinical significance lies in the velocity of fluid transfer. This being a very rapid process, the tractional forces produced are fast and able to tear the retinal tissue.

2.2. Arhegmatogeneous vitreous detachment

The passage of fluid into the retrovitreal space occurs through the *intact* posterior hyaloid by mechanisms still unknown. Arhegmatogeneous vitreous detachment is due to intraocular inflammation, diabetes, vascular disease etc.

Its configuration varies considerably (Fig. 9), depending on the pathological processes at work, as the latter usually cause atypical vitreoretinal adhesions between which the detached hyaloid membrane is taut. The passage is slow to proceed, the hyaloid is slow to detach, and so is therefore the traction. It will cause folds rather than tears in the retina, and should retinal detachment follow it will be arhegmatogeneous. Upon the diagnosis of an arrhegmatogeneous vitreal detachment it is essential always to trace the basic disease responsible for the detachment.

3. THE PARTICIPATION OF VITREOUS IN RETINAL DISEASE

As in other body cavities substances penetrating into the vitreous will sediment within the vitreous space according to their specific weight. Soluble material will accumulate at the bottom, displacing thus the vitreous tracts upwards (Fig. 10). The floating vitreous tracts will then assume an inverse course: instead of sinking down behind the lens they ascend and proceed through the upper parts of the vitreous body towards the posterior pole. Cellular exsudates, e.g. leucocytes and erythrocytes will not collect freely as they do in the anterior chamber, since the vitreous membranelles impede their motility. Instead particles will follow the vitreous tracts (Fig. 11) and collect at their lowest point, usually at their insertion lines. Particles follow-

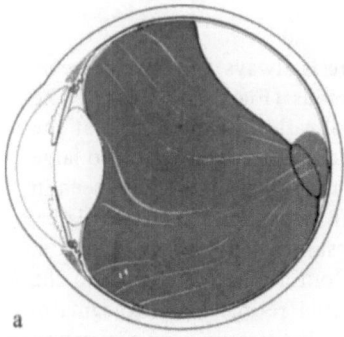 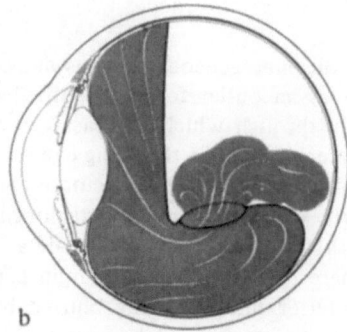

Fig. 7. Rhegmatogeneous posterior vitreous detachment. a) incomplete detachment: the posterior hyaloid still inserted far posteriorly descends obliquely. The prefoveal hole is in a vertical position. b) complete detachment: the insertionline of the posterior hyaloid has migrated anteriorly; the membrane drops. The prefoveal hole is now in a horizontal position. The vitreous tracts are straight, pointing directly towards the prefoveal hole.

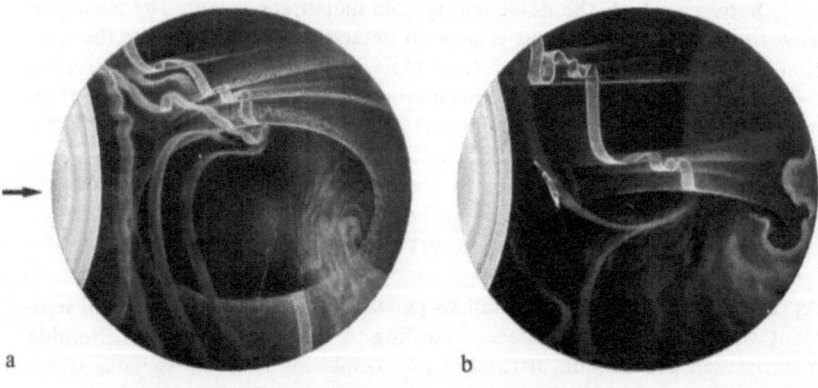

Fig. 8. Biomicroscopy of rhegmatogeneous vitreous detachment.
(male 44 years old). a) incomplete detachment: the prefoveal hole is in a vertical position and thus easily recognizable. Note the prepapillary hole (left) having a much smaller size. b) After completion of the detachment the prefoveal hole is now in a horizontal position. Only the anterior margin is well visible.

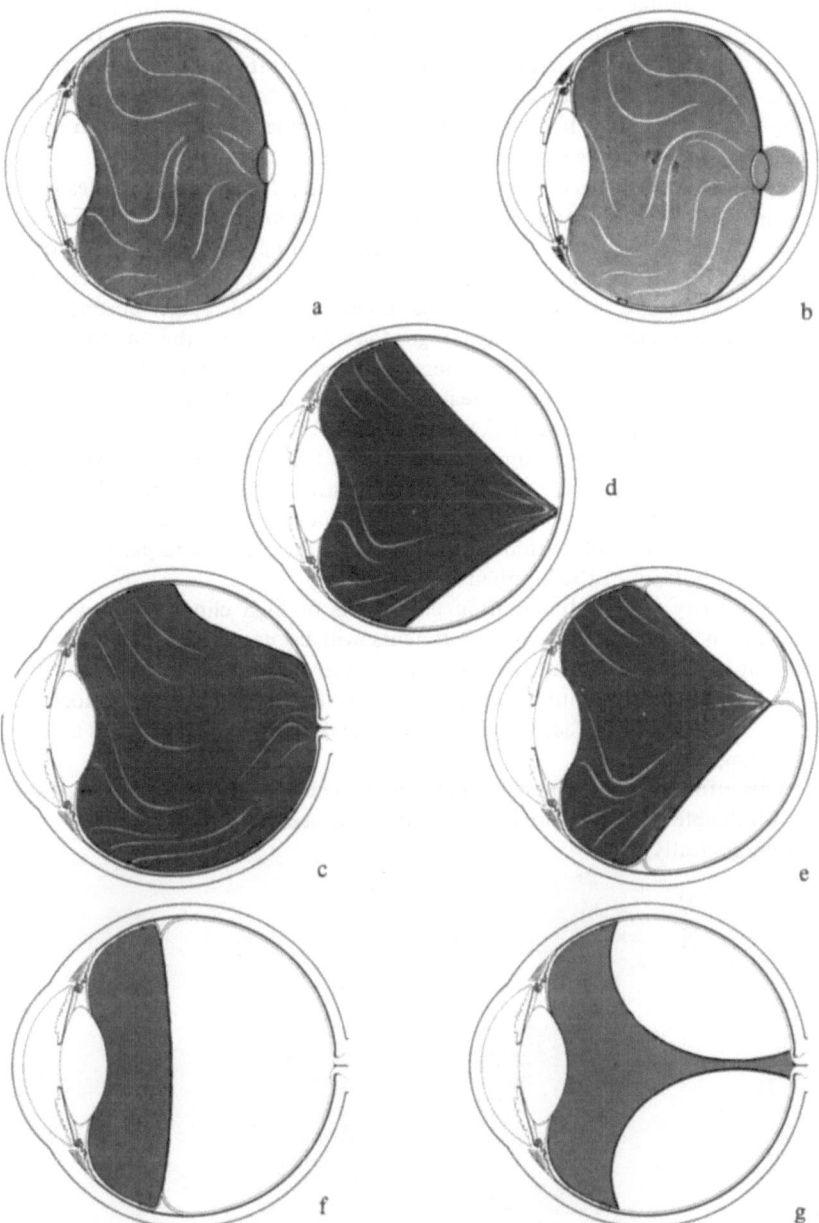

Fig. 9. Arhegmatogeneous posterior vitreous detachments. a) complete detachment: at the prefoveal hole the cortex is not perforated. The vitreous tracts still show their normal S-shaped course. b) complete detachment: at the prefoveal hole the vitreous bulges as a sign of the anatomical weakness of the posterior hyaloid at this location, but does not permeate. c) incomplete superior detachment; d) subtotal detachment with adhesion on the retina; e) shrinking vitreous produces folds on the retina; f) total vitreous detachment causing retinal folds at the posterior border of the vitreous base; g) complete detachment with persisting adhesion at the optic disc.

ing the retrolental tract are found at the lower border of the lens, those in the median tract at the white midline of the pars plana, and those in the preretinal tract at the ora serrata. Beyond the ora serrata no intravitreal sediments can reach the retina, since no vitreous tracts are inserted there. If there are any particles behind the ora, if not originated within that very region, they are a definite sign of posterior vitreous detachment.

The retrovitreal space being a cavity containing fluid only , particles will accumulate at its bottom in a homogeneous deposit with a horizontal upper surface, as a preretinal hyphemia or hypopyon. If the retrospace is filled completely with particles (Fig. 14), the fundus is obattached at its base. If at the prefoveal hole the vitreous bulges posteriorly, as it does sometimes in arrhegmatogeneous detachment, the fundus may remain visible there since the thickness of the opaque retrovitreal layer is decreased. In rhegmatogeneous vitreal detachment particles may penetrate into the vitreous through the prefoveal hole (Fig. 13).

Atypical patterns of sedimentation will be found wherever the vitreous deviates from the onion-peel structure. In children the sediments will follow the radial striation and accumulate perpendiculary to the retinal surface (Fig. 11a + b). In senile vitreous destruction on the other hand particles collect at the bottom of the liquified cavities.

Familiarity with sedimentation patterns is of high clinical importance. Whereas in other body cavities sediments will be detected at the bottom without difficulty, in the vitreous they must be searched for carefully (Fig. 12). They are a clinical sign pertinent to the evaluation of pathological processes. Increase of sediments indicates greater activity, decrease is a sign of healing.

This information permits a very precise guidance of therapy and is particulary valuable wherever the basic pathological process cannot be made out morphologically.

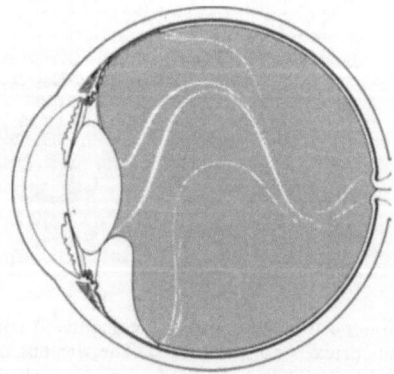

Fig. 10. Sedimentation of soluble material in the vitreous cavity. The floating vitreous tracts ascend behind the lens and proceed through the upper parts of the eye towards the posterior pole (ascension phenomenon of Busacca's).

After presenting some practical applications of vitreous anatomy let me close this paper with a theoretical question: How do the anatomical concepts explained here correspond with the results of previous investigations?

To our great astonishment we find an amazing coincidence. Some findings of earlier anatomists, though gained through methods open to criticism, show the same patterns visible through a slit-lamp in unfixed autopsy eyes (Fig. 15 and Fig. 16). Furthermore, we can also prove a coincidence with former attempts to interpret − however erroneously − the biomicroscopic findings into a general schema of vitreous structure (Fig. 17). In fact, the patterns revealed in autopsy eyes might reasonably be explained in the way of BUSACCA's schema, when observed in the small visual fields of contact glass mirrors. The coincidence of findings obtained through several methods so different from one another increases the confidence in the results of vitreous examination presented here.

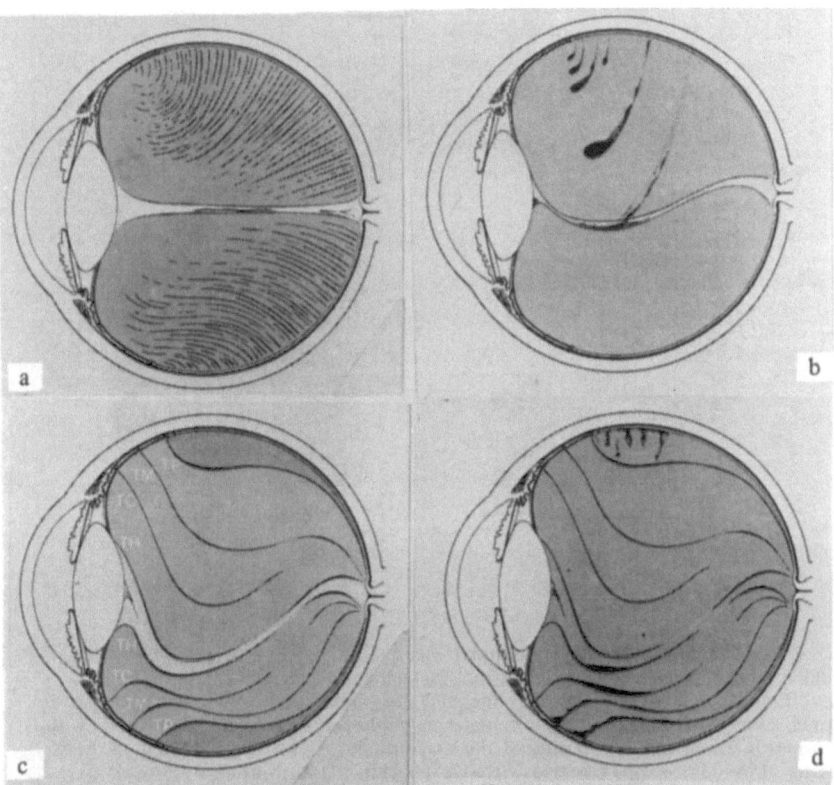

Fig. 11.   Sedimentation patterns of particles in the vitreous cavity.
a) pattern of radial striation in a normal infantile eye; b) penetrating cells follow the radial pattern; c) vitreous tracts in a normal adult eye; TP preretinal tract; TM median tract; TC coronary tract; TH retrolental ('hyaloid') tract; d) particles following the vitreous tracts and accumulating at their lowest point.

99

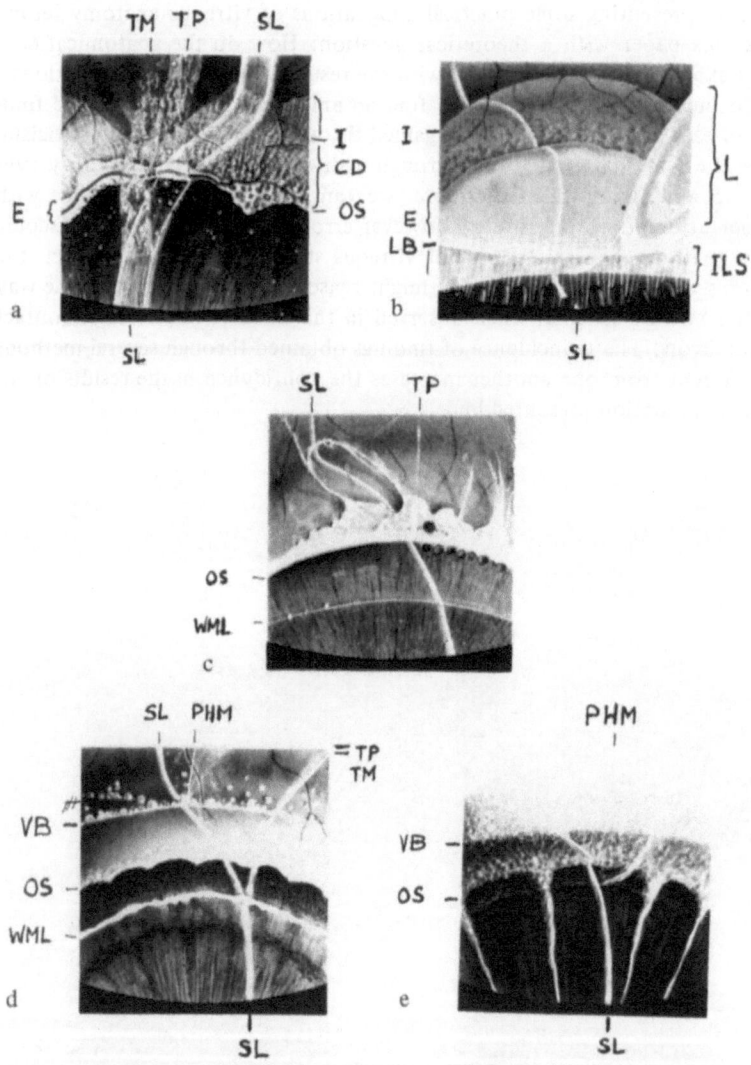

Fig. 12. Sediments in the lower peripheral fundus
(indentation biomicroscopy with a mirror contact lens).
a) cells and precipitates in the preretinal and the median tract in a patient with juxta-
papillary chorioretinitis; b) large exsudates in the lower vitreous base in a patient with
vascular inflammation; c) scarring of the vitreous base after healing of vasculitis; d) deposits of exsudates after posterior vitreous detachment. Infiltration of vitreous tracts,
accumulation behind the vitreous base (preretinal hypopyon); e) complete infiltration
of the retrovitreal space. The retina is visible only where the vitreous has remained attached, i.e. at the vitreous base. TP preretinal tract; TM median tract; SL Slitbeam;
E exsudates; I summit of the indentation protuberance; CD cystoid degeneration;
OS ora serrata; LB lens border; L lens; ILS iridolenticular space; WML white midline of
the pars plana; PHM posterior hyaloid membrane; VB posterior border of the vitreous
base.

100

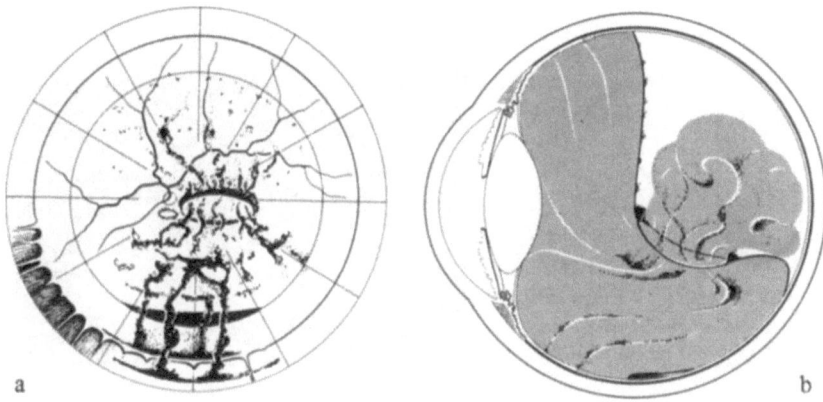

a   b

Fig. 13. Sedimentation in rhegmatogeneous vitreous detachment. a) drawing of the
fundus; b) sagittal section. Sediments accumulate behind the vitreous base; particles
having penetrated through the prefoveal hole accumulate within the vitreous tracts. (see
also Fig. 12d)

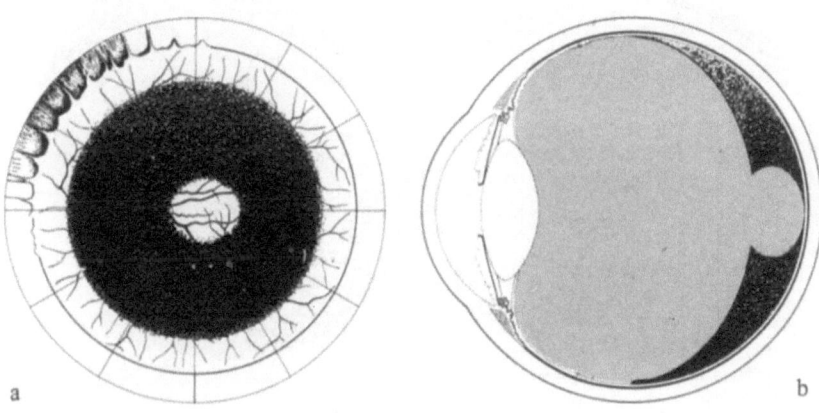

a   b

Fig. 14. Infiltration of the retrovitreal space in arrhegmatogeneous vitreous detachment. a) drawing of the fundus; b) sagittal section. The fundus is obscured except for
the vitreous base and the posterior pole where owing to a bulging of the posterior hyaloid the thickness of the opaque preretinal layer is decreased.(see also Fig. 12e)

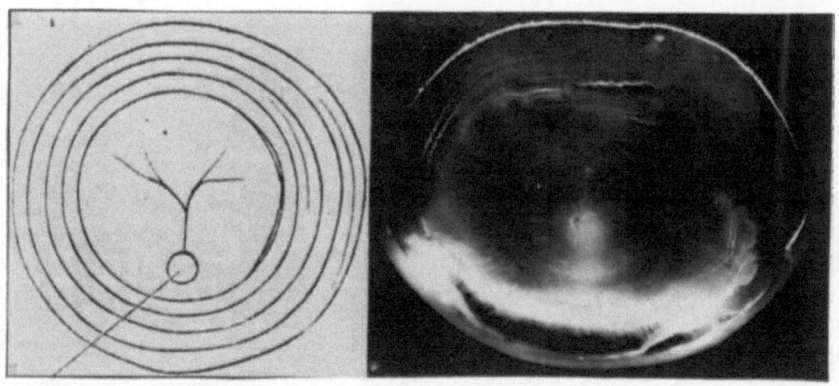

Fig. 15. Juxtaposition of anatomical findings of STILLING (1869) and of optical section through unfixed vitreous (EISNER 1975). The vitreous tracts appear as concentric lines in the periphery. Prevascular fissures produce a radiate dendritic figure in the center.

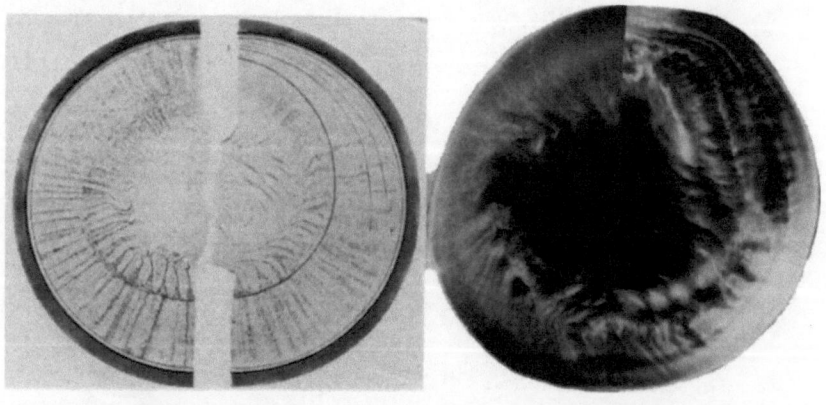

Fig. 16. Juxtaposition of histological findings of SZENT-GYÖRGYI (1971) and of optical section in an unfixed human eye. When using the same direction of section in both methods a similar pattern is observed. The stainable structures (dark) in the histological specimen have the same arrangement as the optically denser structures (light) in the unfixed specimen.

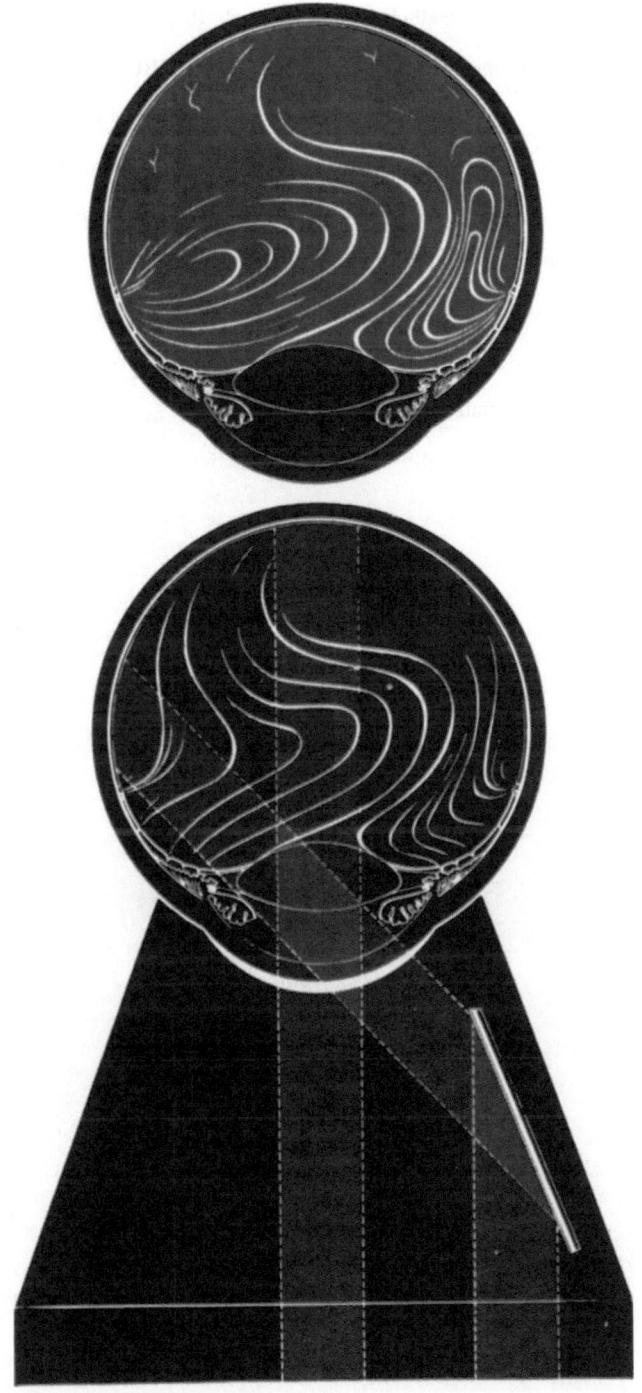

Fig. 17. Juxtaposition of the findings in autopsy eyes with BUSACCA's schema of vitreous structures as observed in biomicroscopy. In the mirrors of the contact glass only small portions of the vitreous are seen at once (left). They might reasonably be interpreted into Busacca's schema (right).

REFERENCES

BUSACCA, A. Biomicroscopie et histopathologie de l'oeil, vol. III. Zürich, Schweiz. Druck- & Verlagshaus AG (1957).

EISNER, G. Autoptische Spaltlampenuntersuchung des Glaskörpers I-III. *Albrecht v. Graefes Arch. Klin. exp. Ophthal.* 182: *1-40* (1971).

EISNER, G. Autoptische Spaltlampenuntersuchung des Glaskörpers IV-V. *Albrecht v. Graefes Arch. Klin. Exp. Ophthal.* 187: *1-20* (1973).

EISNER, G. Zur Anatomie des Glaskörpers. *Albrecht v. Graefes Arch. klin. exp. Ophthal.* 193: *33-56* (1975).

EISNER, G. Biomicroscopy of the peripheral Fundus. Springer-Verlag, Heidelberg, (1973).

STILLING, J. Eine Studie über den Bau des Glaskörpers. *Archiv. f. Ophthal.* 15 Bd 3: *299-319* (1869).

SZENT-GYÖRGYI, A. Untersuchungen über den Bau des Glaskörpers des Menschen. *Arch. mikr. Anat.* 89. *324-386* (1917).

Keywords: Vitreous, Anatomy, Examination, Retina.

Author's address:
Universitäts-Augenklinik
Inselspital
CH–3010 Bern, Switzerland

MACULAR FIBROSIS AND MASSIVE PRERETINAL RETRACTION*

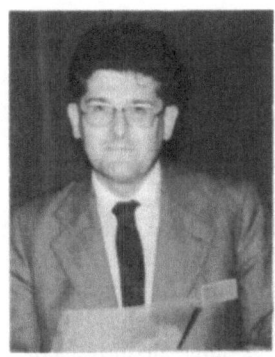

BALDER P. GLOOR

(Basle, Switzerland)

The subject of this presentation is a peculiar disease process which may develop around the vitreo-retinal border structures. It consists pathologically of a cellular proliferation on the inner retinal surface (GLOOR, 1969a, b, c). This is a proliferation of cells in or at the border of a cavity which is usually practically free of cells, except for a few monocytes, which the so-called hyalocytes really are (GLOOR, 1973). I shall try to show on the hand of a few selected cases that there exists any transitional stage between the single postoperative macular pucker or postcoagulative epiretinal fibrosis and massive preretinal retraction. Finally, I shall leave you with some questions which, I hope, could show in which direction pertinent further research on this disease should be guided.

A patient may have had vitreous detachment, formation of several tears and finally a retinal detachment. He may have been operated in appropriate time, even before the macula was detached. He seemed to have a normal postoperative course. When he was discharged from the hospital 10 days following surgery he may have had a visual acuity of 20/20, complaining only of some residual foggyness and fine floaters. Maybe he was controlled every 14 days, but 8 weeks later he comes back telling, that almost of a sudden he lost his sight on the eye operated before. You know too well what you will find: *Massive preretinal retraction*.

The question is, what happened between the moment the patient was discharged with a visual acuity of 20/20 and the disaster we are now looking at. Quite early subjective symptoms are metamorphopsia and blurred vision. Biomicroscopically the first sign will be noted as a paramacular gathering focus on the retina often in the neighbourhood of the larger vessels that curve above or below the macula. Early evidence of this process may be only an area of snail track reflexes. This area then becomes the centre of radiating folds which includes secondarily the macula. The macula itself is seldom the centre of the process. In the area of the pathologic process the retina gets a dirty greyish colour, often before the reflexes appear. The nidus may be tiny or may extend to an area of more than 2 disc diameters in size. The retinal vessels are tortuous and may be pulled towards the centre of the fibroplastic mass. Sometimes these vessels leak in fluorescein angiography,

* This investigation was supported by the 'Schweizerischer Nationalfonds', Grant Nr. 3.859.72.

sometimes they do not. Superficial, fine, flame-shaped haemorrhages are frequently found around the lesion. As the traction folds become thicker, offshoots of this fibroplastic process can cover the macula completely (GLOOR & WERNER, 1967).

Let me show you a few examples:

Case 1: This 61-year-old myopic patient had a visual acuity of 20/20, 10 days after an uneventful cataract extraction. At this time fundus examination showed already a horseshoe tear at 3 h. Two weeks later 4 horseshoe tears were found, 3 of them were photocoagulated and again $2\frac{1}{2}$ weeks later the 4th tear was coagulated also. Three months later a retinal detachment and a new horseshoe tear developed near 12 h. Limitation of this detachment by photocoagulation was unsuccessful, 1 week later an intrascleral plombage was performed and the patient could be discharged with a flat retina and a visual acuity of 0.6. Again $2\frac{1}{2}$ weeks later, the sight of this eye was suddenly closed by a curtain. Massive epiretinal fibroplasia with a huge gathering focus still lying on the detached retina temporal to the macula was found. Two encircling procedures brought no amelioration. At this time the patient was virtually blind and asked for cataract surgery of the other eye. This was performed 5 months following cataract surgery of the first eye. Again 5 months after the uneventful cataract surgery of the second eye, a flat retinal detachment developed in the upper temporal quadrant with 2 horseshoe tears and this was successfully operated by an intrascleral plombage. Four weeks following surgery visual acuity was 1.0; 7 weeks postoperatively again a retinal detachment in the lower temporal quadrant was present. The patient was operated again, but the retina redetached and $2\frac{1}{2}$ weeks later the groove had to be enlarged. In regard to the dubious situation of the right eye the situation of the left eye was re-evaluated and an open sky vitrectomy was performed. The epiretinal masses were dissected from the retina. Histology shows a tremendous infolding process going on in the region of the internal limiting membrane which obviously was cut away from the retina (Fig. 1). Vitrectomy finally did not help. One month following retinal surgery of the right eye the patient could be discharged. Visual acuity was 0.1 and went up in the following 2 weeks to 0.7. In the next weeks he developed a severe epiretinal proliferative process on his right eye which looked terribly threatening. This process was going on during about 2 months, then visual acuity began slowly to increase, the process came to a standstill and today the patient has a visual acuity of 1.0. The 'fibrotic' focuses are still visible, but seem to be quiet.

Case 2: This 47 year-old man with bilateral congenital cataract, which was operated in his youth, is blind in his left eye. He developed massive preretinal retraction following repeated surgery for retinal detachment. The right eye then was photocoagulated prophylactically. Several years later, he showed up with a detachment of the retina of his right eye on the nasal side. No hole could be found. The retina could be reattached by an encircling band and intrascleral buckle on the nasal side. One month later he presented a redetachment at 6 h. Again no hole could be found. The groove was enlarged and the retina could be reattached. $3\frac{1}{2}$ weeks later, massive epi- and retroretinal proliferation developed in a way, I never saw before. There was a flat detachment of the posterior pole and not only the main vessels above

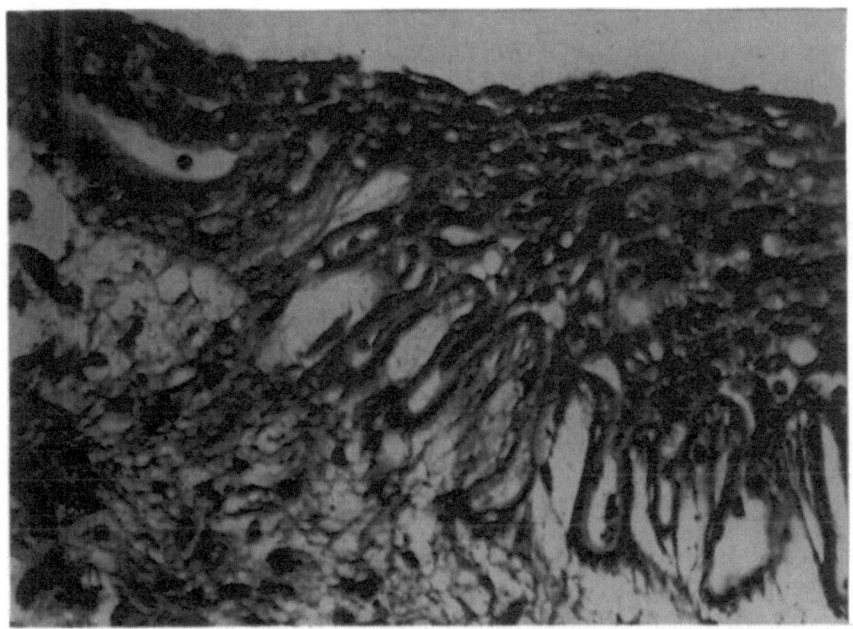

Fig. 1. Epiretinal gathering focus: Extensive cellular proliferations on the retinal surface. Marked wrinkling of the internal limiting membrane.

and below the macula were contracted towards the foveola as usually, but the margins of the optic disc were blurred, the vessels covered by yellow-white snowlike masses, and also behind the retina yellow-white masses of precipitates could be seen. A peculiar type of pre-, probably also intra- and retroretinal cellular proliferation was going on, which at least had some inflammatory components.

Case 3: This 58 year–old lady developed a horseshoe tear and retinal detachment in the superior temporal quadrant 3 months following uneventful intracapsular cataract extraction. Four weeks following successful surgery of the retinal detachment a gathering focus temporal to the macula developed, migrating in the coming weeks close to the macula. Visual acuity dropped from 0.7 to count fingers on 1 meter 2 months later. Four months following surgery a yellowish starfold, also equatorially, developed temporally. In the next months the process came to a standstill, and no further retinal detachment developed.

Case 4: This 57 year-old man had a vitreous detachment with symptoms and developed horseshoe tears at 11 and 1 h in his right eye. Photocoagulation and one week later additional diathermy at the peripheral edges of the holes were applicated. Two months following the photocoagulation some metamorphopsia developed, visual acuity was still 1.25. Metamorphopsia increased and slight folds below the macula could be seen. Visual acuity was still 20/20, but in 2 weeks visual acuity dropped down to 0.1. The nidus increased, migrated towards the macula, pulled the vessels with it and then later left the vessels again.

Case 5: This one eyed patient – he had lost his other eye in an accident – saw suddenly floaters and he went immediately to his ophthalmologist. He found a desinsertion of the retinal ora from $11\frac{1}{2}$ to 4 h, forming a giant tear. When he came to the hospital, practically no fluid was present underneath the retina and the patient could be photocoagulated as an emergency at midnight. Fearing massive preretinal retraction, I put only one row of photocoagulation lesions, leaving a safety distance from the practically dry break. No exsudative reaction occurred, but during the next weeks fluid accumulated and pushed towards the small photocoagulated barrier. After long discussions with Peter Niesel, Franz Fankhauser and Georg Eisner, a second row of photocoagulation lesions was placed to get a safe belt limitating the giant tear. But 3 weeks later the patient developed a very dangerous looking pucker, visual acuity dropped to 0.3, but, and this was extremely relieving, visual acuity went slowly up again and is now 1.0. Only a small rest of the gathering focus is visible.

In the sequence of our clinical examples we came from the worst case to the best, showing any stage between massive preretinal retraction with inoperable retinal detachment and simple pucker of the macula. In the best case visual loss was only temporary.

The fact, that the disease process involves contraction of tissue on the inside of a hollow sphere predetermines the morphology of the evolution. If a detachment develops or not is a matter of chance in the game between the forces pulling the retina and the adhesional forces between the retina and pigmentepithelium. As soon as a break opens in the retina, the battle may be lost.

The proliferative process, once developed, may follow any-one of four courses:

1. The pathologic process may consolidate after a period of time. Oedema and exudation regress. Macular edema and fibrosis may develop into a permanent defect, or they may regress, sometimes with remarkable improvement of visual acuity.

2. Increased proliferation may lead to the development of an epiretinal membrane. The tissue under the greatest tension may be ripped away from the underlying structures, forming intravitreal membranes or strands, often giving better access of the light to the macula.

3. If the adhesions between the contracting proliferative tissue and the retina do not break, a massive thickening of the retina with subsequent splitting in the deeper layers may occur. The ultimate result will be the formation of a retinoschisis or retinal detachment as in 4.

4. When the newly-formed tissue contracts, it may split away from the retina partially, often centrally, forming now a large starshaped intravitreal membrane, inserting with strong footplates on the retina. This is the fully developed form of massive preretinal retraction and retinal detachment with or without break formation. Some peculiar characteristics of this particularly severe type of evolution are: the contracting nidi develop quickly, often only 2 to 3 weeks after surgery; their formation is associated with yellow-gray, dirty retinal edema and cellular proliferation into the vitreous cavity; MACHEMER *et al.* (1975) feel that from a pathogenetic standpoint it is

important that at this time quite often a lot of cells in the vitreous cavity are pigmented. Let us leave open the question, if these pigmented cells are macrophages that have phagocytized pigment, or if these are scattered pigment epithelium cells. The fundus reflex turns from red to grayish-yellow; more than one nidus may arise anywhere from the posterior pole to the equator. After the development of the detachment, many of the original foci appear as yellowish fixed folds.

From the pathologic specimens it became clear, that these membranes, which lie on the retina first and later pull off and then form intravitreal septae are not condensations of preformed fibres of the vitreous, but most of the time newly formed cellular membranes (Fig. 2).

Which type of cells is or are most probably responsible for the formation of these membranes?

We had the impression that a quite similar looking spontaneously occurring disease, the so called spontaneous epiretinal fibroplasia, of which preretinal macular fibrosis, cellophan maculopathy and surface wrinkling retinopathy are synonyms, could give essential hints for the comprehension of the pathogenesis of the postoperative disease (GLOOR & WERNER, 1967).

In spontaneous macular fibrosis ROTH & FOOS (1971), BELLHORN (1975) and FOOS showed that these membranes consist of glial cells proliferating through breaks in the internal limiting membrane. When we produced microlesions in the retina of the rabbit (FOOS & GLOOR, 1975) and in the

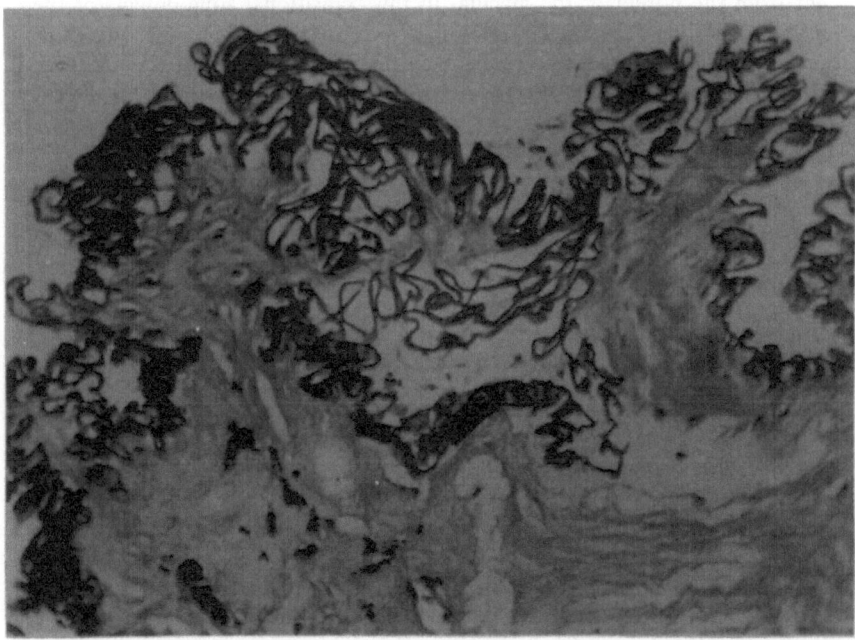

Fig. 2. Epiretinal gathering focus of severe massive preretinal retraction. This tissue was removed 9 months after beginning of massive preretinal retraction. Most extensively wrinkled internal limiting membrane. separated from the retina. Cellular nuclei relatively rare. Cells replaced by hyaline. van Gieson red scar tissue.

cat (GLOOR & DAICKER), outgrowth of the cells through breaks in the internal limiting membrane and forming membranes, was a finding quite similar to what LAQUA & MACHEMER (1974) observed in the monkey in long standing experimental detachment. This was observed mainly in the cat. At this time it is proved, that glial cells are, at least for a large part, responsible for the gathering focuses producing starfolds around the macula and in the periphery. These cells may be astrocytes or Müller cells, of which proliferating potencies are proved (GLOOR 1969a, RENTSCH 1973, ISHIKAWA & IKUI 1974, INOMATA 1975).

To what amount the pigmentepithelium cell is also responsible for producing starfolds and massive preretinal retraction, as put forward by MACHEMER & LAQUA (1975), is an open question (GLOOR, 1969d, 1974, GLOOR & DAICKER).

More important is to find the prerequisites for the development of the disease process in the human. Fig. 3 gives an outline.

A break in the internal limiting membrane and overstimulation of the process of wound-healing could be the preconditions, and retinal necrosis caused by coagulation could be the stimulus. Vitreous detachment could explain the formation of the break in the internal limiting membrane in many cases. How does a break in the internal limiting membrane ILM occur when the vitreous is still attached? Are these then inflammatory processes which create the microlesions? Next question: Why does the process so often start close to the macula? In front of the fovea the vitreous is different from the border of the macula. In this transitional zone defects of the internal limiting membrane could arise more often than in other places. It could be – and some pathologic specimens point in this direction – that in vitreous detachment, not such a clean separation as described by FOOS

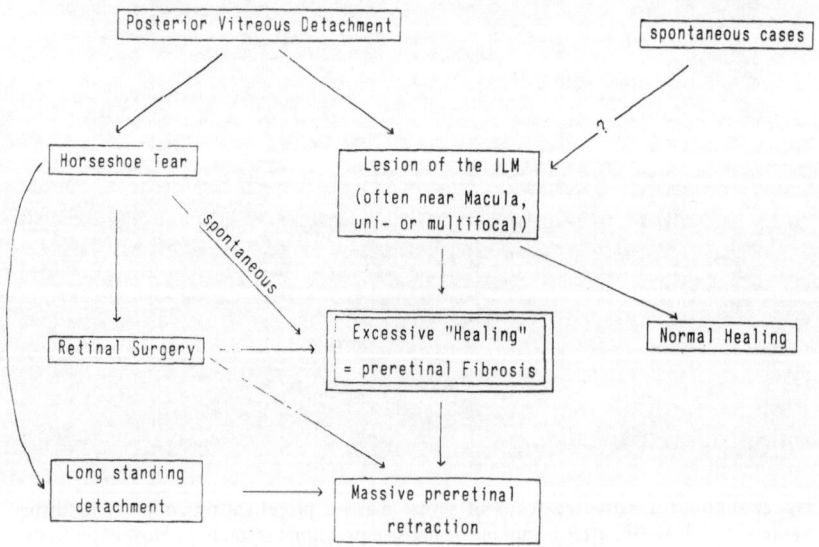

Fig. 3.   Factors involved in pathogenesis of 'preretinal fibrosis'.

(1975) between vitreous and the very thin internal limiting membrane of the macula is occurring. It could be that if the wound created in the internal limiting membrane and the retina heals smoothly, we see no pucker. If there is an overwhelming wound-healing the epiretinal membrane may develop.

Since we reviewed 8 years ago the problem of spontaneous and post-operative epiretinal proliferating processes and massive preretinal retraction, so many experimental and clinical findings came up that I feel that it is now about time to reevaluate the disease process in extremely careful clinical observations, in pathological specimens and in further experiments. When for some time we looked mainly at the similarities of the spontaneous and the postcoagulative disease process, maybe we should now direct our attention much more to the dissimilarities between the two disease processes. For instance, it is of interest that spontaneous cases seem never to turn into massive preretinal retraction. On the other hand there are primary retinal detachments developing extremely fast, which show from the first day already a starfold: The epiretinal membrane responsible for the starfold must have been formed long before the detachment occurred. We have to evaluate the retinal surface and back-face all over the fundus and not only in the macular region. We have to aim biomicroscopically for thickening of the inner surface as well in so called normal eyes as in every stage of retinal detachment before and following surgery. The same applies for the amount and type of cellular infiltration of the vitreous and for localization of membranes and tracks in the vitreous at any stage of the disease process. Unfortunately, vitreous hazyness and cellular infiltration of the vitreous itself make detailed observation of the retinal surface and of the retina in the first days following surgery quite difficult. But with any attempt made, we may be able to differentiate several forms of the disease process, to find clinical groups belonging to one or the other type of pathologically proliferating cells. Our final goal must be to catch the process at the very beginning and to get means for preventing the disaster, which massive preretinal retraction really is.

REFERENCES

BELLHORN, M.B. Ultrastructure and Clinicopathologic Correlation of Idiopathic Pre-retinal Macular Fibrosis. *Amer. J. Ophthal.* 79: *366* (1975).

FOOS, R.Y. Vitreoretinal Juncture – Simple Epiretinal Membranes. *Graefes Arch. Ophthal.* 189: *231* (1974).

FOOS, R.Y. Ultrastructural Features of Posterior Vitreous Detachment. *Graefes Arch. Ophthal.* 196: *103* (1975).

FOOS, R.Y., & GLOOR, B.P. Vitreoretinal Juncture; Healing of Experimental Wounds. *Graefes Arch. Ophthal.* 196: *213* (1975).

GLOOR, B.P. Zellproliferation, Narbenbildung und Pigmentation nach Lichtkoagulation (Kaninchen-Versuche). *Klin. Mbl. Augenheilk.* 154: *633* (1969a).

GLOOR, B.P. Mitotic Activity in the Cortical Vitreous Cells (Hyalocytes) after Photocoagulation. *Invest. Ophthal.* 8: *633* (1969b).

GLOOR, B.P. Biomicroscopy of the Vitreous and of Vitreoretinal Pathology. In: B. Becker & R. Burde: Current Concepts in Ophthalmology, C.V. Mosby, St. Louis, pp 31-48 (1969c).

GLOOR, B.P. Phagocytotische Aktivität des Pigmentepithels nach Lichtkoagulation. (Zur Frage der Herkunft von Makrophagen in der Retina). *Graefes Arch. Ophthal.* 179: *105* (1969a).

GLOOR, B.P. Zur Entwicklung des Glaskörpers und der Zonula. III. Herkunft, Lebenszeit und Ersatz der Glaskörperzellen beim Kaninchen (autoradiographische Untersuchungen mit ^{3}H-Thymidin). *Graefes Arch. Ophthal.* 187: *21* (1973).

GLOOR, B.P. On the Question of the Origin of Macrophages in the Retina and the Vitreous Following Photocoagulation (Autoradiographic Investigations by Means of ^{3}H-Thymidine). *Graefes Arch. Ophthal.* 190: *183* (1974).

GLOOR, B.P. & WERNER, H. Postkoagulative und spontan auftretende internoretinale Fibroplasie mit Maculadegeneration. *Klin. Mbl. Augenheilk.* 151: *822* (1967).

GLOOR, B.P. & DAICKER, B.C. Pathology of Vitreo-Retinal Border Structures. *Trans. Ophth. Soc. United Kingdom* (in print).

INOMATA, H. Wound Healing after Xenon Arc Photocoagulation in the Rabbit Retina. *Ophthalmologica, Basel* 170: *462* (1975).

ISHIKAWA, Y. & IKUI, H. Electron Microscopic Studies on Retinal Repair in the Monkey after Xenon Photocoagulation. *Jap. J. Ophthal.* 18: *334* (1974).

LAQUA H. & MACHEMER, R. Sternfalten bei Netzhautablösung. *Graefes Arch. Ophthal.* 191: *273* (1974).

MACHEMER, R. & LAQUA, H. Pigment Epithelium Proliferation in Retinal Detachment (Massive Preretinal Proliferation). *Amer. J. Ophthal.* 80: *1* (1975).

RENTSCH, F.J. Preretinal Proliferation of Glial Cells after Mechanical Injury of the Rabbit Retina. *Graefes Arch. Ophthal.* 188: *79* (1973).

ROTH, A.M. & FOOS, R.Y. Surface Wrinkling Retinopathy in Eyes Enucleated at Autopsy. *Trans. amer. Acad. Ophthal. & Otol.* 75: *1047* (1971).

Author's address:
Universitäts-Augenklinik
Mittlere Strasse 91
4056 Basle
Switzerland

112

THE USES AND ABUSES OF LIQUID SILICONE

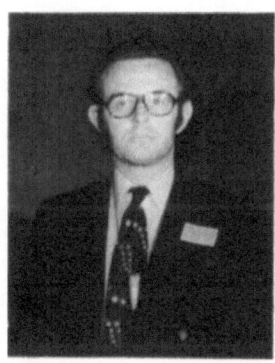

J.D. SCOTT

(Cambridge, England)

The use of liquid silicone in the treatment of advanced retinal detachment problems has been known for the past 13 years, and during this time reports have continued to appear of apparently successful use of this material, to be followed by others of unfavourable results. Many of you, therefore, will know of liquid silicone and its potential use in detachment surgery and some of you will perhaps also already have been influenced by reports of its possible side-effects. However, it is likely that very few of you will have used this material or had a chance to review cases treated in this way.

My talk today is based on the use of silicone fluid in the treatment of more than 350 eyes affected by advanced complications of retinal detachment, and time only permits me to discuss briefly indications and some aspects of technique in the management of these difficult problems.

It is important to review first the early history of the intra-ocular use of liquid silicone. STONE and then ARMALY about 15 years ago reported good tolerance to liquid silicone injected into animal eyes, and ARMALY suggested in 1961 that this material might be used in complicated cases of retinal detachment which were considered otherwise inoperable. In 1962 CIBIS used liquid silicone in the treatment of vitreous pathology reporting few side-effects, and in 1964 described the treatment of massive pre-retinal retraction and giant tears using this material and obtaining a 50% improvement rate after up to two years. Since that time other surgeons have reported less favourable results. CIBIS divided his complications into avoidable ones due to surgical errors made whilst the technique was being learned and late ones due to corneal dystrophy and recurrent detachment. It is perhaps of the greatest significance that the most serious complications described by CIBIS and other workers are those associated with emulsification of the liquid silicone. This appeared to be a common problem with early workers for reasons which we shall come to later.

More recently a Boston group have attempted to show that liquid silicone is toxic to the retina, and have described migration of emulsified silicone into retinal tissues of some of their monkeys with resultant changes in the electroretinogram. They inferred from these observations that the long-term reduction is vision of some patients treated with liquid silicone was due to the toxic effect of the silicone.

It has been my experience that eyes which are successfully treated according to the principles which I am about to describe continue to enjoy their visual improvement and maintain normal electroretinograms for up to five years. One can only assume from these findings that at least as far as tolerance to liquid silicone is concerned monkeys really are different to man.

There are three main varieties of retinal problem which I wish to discuss: massive vitreous retraction, giant equatorial retinal tears and primary macular holes.

Massive vitreous retraction is perhaps the most serious complication encountered in retinal detachment surgery and certainly accounts for most of the eventual failures in treatment. It immobilises the detached retina by fibrous membranes so that conventional surgery by scleral buckling fails to restore the retina permanently to its normal position.

Clinically the condition can be recognised in two distinct stages and silicone fluid is used in the treatment of the later disease. In the late stage fibrous membranes can easily be seen and their effects are much more obvious than in the early period of the disease. I should like to say a little about the early stages for they are often overlooked so that inappropriate treatment inevitably leads to progression to the late stages.

In the early development of the disease fibrosis is occurring on the surface of the retina immobilising the retina and vitreous in a subtle way. Close examination, however, will show the effects of this early fibrosis. If it occurring in the area of retinal tears these will be distorted in a characteristic manner. Horseshoe tears may be rounded or show rolling of their posterior edges and perhaps a retraction of the operculum. Normal peripheral retinal mobility will be reduced by the membrane, and as progression occurs retinal wrinkling will be seen focussed around a central spot where fixed folds will occur as the membrane contracts in the later stages. With fixation of the retina vitreous mobility is lessened so that on the slit-lamp normal vitreous excursions are reduced in all phases.

Most interesting of all perhaps is the appearance in the vitreous of huge numbers of large pigmented cells scattered throughout the gel. Closer examination shows these cells to be present in the retinal tissues as well as on its surface, and under the microscope are found to be pigmented macrophages. These cells are also present in sub-retinal fluid and are now known to be free pigment epithelial cells which have changed into macrophages and migrated through the retina into the vitreous. They are intimately concerned with the formation of vitreous membranes and are very likely to be the prime mover in the process of vitreous fibrosis.

Treatment of the early immobilisation stage of massive vitreous retraction is by conventional buckling surgery with cryotherapy and with the drainage of sub-retinal fluid. The surface membranes interfere with spontaneous drainage of fluid, and the closure of tears by the buckles with drainage must be carried out if progress to the contractual stage is to be prevented.

Such progress, however, often does occur, due either to failure of the conventional surgery or to complications of it, and indeed may rarely occur as a primary phenomenon where no previous surgery has been done.

The change to the contracted stage of massive vitreous retraction is characterised by the development of three further signs, and these are:

114

visible membranes, retinal puckering and narrow posterior retinal folds. They are all the effects of contraction of the membrane lying on the surface of the retina. However, if the membrane occurs in an eye in which the vitreous has detached then a characteristic appearance is seen. It occurs rarely, but when seen presents a difficult problem in treatment, for the fibrosis is found peripherally on the surface of the retina, and where the posterior hyaloid membrane leaves the retina, which is usually at the equator in the phakic eye, fibrosis too leaves the retina and a membrane stretches across the eye composed peripherally of retina and epiretinal membrane, and centrally of fibrosed hyaloid membrane. The problem with these membranes is that they are attached to the opercula of the tears and therefore elevate them beyond the reach of any conventional buckle. Treatment is by liquid silicone, but before injection it is necessary to divide the attachment of the membrane to the tear by vitreous scissors and then to divide the membrane across the eye to allow the retina some relaxation. The liquid silicone will be necessary to force the retina flat onto the encircling buckle and thus to completely close the tear.

Treatment of massive vitreous retraction in the contractual stage when the vitreous has not previously detached is comparatively more straightforward, provided it is carried out at the correct stage of development of the disease. The correct time is as soon as the diagnosis of the contractual stage has been made. Using the criteria already described liquid silicone should again be employed. It is no use having another go with conventional buckles for the contracting membranes will not allow the retina to remain flat and will certainly contract further producing a retraction detachment. It is even worse to wait until such time as the detachment is so hopelessly involved in membrane formation that even liquid silicone will fail to reposition the retina.

The reason for this important timing is that in the early days of the contractual stage the membrane only involves the peripheral retina, so that correct placement of the liquid silicone will detach the immobilising membrane from the posterior retina and a good visual result will often be obtained. If surgery is postponed so that posterior retina is involved, not only will it often be impossible to close the tears and thus prevent silicone from passing through into the sub-retinal space, but the membrane may not be detachable from the posterior retina and a poor visual result will occur. In addition fibrosis will often be found within and beneath the retina in the late contractual phases and this is quite untreatable.

The technique of liquid silicone injection is very difficult and involves vitreous manipulation under indirect ophthalmoscopic control. It cannot be done with the direct ophthalmoscope and is very difficult indeed under the microscope, because rapid and large changes of field are used in manipulating the syringe and vitreous scissors, and this is exceedingly difficult with existing microscope technique.

Early workers in the field used liquid silicone as a vitreous implant without reference to manipulation of vitreous membranes, and its was only CIBIS and later OKUN who attempted to use silicone to detach membranes from the retina: it is perhaps one of the great tragedies of our time that Paul CIBIS died so early in his career for it was his innovation that gave us an idea of what could be done with these membranes. Had he lived we might be much further towards the solution of the treatment of massive vitreous retraction.

His idea was that there was usually a gap between the membrane and the retina and the silicone should be injected behind this membrane and thus dissect it away from the retina as the silicone bubble expands. Although this situation is seen in some retinas affected by massive vitreous retraction it is more common for there to be no gap posteriorly, so that for these eyes a rather different approach must be used. The technique depends on the stretching of the posterior gel, or the membrane if it has extended to the posterior pole of the eye, so that it can be incised and then detached from the retina. The stretching is done by injecting as much liquid silicone as possible. The injection is commenced in the mid-vitreous region and continued as sub-retinal fluid is drained. If there is only a relatively shallow detachment before the injection it is necessary to withdraw vitreous fluid before the first injection is begun. The injection then replaces vitreous fluid aspirated. Next sub-retinal fluid is drained and a further injection carried out with the needle inserted into the first silicone bubble. Thus enough liquid silicone is injected to press anteriorly on anterior gel and posteriorly on epiretinal membrane or posterior gel depending on the extent of the disease. Of course this posterior gel is continuous with the equatorial membrane and has the advantage that it is much easier to divide when stretched and this is done with the injection needle. Indeed it very often happens that the posterior gel spontaneously splits when under pressure from the liquid silicone and further injection forces silicone between retina and gel. Further splitting of the gel then occurs so that as the retina flattens completely the gel retracts peripherally and a successful result can be expected with good vision. If the membrane has extended posteriorly requiring division before the silicone will pass between membrabe and retina, an important step must be carried out to ensure a good visual result. The membrane is fibrotic and continuous so that as it separates from the retina it will pass forward and come to lie behind the lens; if it is allowed to do this without modification the membrane will usually be so opaque as to obscure vision. It is therefore important that when the membrane has separated so that it lies at the mid-vitreous level it should be divided with vitreous scissors as widely as possible to prevent obstruction of vision.

Although I have emphasised the role of silicone in separating membranes from the retina it must be remembered that very often retinal tears are still unclosed when massive vitreous retraction is present and these tears must be closed. Sometimes previous surgery has already provided buckles which are in correct position but have failed to close the tear because of retinal membrane formation, sometimes new buckless will be necessary and these new buckles must be as high as possible for the commonest cause of failure of liquid silicone surgery is the inability to close a retinal tear allowing the silicone to pass into the sub-retinal space. When this occurs of course all is lost and the eye is incurable.

A few words now about giant equatorial tears. The vitreous of eyes affected by giant equatorial tears is characterised by the splitting of cortical gel behind the equator. The main mass of gel is attached to the anterior edge

116

of the tear and not, as has been described in some previous work, to the posterior edge. Instead a thin layer of cortical gel is spread over the posterior retina extending anteriorly as far as the posterior edge of the giant tear. The main mass of gel is not only attached to the anterior edge of the tear but also to the equator elsewhere and is frequently associated with satellite retinal tears. Giant tears of the retina which have not extended beyond the apices of the tear can probably be regarded as flat tears with rolled posterior edges and treated conventionally with buckles designed to close the apices of the tear only. However beware the localised giant equatorial tear for it will develop massive vitreous retraction very easily indeed and when it does it is extremely difficult to treat.

In order to understand the manner in which massive vitreous retraction affects eyes with giant equatorial tears it is necessary to look a little further into the vitreous. Over the extent of the tear the gel is split by the retraction of the posterior edge with the main mass of gel attached to the anterior edge. At the apices of the tear the two divided areas of gel unite but the main mass of gel remains separated from the retina posteriorly leaving a thin layer still attached to the posterior retina. Fibrosis within these membranes produces a characteristic appearance in which retraction of the posterior edge of the tear occurs accompanied by a contraction of the surface of the gel attached to the anterior edge of the tear. The retina at the equator elsewhere is puckered and contracts by the trans-vitreal traction from the membrane and the circumferential sphincter-like contraction of the fibrosing gel on the surface of the equatorial retina. The anterior edge of the tear elevates so that in time it lies in the same plane as the transvitreal membrane and the apices of the tear become squared off. The apices of the tear are the basis for the great difficulty in closing these tears for they form the points at which the retraction of the anterior edge of the tear is transferred to the posterior edge which is also contracting. The result of all this retraction is to create a huge elevation of the apices of the tear. If this happens then the situation is incurable.

Fortunately it is possible to predict this situation and to take steps to avoid it. If in the presence of a giant retinal tear the retinal detachment extends beyonds the edges of the tear itself then massive vitreous retraction can be expected to quickly supervene. If the main mass of gel has a posterior surface which is smooth and not fully mobile then fibrosis is occurring, and of course if any of the other signs of the contracting stage of massive vitreous retraction are present then urgent surgery must be carried out.

In addition to placing as high radial buckles as possible at the apices of the tear and extending these well posteriorly, it will be necessary to divide the trans-vitreal membrane. Although this will considerably reduce the retraction of the anterior edge of the tear at its apices it will usually not be enough, for the circumferential sphincter-like effect will still be present. The only way to successfully treat this situation is by means of liquid silicone combined with an encircling band. The liquid silicone will have several actions; it will force the retina back onto the buckle against the forces of the circumferential retraction, it will help to close the apices of the tear against the radial buckles, it will help to delineate the trans-vitreal membrane during its division with vitreous scissors and it will press the posterior edge of the tear into position unfolding it and perhaps allowing separation of the posterior membrane so that the retina may flatten smoothly.

The method or injection is rather different from that for massive vitreous retraction complicating a small tear, in that it must be begun anteriorly. In this way the trans-vitreal membrane will be delineated early and more easily divided. After division the silicone will pass posteriorly and retinal flattening will occur. However, it cannot be emphasised enough that the correct time to operate is as soon as the membrane is retracting forward, not after it has formed a tight sheet across the eye just behind the lens. If surgery is delayed so that this happens it will fail.

Now I wish to talk briefly about macular holes. As primary causes of retinal detachment they are very rare, accounting for about 10% of macular holes. Most primary macular holes occur in highly myopic and produce a characteristic distribution of fluid. The detachment is usually shallow and does not extend to the ora serrata, it rises only slightly above the horizontal meridian and is mostly confined to the lower half of the retina. Traditionally conventional buckling has been applied to macular holes with diathermy or cryotherapy treatment. Part of the rationale of this approach has been the idea that macular holes result in severe loss of vision so that it does not matter if further destructive lesions are produced. However careful analysis of the vision of eyes affected by flat macular holes has shown that fullthickness holes are compatible with a visual acuity better than 6/60 in most cases, one-fifth seeing better than 6/36. It would therefore appear indefensible to treat such holes with diathermy or cryotherapy. An alternative is to close the hole from the inside using liquid silicone. Vitreous fluid passes easily through a macular hole whereas liquid silicone does not, however in order to close the hole a great deal of fluid must be injected, enough in fact to allow the anterior surface of the bubble to press against the gel behind the lens and posteriorly against the macular hole. In a highly myopic eye this may be as much as 12 mls. There is rarely enough sub-retinal fluid to allow this volume of injection so that space is created for the silicone by aspiration of intra-vitreal fluid. Using a wide-bore needle through the pars plana fluid is withdrawn in $1\frac{1}{2}$ ml. steps, after each of which a similar quantity of liquid silicone is injected. Each successive aspiration is from vitreous fluid surrounding the silicone bubble and each injection is into the previous bubble so that multiple bubbles are not formed. This sequence is continued until the silicone is seen to press against the macula: at this stage sub-retinal fluid may be released if it is possible. If it is not, then a further attempt should be made to remove the last drops of vitreous fluid for the macular hole may be uncovered when the patient stands up and the silicone bubble floats upwards. Usually it will not be and all should be well. The long-term visual results of this procedure are very encouraging and far superior to those in which the macula is scarred by treatment.

Finally I should like to say a little about complications. The commonest problems encountered in the long-term follow-up of patients treated with liquid silicone is cataract. The reason for this is usually a worsening of the lens opacities seen before surgery and the effect may well be similar to that found after intra-vitreal gas injection, that is an interference with ionic exchange across the posterior surface of the lens with subsequent loss of transparency. Removal of the cataract is by the extracapsular method and is usually uneventful.

A more serious problem has occurred in two patients and that is emulsification of the silicone. Mention has already been made of the experience of early workers in this field who used liquid silicone in small amounts and very commonly noticed complications from silicone emulsification. The reason for this is probably that the silicone bubble was mobile in the eye and mechanical activity at the edge of the bubble allowed smaller bubbles to break off and enter the anterior chamber. Glaucoma may follow with irretrievable loss of vision. In my two patients the silicone bubble was mobile. In one case the vision was lost from glaucoma, in the other the silicone was removed and the eye recovered. The lesson to be learned from this is inject a large enough bubble that is static within the eye.

Large bubbles of silicone may sometimes enter the anterior chamber and usually cause no problem apart from the effect on vision. If the bubble becomes so big as to completely fill the chamber then glaucoma may follow, but this does not always occur.

Complications then have been few and many successfully treated eyes continue to see up to ten years following surgery. One patient has even taken up oil painting having previously seen light perception only and four years after successful surgery for massive vitreous retraction is still painting with a visual acuity of 6/24.

In summary then I wish to repeat five main points:

Liquid silicone is the only possible treatment for the contractual stage of massive vitreous retraction.

Giant retinal tears are rapidly affected by massive vitreous retraction and need liquid silicone when the detachment spreads beyond the apices of the tear.

Primary macular holes treated by liquid silicone have a good visual prognosis comparable to that expected from a flat macular hole.

Liquid silicone is not a vitreous replacement but a means of separating membranes from the retina and an internal tamponade.

Liquid silicone is not toxic to the human retina.

Author's address:
Department of Opthalmology
Addenbrooke's Hospital
Hills Road
Cambridge
England

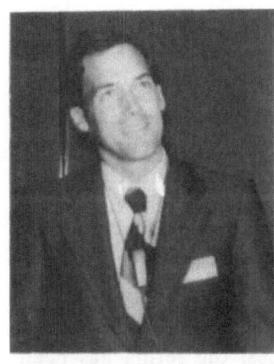

PARS PLANA VITRECTOMY:
INDICATIONS AND RESULTS

STEPHEN J. RYAN*

(Los Angeles, California, USA)

Pars plana vitrectomy has opened a number of previously untreatable ocular disorders to successful surgical management. MACHEMER (1971, 1972), DOUVAS (1973) and others (O'MALLEY & HEINTZ 1972; PEYMAN & DODICH 1971; FEDERMAN et al. 1974; KLÖTI 1973; SCHEPENS 1972; KRIEGER et al. 1973; KAUFMAN 1975) have introduced effective instrumentation to further the technique pioneered by MACHEMER (1971, 1972). This pars plana approach can be utilized for the removal of vitreous, lens, or virtually any other intraocular tissue. In addition to intravitreal sheets and preretinal membranes, membranous cataracts and other anterior segment abnormalities can now be surgically approached with vitrectomy technique.

The indications for vitrectomy very much influence the results in any series. On analysis of our initial cases, the authors had a 20% success rate, whereas, at the time of tabulation of these cited results, an 80% success rate was achieved. In the analysis of our results 'success' never refers to a morphologic or anatomical cure, but rather demands functional improvement; i.e., the postoperative visual acuity must be maintained as significantly improved when compared to the preoperative acuity. The initial poor results were in part related to a lack of surgical experience and repeated instrument malfunctions. However, the single most important factor influencing the visual results was case selection. Case selection still remains the most important factor in the determination of successful results. The initial failures were for the most part juvenile onset diabetics with traction detachments and poorly perfused retinas. In such cases technically successful operations without complication and producing anatomic cures are listed as failures since there was no functional improvement. Better results are achieved with adult-onset diabetics, and particularly, vitreous hemorrhages in the non-diabetics.

While one's success rate improves with better surgical technique and instrumentation, case selection can remain a counter-balancing factor. On the one hand, ideal cases for the optimal success rate can be selected, but now we continue to push back the frontier so that we progressively become more bold and operate more difficult cases than previously. Traction retinal

* Dr. Ryan is a recipient of the Louis B. Mayer Scholar Award from Research to Prevent Blindness, Inc., New York City

detachments, not just vitreous hemorrhage, are now becoming an indication for vitrectomy. Such indications decrease the success rate. Our pooled results for vitrectomy reported in the American Journal of Ophthalmology (MICHELS & RYAN 1974) and a subsequent overlapping series have been published elsewhere (MICHELS & RYAN). Current independent series in Los Angeles and Baltimore reflect similar percentages and statistics. However, the follow up is not long enough in the more recently operated cases. Therefore, this manuscript is based on these previously reported series.

Visual acuity following technically successful vitrectomy is limited by the functional capacity of the retina, especially the macula. However, the potential level of retinal function in the presence of dense vitreous opacities cannot be determined with certainty. In most cases, the retina has been affected to some degree by the underlying disease. The visual acuity and fundus appearance prior to vitreous hemorrhage is of great help. The presence and quality of light projection is probably the most reliable preoperative clinical test. It must be emphasized that we have observed many false positives and false negatives with this test. Preoperative evaluation with bright flash ERG to determine whether the retina is attached and functional performed in combination with A and B scan ultrasonography is quite helpful. All too frequently, however, the final decision regarding recommendation of vitreous surgery remains equivocal. In offering surgical intervention

TABLE 1

Indications for pars plana vitrectomy*

I.   Blindness due to nonresolving vitreous opacities
     A. Vitreous hemorrhage
        1. Diabetes
        2. Non-diabetic
     B. Other vitreous opacities

II. Trauma
     A. Certain penetrating injuries
     B. Non-magnetic intraocular foreign bodies

III. Retinal detachment
     A. Recent traction detachment involving the macula
     B. Certain giant tears
     C. Severe vitreous traction preventing successful conventional retinal surgery

IV. Vitreous biopsy

V.   Anterior segment 'reconstruction'
     A. Membranous cataract
     B. Pupillary membrane
     C. Persistent hyperplastic primary vitreous (PHPV)

VI. Other
     A. Vitreous incarceration with persistent Irvine-Gass syndrome
     B. Aphakic vitreous 'touch' with corneal edema
     C. Aphakic pupillary-block glaucoma
     D. Glaucoma, other
        1. Hemolytic
        2. Phakolytic, due to retained lens material
     E. Endophthalmitis

122

to the individual patient, a full discussion of the significant risks and potential benefits of surgery is presented. The total patient, including life expectancy, must be considered and be balanced against the importance of sight to these desparate patients – the majority of whom are legally blind and physically dependent secondary to their marked visual deprivation.

Our indications for vitrectomy remain essentially unchanged from those previously reported (see Tables 1 and 2). This 100-case series is chosen because of the statistical convenience for the reader and authors, but most importantly because these trends have continued in our more recent cases.

Our success rate in vitreous hemorrhage in non-diabetic patients exceeds 80%, but in diabetic patients with vitreous hemorrhage, the overall success rate has been approximately 60 to 70 percent (see Table 3) (MICHELS & RYAN, 1974). Postoperative visual acuity varied from 20/20 to 3/200. In diabetic patients with vitreous hemorrhage alone, there was a 90% success rate, whereas, those that have traction detachments as well as hemorrhage have a much lower success rate – approximately 40% (see Table 5). It is important to emphasize that relatively few of the diabetics achieve 20/50 or better vision. Only 5 of 22 diabetics with improved vision achieved 20/50 or better visual acuity (see Table 5).

Non-diabetic vitreous hemorrhage includes those cases of branch vein occlusion with vitreous hemorrhage, Eales' disease, the proliferative sickle retinopathies, and other causes of proliferative retinopathy. The 80% success rate again is tempered by the fact that none of the 8 success achieved 20/50 or better visual acuity. This again reflects the fact that the macula can be damaged by the underlying disease process or that the retina can be poorly perfused or be detached, etc. The underlying disease remains the limiting factor to visual recovery.

TRAUMA, PENETRATING INJURIES, INTRAOCULAR FOREIGN BODIES

Pars plana vitrectomy technique offers a new approach to the management of certain penetrating injuries and non-magnetic reactive intraocular foreign

TABLE 2

Indications for vitreous surgery: 100 consecutive cases

Complications of diabetes	51
Vitreous opacities (non-diabetic)	10
Trauma	
penetrating	8
intraocular foreign body	5
Anterior-segment 'reconstruction'	8
Endophthalmitis	4
Retinal detachment	4
Persistent Irvine-Gass syndrome	3
Vitreous biopsy	2
Aphakic pupillary-block glaucoma	2
Other	3
	100 eyes

bodies. Penetrating injuries can produce a wide variety of mechanical damage acutely as well as subsequent complications by fibrous ingrowth, vitreous traction band formation, and complicated retinal detachment. The vitrectomy technique is useful to remove a cataractous lens, excising vitreous and blood from the anterior segment, permitting treatment of retinal breaks or detachment before organization results in inoperable damage to the retina.

While vitrectomy can prevent certain complications of late vitreous organization, it must be noted throughout that this is a potentially hazardous procedure and should be reserved for cases where conservative management is most likely to fail. We advocate vitrectomy in eyes with an admixture of vitreous and lens material in which severe inflammation and organization is almost certain to follow. In eyes with dense hemorrhage and evidence of retinal detachment, vitrectomy can be used to clear the opacities permitting treatment of the retinal break or detachment. Likewise, it is of value in double perforating ocular injuries and the removal of reactive intraocular foreign bodies. We favor following cases with clear media in which traction bands develop and result in retinal detachment. It is our opinion that frequent observation is required in these eyes because the retina may be involved in a fibrous scar making contraction and subsequent successful reattachment difficult, if not impossible. Clear media allow one to follow vitreous traction and its effect on the retina so that the surgeon can determine the optimum time for intervention and the role of vitrectomy and scleral buckling in such cases. The Kasner approach of 'exploratory vitrectomy' is also employed in trauma. If an eye is scheduled for enucleation following trauma but there is a faint hope of salvage of the eye, the opacities are removed to permit observations of the posterior segment to determine whether or not the eye is salvageable. If not, enucleation will be performed at the same sitting. Otherwise, an extensive procedure will be performed in an attempt to save the eye.

It can be extremely difficult to remove all the cortical vitreous following trauma since this frequently occurs in the younger patient and as a result there may be a subsequent puckering of the retina although trans-vitreal sheets are absent.

It should be emphasized that there is barely six years follow up available from the earliest cases of pars plana vitrectomy and, thus, the question as to how long the eye will function well after vitreous excision remains a subject for speculation. For these reasons, conservatism in the management of the traumatized eye is urged. We do not advocate vitrectomy as a prophylactic measure to prevent possible traction band formation.

The pars plana vitrectomy technique combined with specialized intraocular forceps has dramatically altered the approach to certain reactive intraocular foreign bodies, especially the non-magnetic foreign body. MACHEMER has also pioneered this technique. Non-magnetic foreign bodies may pose a threat to the eye on the basis of several mechanisms: 1) Mechanical damage by the injury; 2) Toxicity from the foreign body; 3) Infection; and 4) Secondary changes in the vitreous leading to retinal detachment. Previously, there was no satisfactory method to permit direct visualization in extraction of the foreign body. An extensive incision may be required to remove large foreign bodies. The normal configuration of the anterior segment can be maintained in the face of scleral collapse with the extreme hypotony by a double Fleringa ring.

The foreign body is mobilized with the vitreous instrument and then removed with a forceps via the separate incision through the pars plana with utilization of the specific two instrument technique (HUTTON *et al*, 1975; MICHELS, 1975). The fiberoptics sleeve of the vitrectomy instrument provides optimum reflex-free illumination. Any retinal breaks may be treated with cryotherapy with or without scleral buckling. A gas bubble in the vitreous cavity again provides effective internal tamponade. The results of vitreous surgery for the complications of ocular trauma have been encouraging (see Tables 3 and 4).

TABLE 3

Vitrectomy results · postoperative change in vision: 100 eyes

	Improved	*Same or Decreased*
Complications of diabetes	31	20
Vitreous opacities (nondiabetic)	8	2
Trauma		
Penetrating	5	3
Intraocular foreign body	2	3
Anterior-segment 'reconstruction'	8	0
Endophthalmitis	3	1
Retinal detachment	0	4
Persistent Irvine-Gass Syndrome	2	1
Vitreous biopsy	2	0
Aphakic pupillary-block glaucoma	1	1
Other	2	1
	64	36

TABLE 4

Results: visual acuity after vitreous surgery in 64 eyes showing improved vision

	20/20-20/50	20/50-20/200	20/300-3/200
Complications of diabetes	5	10	16
Vitreous opacities (non-diabetic)		6	2
Trauma			
Penetrating	1	2	2
Intraocular foreign body	2	..	–
Anterior-segment 'reconstruction'*	4	2	..
Endophthalmitis	2	1	..
Persistent Irvine-Gass syndrome	1	1	..
Vitreous biopsy	1	1	–
Aphakic pupillary-block glaucoma		1	..
Other	2	..	–

* Patient with bilateral persistent hyperplastic primary vitreous is too young to measure acuity.

125

RETINAL DETACHMENT

This was perhaps the major indication leading to the development of vitrectomy by a retinal surgeon — Dr. MACHEMER. We have had experience, but not a good success rate to date. The four cases (see Tables 2 and 3) had either massive periretinal proliferation (MPP) otherwise termed massive vitreous retraction (MVR). We have operated traction retinal detachments and operated successfully those detachments after penetrating injuries. In the diabetic traction detachments (see Table 5), we have had only one out of six successful cases. The role of vitrectomy in giant tears has been emphasized. MPP or MVR remains a major problem. In our hands, at this time, we have not successfully operated this disease (MPP) via vitrectomy.

ANTERIOR SEGMENT RECONSTRUCTION

Vitrectomy instrumentation and techniques can be applied to multiple surgical problems and complications of the anterior segment. This approach has been particularly important in eyes with an occluded or inadequate pupillary space due to membranous or secondary cataract, vascularized membranes with secluded and updrawn pupils and persistent hyperplastic primary vitreous (PHPV). The vitrectomy instrument can open the pupillary space by excising dense fibrous material that may be too difficult to cut with a knife, a Holth punch, or with scissors. The vitrectomy instrument can be introduced through the limbus or the pars plana, depending on the indication, visibility, and potential complications. Iris tissue and soft pliable membranes can be easily excised. Tough membranes that cannot be aspirated into the port frequently require a second instrument, usually a knife to cut the membrane or impact the membrane into the cutting port. Anterior segment reconstruction and surgery provide the highest success rate of all indications for surgery with vitreous instruments. This simply reflects the healthy retina and macula in such eyes as opposed to the damaged retina found in the other indications. This 100% success rate to date is noted in Tables 3 and 4.

Secluded pupils may require surgery to create an adequate pupillary space or to relieve iris bombe with secondary glaucoma. Again, the two cases operated in this manner have been most successful. PHPV is a monocular congenital anomaly characterized by microphthalmos and retrolental

TABLE 5

Results of vitreous surgery: diabetic eyes (51)

Indication for Surgery	Total Eyes	Vision Improved	Vision after Surgery		
			20/20-20/50	20/60-20/200	20/300-3/200
Vitreous hemorrhage	24	22	5	10	7
Traction detachment involving macula	6	1	–	–	1
Hemorrhage and detachment	21	8	–	–	–

fibrovascular membrane with traction on the ciliary processes. The surgical indication and goal in this procedure is not to restore normal vision (because of monocular aphakia and deep amblyopia) but rather preservation of the eye. In the microphthalmic eye, there can be progressive shallowing of the anterior chamber and resultant secondary angle closure glaucoma. Thus, the prevention of secondary glaucoma and loss of the eye is the rationale for surgical intervention.

OTHER VITREOUS COMPLICATIONS IN THE ANTERIOR SEGMENT

More recent data is included in this group so that a more meaningful experience can be employed for discusssion. Pars plana vitrectomy can be employed in 'vitreous touch' with corneal edema, vitreous incarceration in a cataract wound (Irvine-Gass syndrome), and aphakic pupillary block.

VITREOUS TOUCH WITH CORNEAL EDEMA

Corneal damage is most likely to occur if there are pre-existent guttata and vitreous may then contact the already compromised corneal endothelium. The instrument tip is placed in the pupillary space with the cutting port directed anteriorly. The vitreous is gently aspirated into the cutter without collapse of the cornea. The vitreous peels off the corneal endothelium and all visible vitreous can be removed from the anterior chamber. This can be difficult because of the associated corneal edema related to the vitreous touch. There should be strict criteria for vitrectomy in aphakic bullous keratopathy. Progression of the area of corneal decompensation must be documented. On the one hand, success cannot be achieved in endstage aphakic bullous keratopathy since the endothelium has been irreversibly damaged. On the other hand, vitreous touch has been observed in some individuals for 20 years without decompensation of the cornea. Strict criteria for progression dictates that the initial area of decompensation be central and circumscribed so that documentation can be obtained. We have successfully operated two such cases with recovery of the corneal endothelium and clearing of the corneal edema after documenting progression of the area of corneal decompensation.

CYSTOID MACULAR EDEMA WITH VITREOUS INCARCERATION (IRVINE-GASS SYNDROME)

This maculopathy can be associated with a number of vascular disorders and following various types of ophthalmic surgery. The etiology remains unknown. The Irvine-Gass syndrome is a common occurrence which usually clears spontaneously. Previous attempts have been made by ILIFF and others to cut vitreous bands. The pars plana vitrectomy technique is particularly appropriate for cutting the broad incarcerated vitreous sheets in selected cases with cystoid macular edema persisting for more than one year. We have operated five such cases with successful removal of vitreous from the wound in four. Of the five cases, one eye showed dramatic visual improvement; in two, the vision remained unchanged; and in the remaining two, the follow up is too short for interpretation of results.

APHAKIC PUPILLARY BLOCK GLAUCOMA

Vitreous may obstruct the pupillary space and iridectomy sites in aphakic eyes resulting in aphakic pupillary block. When the pupillary block cannot be relieved by medical therapy, then surgery may be indicated. Incision of the hyaloid often relieves the obstruction, but may be complicated by vitreous to the corneal wound. If reformation of the hyaloid occurs, then pupillary block may recur. The hyaloid can be readily cut and with this, four eyes have been operated with dramatic deepening of the chamber and without complications. The technical results have been encouraging. However, there are additional surgical risks to those of conventional surgery and longer follow up is necessary to evaluate this.

HEMOLYTIC GLAUCOMA

Vitreous hemorrhage may occasionally be complicated by hemolytic glaucoma. Macrophages filled with hemoglobin blood breakdown products can obstruct the outflow channels. If hemolytic glaucoma occurs after vitrectomy and the intraocular pressure cannot be satisfactorily controlled, the remaining blood can be washed from the eye using a two-needle technique with infusion and suction through the peripheral cornea.

PHACOLYTIC AND PHACOANAPHYLACTIC GLAUCOMA

Retained lens material following cataract surgery may elicit an inflammatory response with obstruction of the trabecular outflow channels. Retained lens cortex is usually absorbed without complications. The retained nuclear material generally does not absorb spontaneously and often elicits a marked inflammatory response. The pars plana technique again provides a useful method to remove lens material from the vitreous cavity. The cortical material is easily aspirated. However, nuclear material may be more difficult. In this situation, suction can be used to grasp the nucleus, bring it to the pupillary space where it can be mechanically crushed with a second instrument if necessary. This technique has been used successfully to treat phacolytic glaucoma caused by retained cortical material in the vitreous. Also, a lens nucleus has been successfully removed from the vitreous cavity with considerable local inflammation and secondary glaucoma.

Thus, vitrectomy, while a relatively new technique, is one of the most exciting horizons in modern ophthalmology. The surgical indications consist of diabetes, non-diabetic vitreous hemorrhages and opacities, trauma — penetrating and intraocular foreign bodies, selected retinal detachments, and anterior segment reconstruction. Our indications and results have been reviewed and provide optimism for this rapidly expanding field.

REFERENCES

DOUVAS, N.G. The cataract roto-extractor. *Trans. Amer. Acad. Ophthal. & Otolaryng.* 77: *792* (1973).

FEDERMAN, J.L., L.K. SARIN & W. ANNESLEY et al. Suction Infusion Tissue Extractor (SITE). Presented at meeting of the Retina Society, Montreal, Canada, Sept. (1974).

HUTTON, W.L., W.B. SNYDER & A. VAISER. Surgical removal of nonmagnetic foreign bodies. *Amer. J. Ophthalm.* 70: *838-843* (1975).

KAUFMAN, H. Vitrectomy from the anterior segment. *Ophthal. Surg.* 6: *58* (1975).

KLÖTI, R. Vitrektomie I. Ein neues instrument fuer die hintere vitrektomie. *Graefe Arch. Ophthal.* 187: *161* (1973).

KRIEGER, A.E., B.R. STRAATSMA & J.R. GRIFFIN et al. A vitrectomy instrument in stereotaxic intraocular surgery. *Amer. J. Ophthal.* 76: *527* (1973).

MACHEMER, R., J.M. PAREL & H. BUETTNER et al. A new concept for vitreous surgery. I. Instrumentation. *Amer. J. Ophthal.* 73: *1* (1972).

MACHEMER, R. A new concept for vitreous surgery. II. Surgical technique and complications. *Amer. J. Ophthal.* 74: *1022* (1972).

MACHEMER, R., H. BUETTNER & E.W.D. NORTON et al. Vitrectomy: A pars plana approach. *Trans. Amer. Acad. Ophthal. & Otolaryng.* 75: *813* (1971).

MACHEMER, R., J.M. PAREL & F.W.D. NORTON et al. Vitrectomy: A pars plana approach. Technical improvements and further results. Trans. Amer. *Acad. Ophthal. & Otolaryng.* 75: *462* (1972).

MICHELS, R.G. & S.J. RYAN Pars plana vitrectomy: 100 consecutive cases. *Amer. J. Ophthal.* 80: *24* (1975).

MICHELS, R.G. & S.J. RYAN Vitrectomy in diabetes and other disorders. In: Current Concepts of the Vitreous including Vitrectomy. K. GITTER, (ed.), St. Louis, C.V. Mosby (in preparation).

MICHELS, R.G. Surgical Management of nonmagnetic intraocular foreign bodies. *Arch. Ophthalm.* 93: *1003-1006* (1975).

O'MALLEY, C. & R.M. HEINTZ Vitrectomy via the pars plana. A new instrument system. *Trans. Pac. Coast. Ottophalmol. Soc.* 53: *121* (1972).

PEYMAN, G.A. & N.A. DODICH Experimental vitrectomy: Instrumentation and surgical technique. *Arch. Ophthal.* 86: *548* (1971).

RYAN, S.J. Pars plana vitrectomy: Instrumentation. *Trans. Amer. Acad. Ophthal. & Otolaryng.* (in Press).

SCHEPENS, C.L. Vitreous surgery: Tissue removal. In: Retina Congress R.C. PRUETT & D.J. REGAN (eds). New York, (1972).

Authors' address:
The University of Southern California
School of Medecine
Department of Ophthalmology
Los Angeles, California
USA

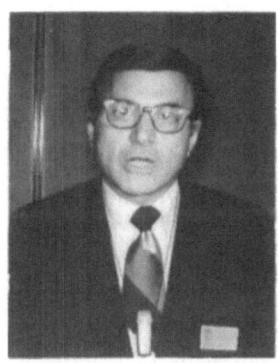

ROTO-EXTRACTOR INSTRUMENTATION, INDICATIONS TECHNIQUES AND RESULTS

NICHOLAS G. DOUVAS

(Port Huron, Michigan, USA)

This paper discusses vitrectomy instrumentation design requirements, a description of the Roto-Extractor (DOUVAS 1975) results and analysis of 100 consecutive Roto-Extractor cases.

All vitrectomy instruments must have certain basic requirements. The instrument must have the capacity to cut and there are three types of cutting instruments. One is the mortar and pestle or a grinding, shear principle. This type of instrument has an axial thrust that is pushing the rotating male cone element against a fixed female component. One version of this principle has a fixed hole matching a rotating hole. This grinding shear must of necessity work slowly. It has a short duty cycle because the aspiration hole is closed about two-thirds of the time. The other instrument working this principle incorporates an auger that is still working on an axial thrust with a spring load to accomplish a grinding shear. The difference is

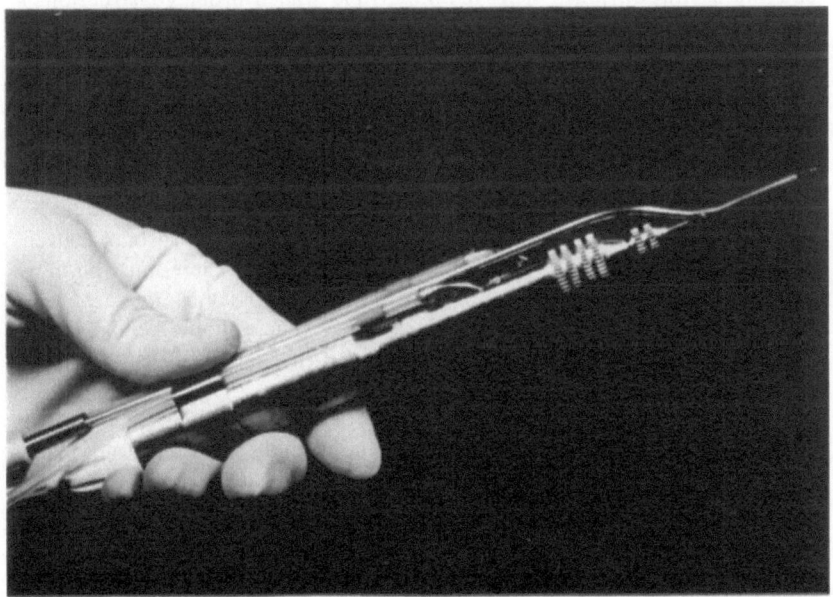

Fig. 1. Roto-Extractor handpiece with fiber-optic light pipe.

that with this auger principle, there is a continuous feed because the cutter opening is never fully closed. Therefore, the instrument does not fully cut free at one time unless there is back flushing.

The next principle is a circular scissor principle such as is exemplified by the Roto-Extractor (Fig. 1). The vitrectomy tips are of a triple walled construction with a double edged cutter blade within that is flaired, not only posteriorly but to the side to create a spring form that provides the scissor-like contact with the inner cutting aperture edges. The cutting blade may be rotated up to 1,000 rpm in a continuous direction or be oscillated clockwise without making more than a 360 degree turn.

The next principle is a guillotine-like cutting principle. There are two types of guillotine-like principles that cut either internally or externally with the blade going in an axial direction.

All instruments must provide an adequate infusion without a jet stream force. There must be an adequate controlled vacuum with back-flush or reverse injection ability by one means or another. The surgeon should be in full control of cutting at all times and preferably by foot control.

Mandatory vitrectomy instrument requirements consist of ability to aspirate without cutting and cutting without aspiration. To me this is very important. Others do not feel that it is important. It is equally important to have the ability to cut totally free of tissue at the aspiration port surface opening. Some of the continuous feed instruments lack this ability.

Instrument reliability is paramount. If there are minor repairs needed, it should be possible for the surgeon to make them. A modular construction with fast factory repair and replacement is most important.

Desirable features of vitrectomy instrument design should insure that there be no internal liquid or vacuum short circuited between the infusion and the aspiration ports. This requires triple walled probe construction. I feel that there should be an optional oscillatory double cutting edge ability at least for the rotary type of instrument. There should be no exposed moving parts within the infusion port. There should be interchangeable probe tips with the same diameter and there should be ability to vary cutting aperture openings because of tissue bridging effects. Because of varying tissue character, some tissue can be impacted in a small opening whereas other tissue is best impacted with a larger opening. There should be an ability to vary the cutting speed and vacuum pull to sustain a given minimal vacuum without circulating nurse assistance. There must be minimal interruption of suction during cutting so that tissue (i.e. luxated lens material) is not lost when the cutter is activated. There should be high speed cutting for small tissue slicing and avoidance of spaghetti-like tissue cuttings to prevent instrument clogging.

There should be a fiber-optic light pipe or sleeve, a trocar, cannula and an infusion tube that can be locked into the cannula so as to permit globe pressurization during indirect ophthalmoscopy or cutting tip change. The infusion contact lens with an optional gimballed assistant's handle (Fig. 2) for use when the surgeon has both hands occupied with two instruments within the eye is of benefit. The rack and pinion syringe drive of Charles (Fig. 3) has the distinct advantage of permitting one hand aspiration. Manual aspiration with proprioceptive feedback to a competent assistant will never

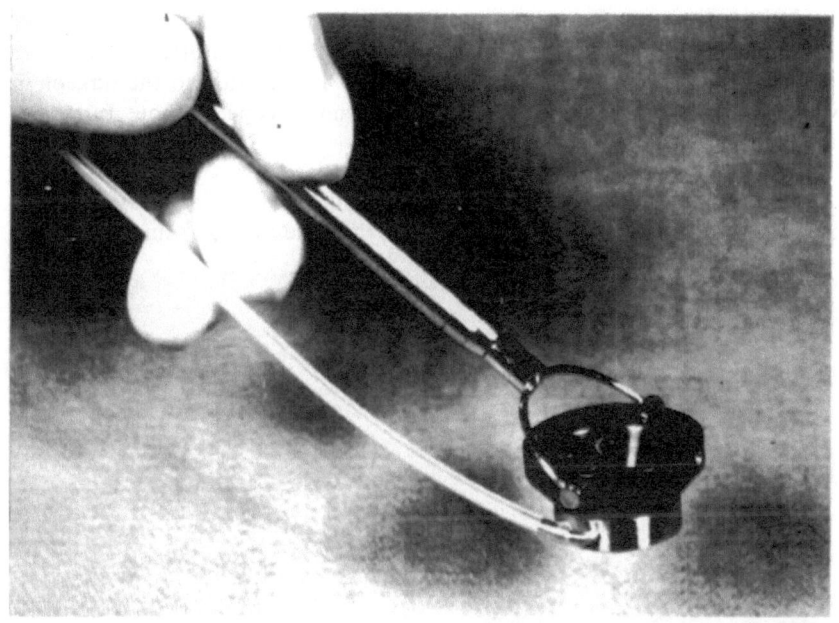

Fig. 2. Gimballed assistant's infusion contact (removable) lens holder.

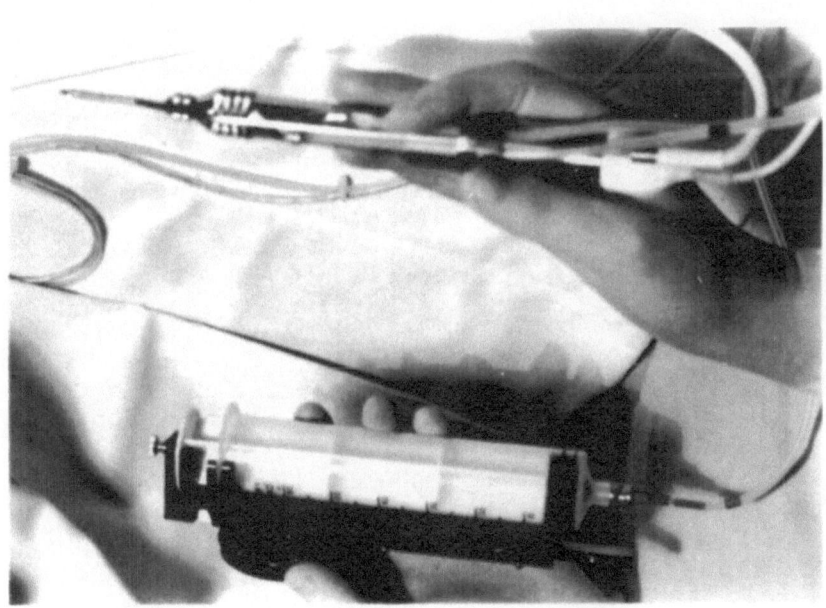

Fig. 3. Rack and pinion syringe drive of Charles used with Roto-Extractor handpiece.

be exceeded by any automated instrument because the human mind is a computer that is tough to beat (Fig. 4). If one employs an automated system, it must attempt to provide equal control and information to the surgeon while the surgeon maintains his eyes at the microscope, without turning around to look at dials.

Some of the undesirable vitrectomy instrument designs will now be discussed. Although others may disagree, the following are my ideas on this subject. Instruments which are unable to aspirate without simultaneous

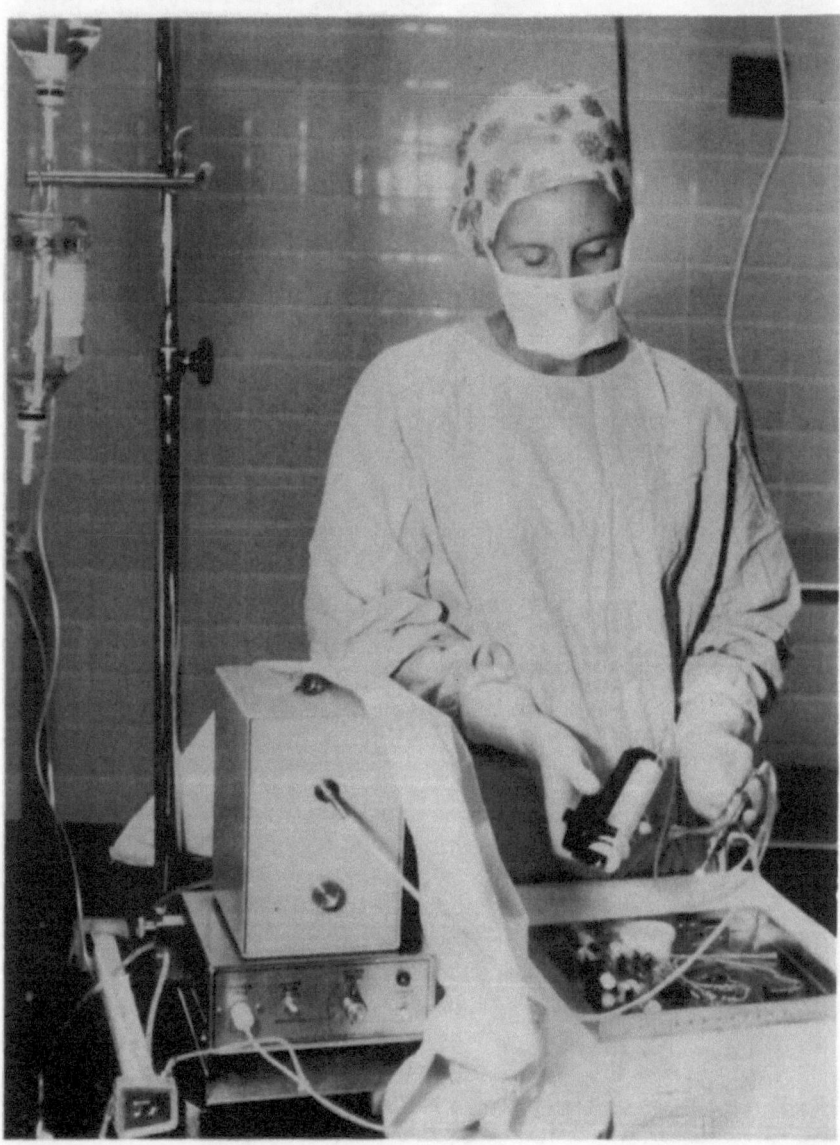

Fig. 4. Roto-Extractor surgical assistant with instrument system components – (foot pedal not shown).

cutting are undesirable. There are many times when aspiration alone is highly desirable.

Finger control of suction or cutting is also included as an undesirable instrument design. There is loss of finger agility after prolonged surgery that precludes delicate maneuvers close to the retina. Probe tip rotation of 180 degrees or more necessitates an awkward hand position with some finger controlled instruments. Furthermore, a pressure gradient may exist when the finger is off the vacuum hole. If the eye is pressurized above atmospheric pressure, this pressure will force fluid and tissue material into the cutter opening with inadvertent tissue incarceration.

A .6 mm. external piston-like movement at the end of a reciprocating guillotine-like instrument precludes working close to the retina.

The continuous auger feed principle with uninterrupted aspiration prevents cutting totally free of tissue. There is always tissue wound or incarcerated into the instrument. Consequently, backflushing and reverse cutting are required to cut free of tissue. The back flush ability exists in only one of two available instruments using this auger principle.

Distant and separate fiber-optic light probe systems may result in inadequate visibility at the end of the cutting probe because of difficulty in aligning the fiber-optic light in a heavily organized eye. Distant and separate infusion may result in instrument clogging because of inadequate vehicular fluid necessary to carry tissue cuttings through the aspiration passages in a heavily organized eye.

DESCRIPTION OF DOUVAS ROTO-EXTRACTOR

The Roto-Extractor cross-section diagram is illustrated in Fig. 5. The instrument has interchangeable probe tips of end-core and side cutting design. The trephine end-core cutter (Fig. 6) is used for preliminary phacofragmentation and hydrolysis. There are two sizes of side cutters — a .6 mm. side cutter and a .4 mm. (Fig. 7). The .4 mm. cutter can be stopped in a half closed position and effectively narrowed to a .2 mm. opening when necessary be-

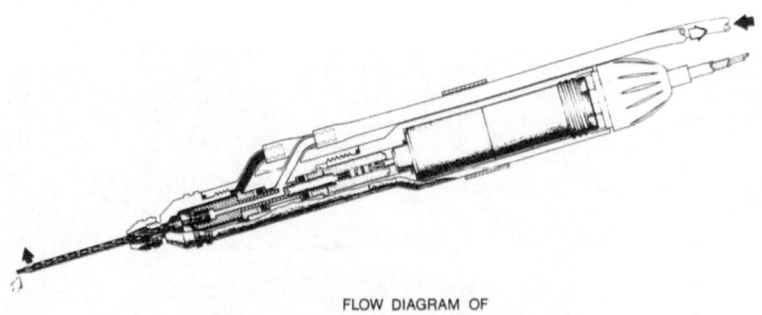

FLOW DIAGRAM OF

ROTO-EXTRACTOR HAND PIECE

WITH MOTOR CARTRIDGE, CUTTER SET, CABLE, AND TUBING

Fig. 5. Roto-Extractor handpiece flow diagram with motor cartridge, cutter set, cable and tubing.

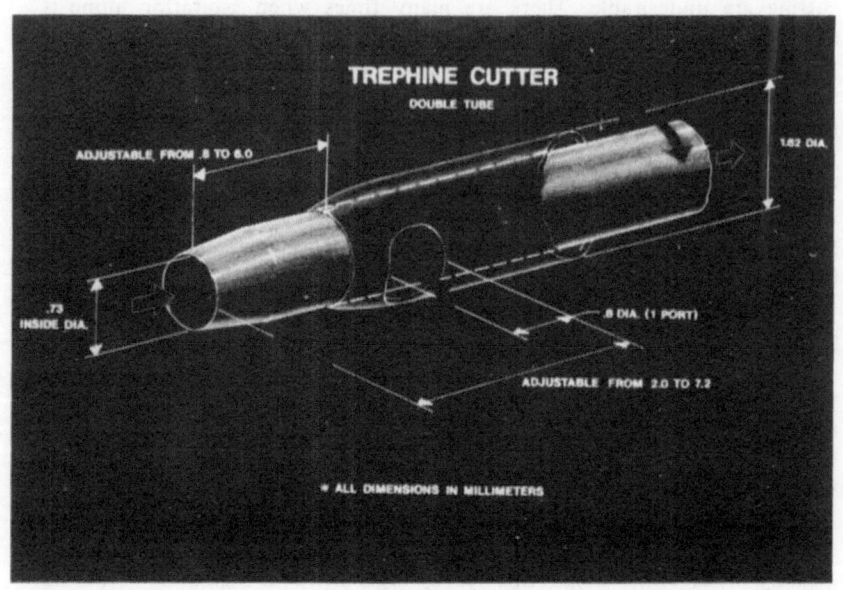

Fig. 6. Diagram – double-walled trephine end-core cutter.

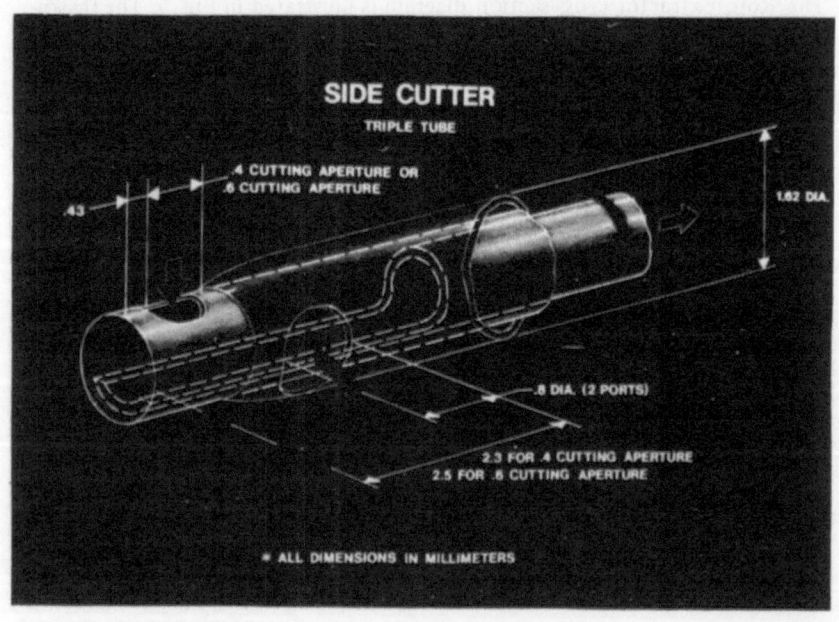

Fig. 7. Diagram – triple-walled side cutter.

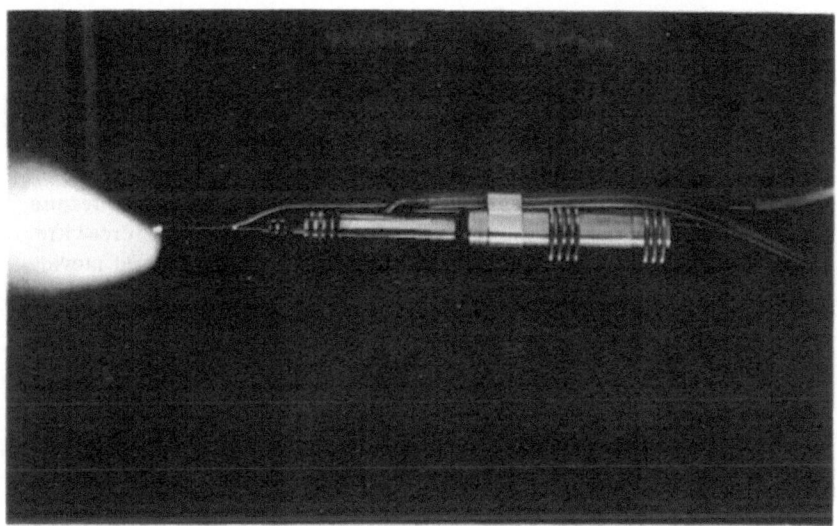

Fig. 8. Roto-Extractor fibro-optic illumination.

fore impacting a thin strand that otherwise could not be impacted because fluid seeps around the edges of the larger cutting aperture. The fiber-optic light illumination with the Roto-Extractor handpiece is shown in Fig. 8.

A high speed clockwise or optional clockwise — counterclockwise oscillatory double cutter edge rotation is of value. The single speed continuous single direction is faster, smoother and most effective when used with the trephine end-core cutter for initial lens fragmentation and honeycombing. It does permit a faster vitrectomy when there is little resistance to cutting and it promotes longer motor life. The oscillatory cutting action is safer when removing iris which otherwise may have a propensity to become wrapped in case of cutter malfunction; it frequently permits more effective cutting of taut anterior lens capsule which tends to slide off a cutter moving in a single direction. The .4 mm. protected side cutter is usually more effective than the .6 mm. or .8 mm. probe tip because of bridging or saddle effect. Every tissue has a different characteristic and one size cutter works better in one case and another in another. Taut vitreous bands are often effectively cut with the oscillatory mode when little progress is being made with single direction cutting. The oscillatory mode is not effective with the trephine end-core cutter for lens fragmentation because it tends to cause a firm lens to rock back and forth. Sometimes in using the oscillatory mode while impacting dense aftercataract lens membrane, a rocking effect results that prevents full impaction and cutting at full speed but after slowing the motor to two-thirds cutter speed, one is able to make progress because of increased capability to impact more deeply within the instrument.

The advantage of the triple-tubed cutters have already been alluded to, namely the prevention of internal liquid or vacuum short circuiting so that vacuum efficiency at the aspiration port is increased so as to better impact cataractous material or vitreous for cutting and aspiration. A vacuum pull

137

across a two tube bearing seal cannot occur so as to impact vitreous or cataract into the infusion port where it may be wrapped or caught on an exposed rotating or oscillating type of shaft. In a two tube system, obviously, the bearing seal between infusion and aspiration chambers has to be less than perfect, otherwise, the moving element cannot move. As long as a two tube instrument is new and fits well, this apparently is not much of a problem. With wear, it may be a problem. Increased intraocular pressure resulting from contact lens manipulation during vitrectomy may force vitreous into the infusion port where it may be caught on an exposed moving element in a two tube system.

The system component arrangement of the Roto-Extractor (Fig. 9) consists of two infusion pressure bottles, a control console, a hand piece with manual aspiration and a dual foot pedal. The left side of the pedal permits cutting only. A sequential pedal on the right side initially activates the solenoid that opens the high infusion bottle to permit higher flow. Further right pedal depression activates cutting. The console showing the tubing with the 'tee' check to the low infusion bottle and the high infusion bottle tubing going to the solenoid clamp control is seen in Fig. 10. There is a speed control knob and a cutter mode switch for either continuous cutting direction or an oscillatory mode of clockwise, counterclockwise cutting. An off – on switch is also present on the console front panel.

The instrument is housed in a sterilizing case with the various cutting tips, two wrenches for cutter changing and spindle body servicing when needed. The fiber-optic light pipe is positioned along the periphery of the box and an irrigated Goldman contact lens is contained in a small white case (Fig. 11). The Roto-Extractor may be gas sterilized on a cold cycle or flash autoclaved for successive case use if the motor-cartridge and the white case containing the Goldman contact lens are removed from the sterilizing box. Although the fiber-optic light pipe can be autoclaved, it has a longer life when gas or cold solution sterilized. The contact lens can be cold solution or

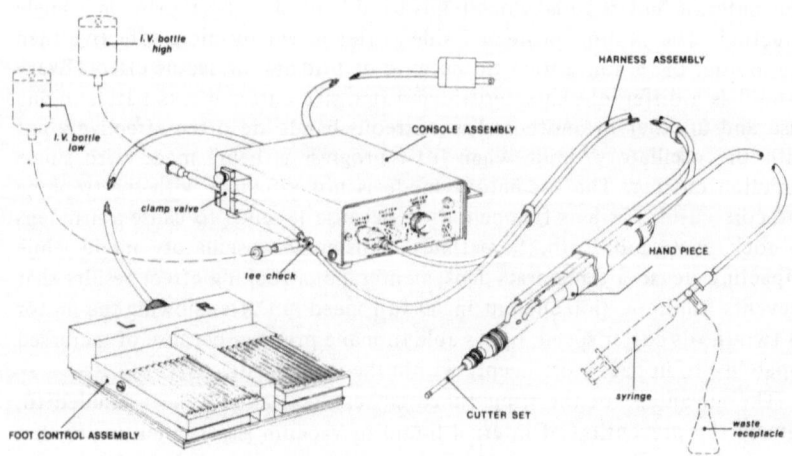

Fig. 9. Roto-Extractor system component arrangement.

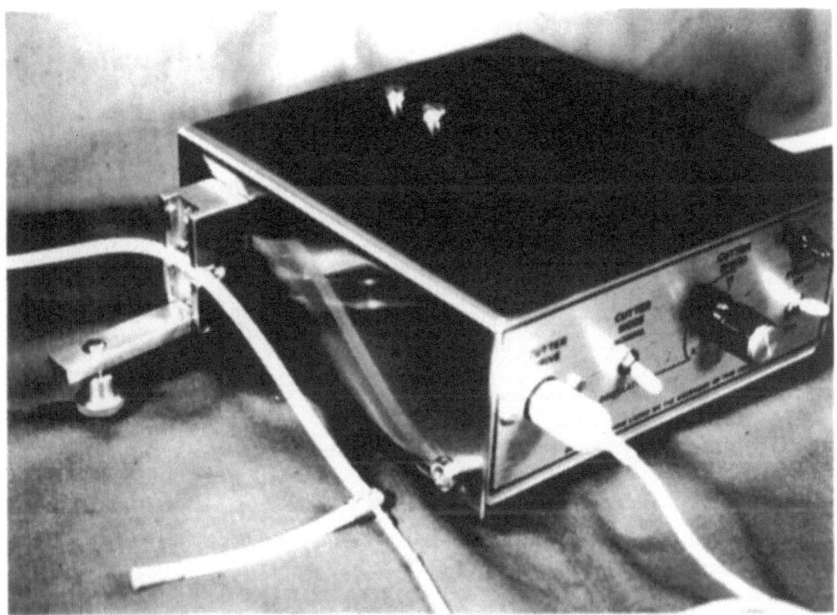

Fig. 10. Roto-Extractor electronic console with 'tee' check for low infusion bottle and solenoid clamp for high infusion bottle.

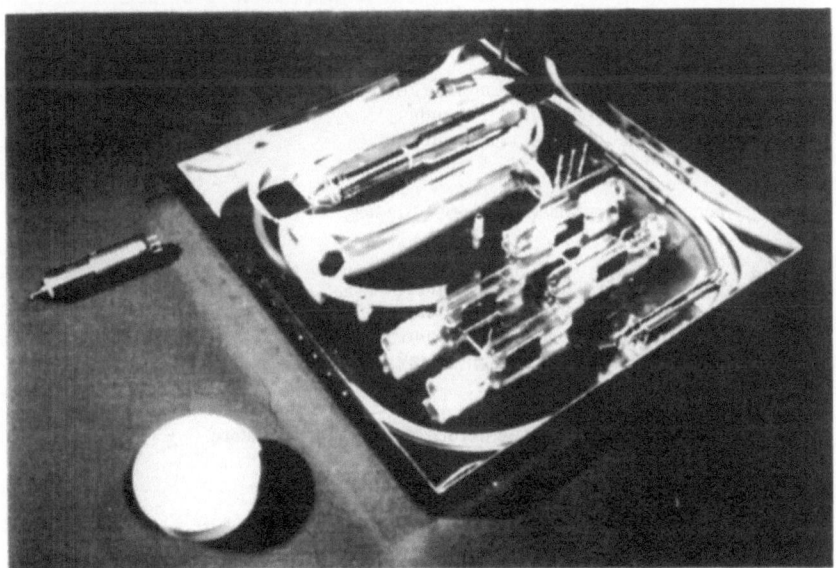

Fig. 11. Roto-Extractor sterilizing box with contact lens container, motor cartridge removed for fast flash autoclaving.

139

TABLE I

100 CONSECUTIVE ROTO-EXTRACTOR OPERATIONS WITH VITRECTOMY

1. Congenital and Development Cataract   Cases
    a) Primary surgery – limbal incision   4
    b) Previous surgery – limbal incision   3
    c) Primary surgery – pars plana incision   5
                                                                 (12)

2. Traumatic Cataract
    a) Primary surgery – limbal incision   7
    b) Previous surgery – limbal incision   10
                                                                 (17)

3. Cataracta Complicata secondary to Uveitis
    a) limbal incision   1
    b) pars plana incision   2
                                                                 (3)

4. Massive Anterior Chamber Hyphema with Glaucoma   2
                                                                 (2)

5. Complications of Intracapsular Cataract Extraction
    a) Bullous keratitis with vitreous touch   5
    b) Updrawn pupil after vitreous loss   3
    c) Miotic pupil with cloudy vitreous   1
    d) Iris-ciliary body implantation cyst   1
    e) After cataract membrane   2
    f) Pupillary block glaucoma   1
    g) Totally luxated lens with phacolytic glaucoma   2
    h) Subluxated senile cataract with vitreous   1
    i) Inadvertent vitreous loss   2
    j) Aphakic glaucoma filtering op. with vit.   1
                                                                 (19)

6. Complications of Phaco-Emulsification
    a) Vitreous into anterior chamber   1
    b) Opaque after-cataract membrane   1
                                                                 (2)

7. Persistent Hyperplastic Primary Vitreous   1
                                                                 (1)

8. Traumatic Massive Vitreous Hemorrhage
    a) Contusion – P. P. Vitrectomy   1
                     P.P. Lensectomy & Vitrectomy   1
    b) Perforating P. P. Lensectomy & Vitrectomy   3
                                                                 (5)

9. Vitreous Opacification & Retinal Detachment secondary
    to Uveitis (L & V); (V) P. P.   2
                                                                 (2)

10. Massive Unabsorbed Vitreous Hemorrhage P. P. secondary
    to Branch Vein Occlusion (L & V); (V)   2
                                                                 (2)

11. Massive Unabsorbed Vitreous Hemorrhage secondary to
    Hypertension – P. P. Vit.   1
                                                                 (1)

140

TABLE I *(continued)*

12. Diabetic Vitreous Hemorrhage – unabsorbed
    a) Pars plana vitrectomy   10
                                                                     (10)

13. Diabetic Vitreous Hemorrhage and Cataract
    a) Pars plana lensectomy & vitrectomy   24
                                                                     (24)

   P. P. = pars plana
   L   = Lensectomy
   V   = Vitrectomy

gas sterilized, but the tubing should be gas sterilized or autoclaved. The motor does not have to be sterilized if care is taken in its insertion into the motor housing (Fig. 12). If the motor was gas sterilized for the first case, its sterility can be maintained with proper technique between successive operations while the sterilizing box and its contents are flash autoclaved.

Table I outlines 100 consecutive Roto-Extractors operations and provides an idea as to indications and results of these 100 cases, which are subdivided into 13 categories. There are 12 cases of congenital or developmental cataracts done either by limbal incision (DOUVAS, 1973) approach or a pars plana approach. Pre and post-op photographs of an example of congenital cataract are shown in Fig. 13. There were also cases that had had previous surgery that were approached by a limbal incision. Fig. 14 illustrates a patient who had had two previous operations before being improved

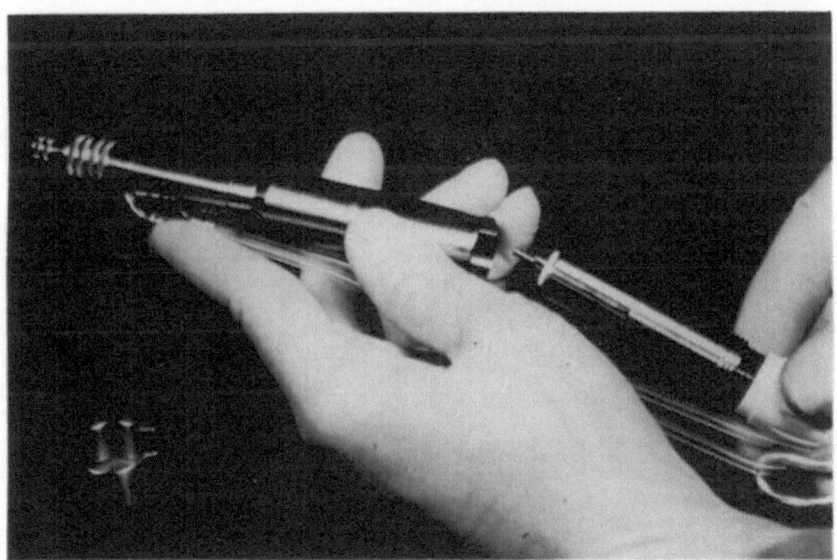

Fig. 12. Insertion of motor cartridge into Roto-Extractor handpiece motor housing.

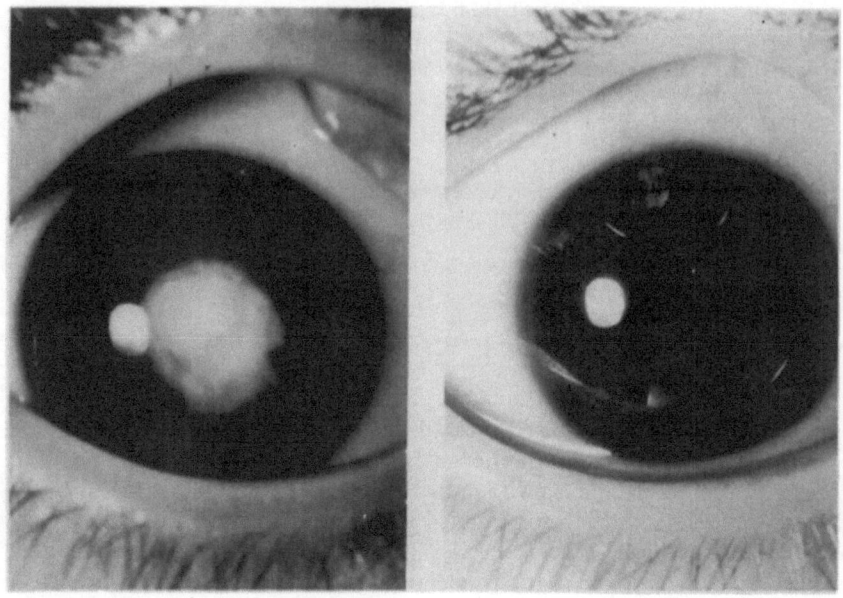

Fig. 13. Congenital cataract – (left) preoperative appearance; (right) postoperative appearance.

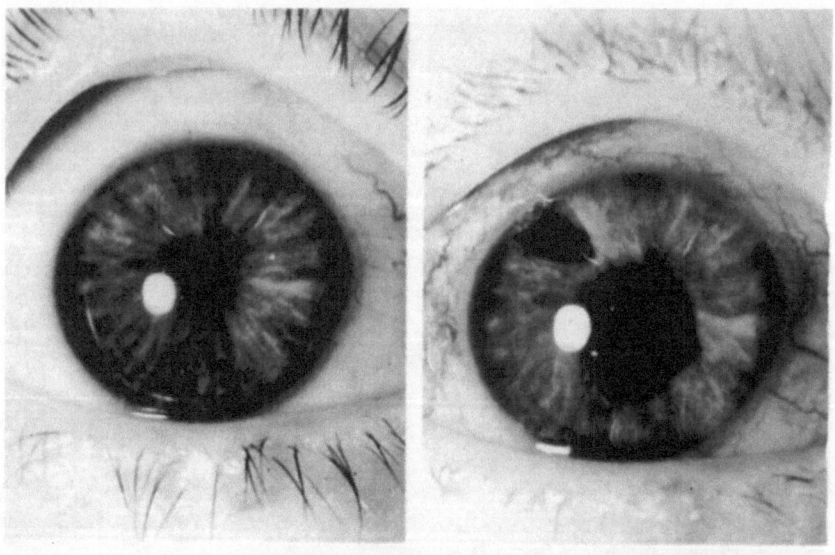

Fig. 14. Previously operative (two times) congential cataract (left); post-operative Roto-Extraction appearance (right).

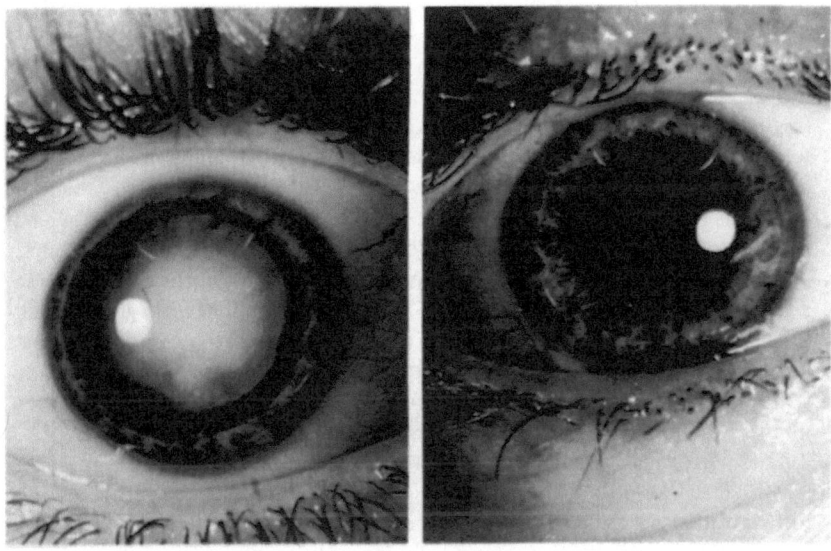

Fig. 15. Traumatic cataract 28 year old patient – (left) pre-operative appearance; (right) post-operative 9th day appearance.

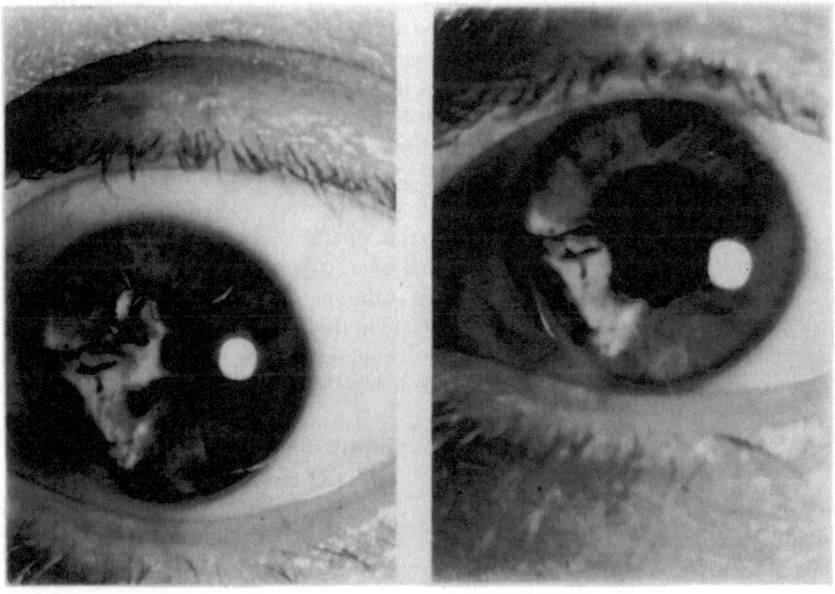

Fig. 16. Dense traumatic after-cataract membrane – (left) pre-operative; (right) post-operative appearance.

143

from 20/70 to 20/20. Much of the lensectomy was accomplished through a peripheral iridectomy.

In doing primary lensectomy on congenital, developmental cataracts, cataracta complicata and presenile cataracts under age 40 preliminary lens fragmentation and hydrolysis is performed with the trephine end-core cutter. The capsular bag is entered through a small knife opening in the anterior capsule near the dilated 12 o'-clock pupillary border if a limbal approach is used. An equatorial sclerotomy knife opening into the lens is made if a pars plana approach is used through a limbus parallel sclerotomy 3.5 to 4.5 mm. posterior to the surgical limbus. Repeated coring cutter thrusts are made across the lens within the capsular bag in conjunction with gentle back flushing of Ringer's solution by the assistant through the central trephine lumen so as to hydrate the lens while high speed continuous rotary cutting is used. This fragmentation and hydration of the lens may persist for five minutes or more in order to soften and mature the lens prior to aspiration. This is performed within the capsular bag so that one doesn't have to chase lens material all around the anterior chamber. The posterior capsule is carefully avoided so as to obviate lens material luxating posterioly. After lens fragmentation, aspiration is started, taking only what comes easily with the trephine prior to switching to a side cutter. Lensectomy is carried out within the capsular bag so long as possible. Ultimately, the entire lens within the pupillary area is removed – namely, the anterior capsule and cortex, nucleus, posterior cortex and capsule in conjunction with a shallow or deep vitrectomy as may be indicated.

In the young patient during the first or second decade of life the limbal approach is preferred. The posterior capsule is removed in conjunction with a shallow anterior vitrectomy because of the high incidence of dense after – cataract membranes following conventional irrigation – aspiration techniques. During the second or third decade of life where a lens may be more rigid and firm, a pars plana approach is selected because inadvertent posterior lens fragment luxation can be easily followed and removed.

Pars plana lensectomy has been limited to senile cataracts with nuclear sclerosis not exceeding grade II on a scale of IV wherein vitrectomy is the primary surgical indication. Pars plana lensectomy with preliminary ultrasonic phaco-emulsification reduces the operative time required in cases where nuclear sclerosis exceeds grade II on a scale of IV.

A total of 17 cases of traumatic cataract underwent Roto-Extractor lensectomy of which 7 were performed via the limbal incision. Fig. 15 illustrates the pre and post-op appearance nine days after surgery of a 28 year old. Cases with previous surgery and dense after-cataracts were performed, as shown in Fig. 16.

Cataracta complicata secondary to uveitis totalled 3 cases. Fig. 17 illustrates what proved to be a very dense cataracta complicata in a 43 year old which was removed almost entirely within the capsular bag without posterior lens luxation. The procedure was lengthy and tedious. A pars plana approach was utilized because of previously known vitreous uveitic opacification.

There were 2 cases of traumatic anterior chamber hyphema with secondary glaucoma. Fig. 18 shows the post-op appearance of one of the eyes

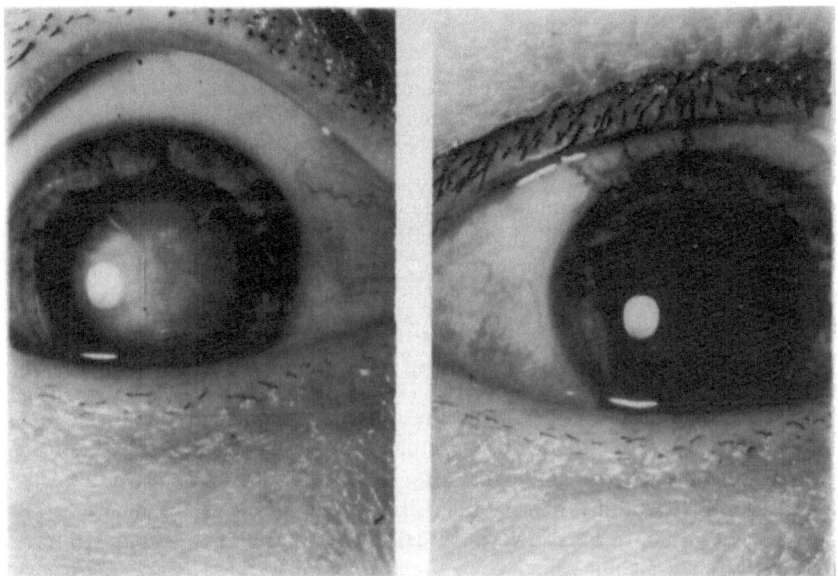

Fig. 17. Dense cataracta complicata secondary to uveitis – (left) pre-operative; (right) post-operative appearance.

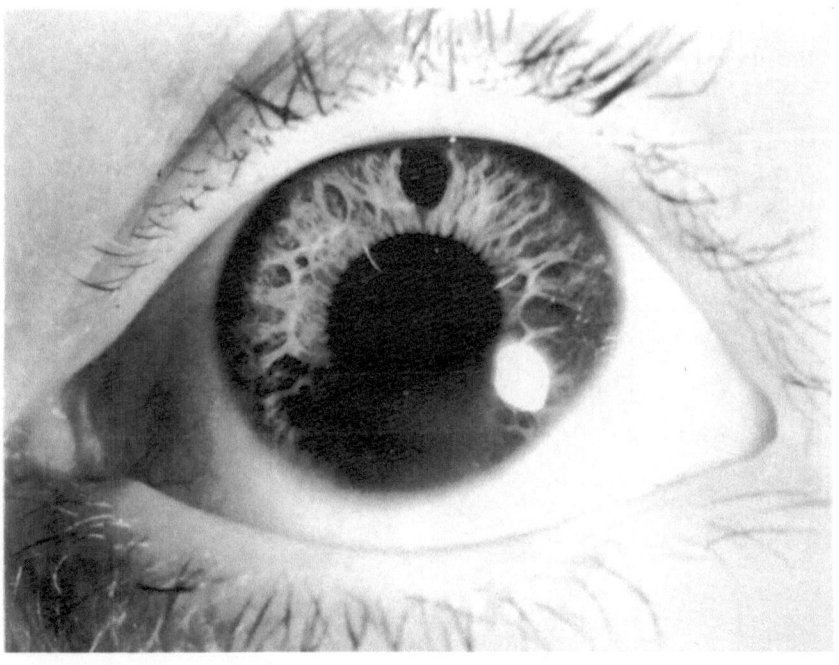

Fig. 18. Anterior chamber hyphema with secondary glaucoma – post-operative appearance with residual corneal blood staining.

145

which still has blood staining of the cornea inferiorly. No lens opacities developed.

There were 19 cases with complications following cataract extraction.

Fig. 19 is an aphakic one-eyed patient complaining of flashes and floaters whose other eye was lost because of a totally detached retina, who was under treatment with Phospholine Iodine. She had a miotic tented pupil that would not dilate. A murky horsetailed vitreous herniated through the miotic pupil, which precluded visualization of her retina. Although initial visual acuity after cataract surgery was 20/25, vision subsequently reduced to 20/200 with increasing opacification of the horsetailed vitreous. The surgical plan was to remove the murky vitreous and enlarge the pupillary opening by performing an iridectomy via a limbal incision. The anterior chamber angle was first swept with a fine Bonn iris hook and a vitreous strand was caught and pulled from the wound. The anterior chamber was then re-entered with the Roto-Extractor (.4 mm. side cutter) and briefly pulsed in an oscillatory mode to create a sector iridectomy. An anterior microsurgical vitrectomy was then performed and indirect ophthalmoscopy revealed the retina to be attached. Visual acuity improved to 20/25 within one week and what must have been a relative pupillary block glaucoma was relieved. She no longer requires glaucoma therapy.

The next illustration is an updrawn pupil in a 28 year old aphakic eye (Fig. 20) that was complicated by massive unabsorbed vitreous hemorrhage and vitreous incarceration into the wound. A pars plana vitrectomy and iridectomy was performed with good visual result. The correct manner of

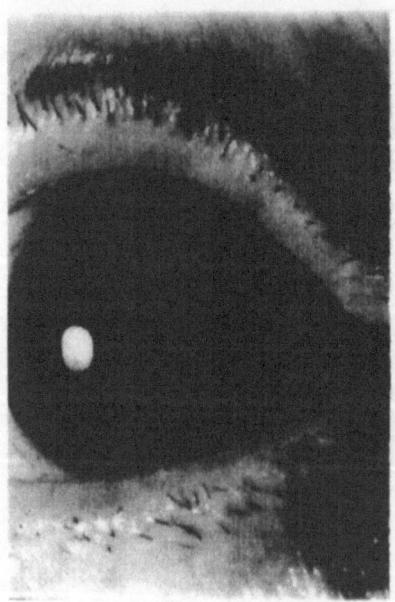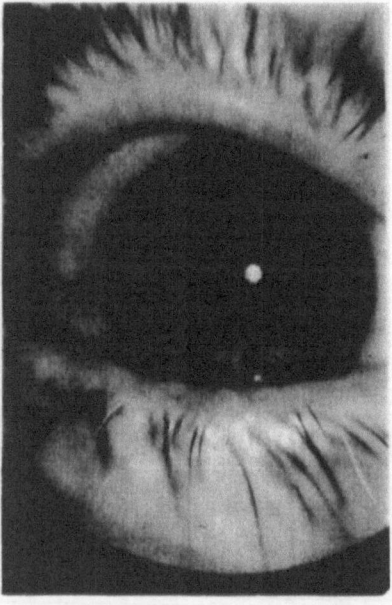

Fig. 19. Aphakic glaucoma with miotic pupil filled with mushroomed opacified horsetailed vitreous – (left) pre-operative tented pupil; (right) post-operative clear red reflex with sector iridectomy.

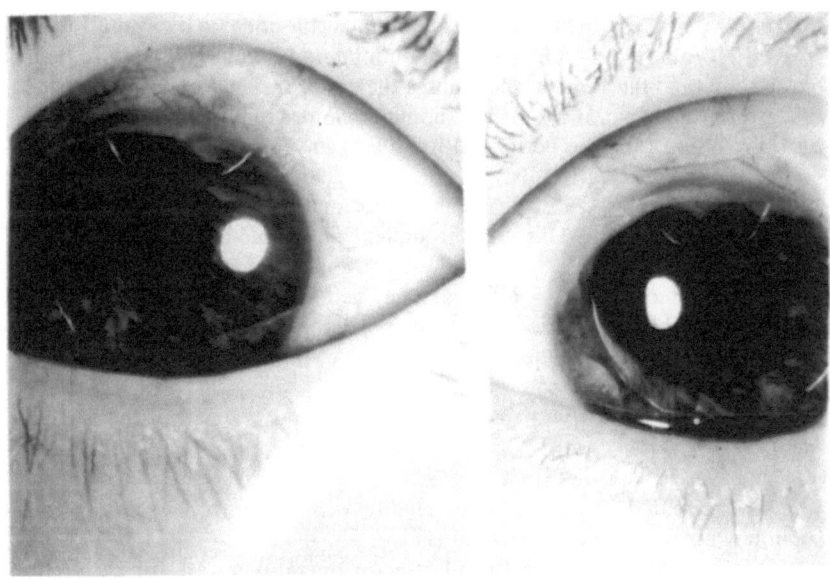

Fig. 20. Aphakic updrawn pupil following vitreous loss – (left) pre-operative; (right) post-operative appearance.

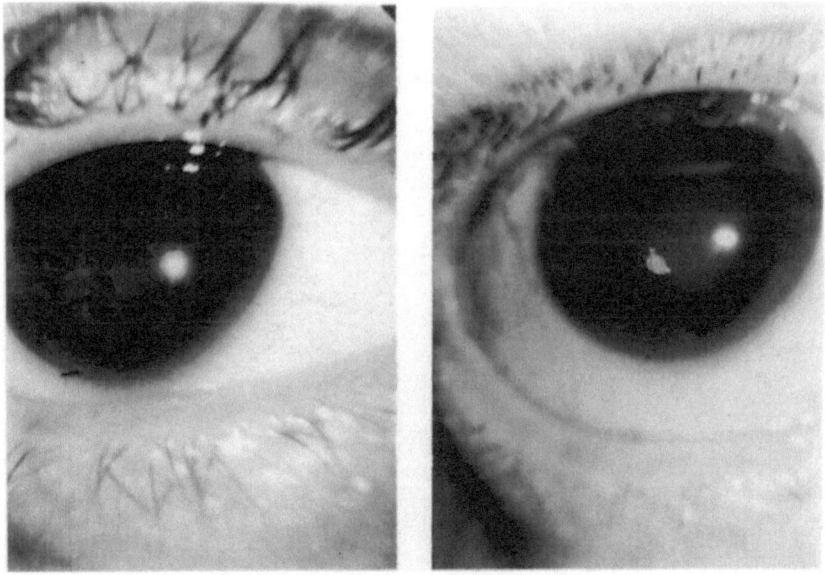

Fig. 21. Phacoemulsification after-cataract membrane – (left) red reflex; (right) post-operative Roto-Extraction red reflex.

tent impacts the iris tissue into the 0.4 mm. cutter opening by aspiration to create a 'Morning Glory' effect with only minimum vacuum necessary to hold onto the iris and the surgeon then pulses the cutter in the oscullatory cutting mode for a single cut of iris. There should be no residual vacuum pull on the iris, nor should there be peripheral iris tug or any tendency to wrapping or pulling that might create a dialysis.

Fig. 21 illustrates a post-phacoemulsification complication and the post-Roto-Extractor result. This patient underwent phaco-emulsification elsewhere with vitreous loss that required conversion and vitrectomy by the Weck sponge technique. An after-cataract membrane persisted which had a small central opening. The peripheral remaining capsule was opaque and precluded adequate visualization of an underlying bullous retinal detachment.

The Roto-Extractor was employed prior to surgical repair of the detachment.

There was 1 case of PHPV (Fig. 22) where an inadvertent sector iridectomy was created. This can occur readily with uncontrolled cutting and suction while working close to the iris.

5 of the 100 consecutive Roto-Extractor operations were for traumatic vitreous hemorrhage. 2 resulted from contusion alone; 1 was approached with vitrectomy alone and 1 with vitrectomy and lensectomy. 3 traumatic perforating cases produced vitreous hemorrhage. 2 cases of vitreous opacification and retinal detachment secondary to posterior uveitis were operated. There was 1 case of massive unabsorbed vitreous hemorrhage secondary to

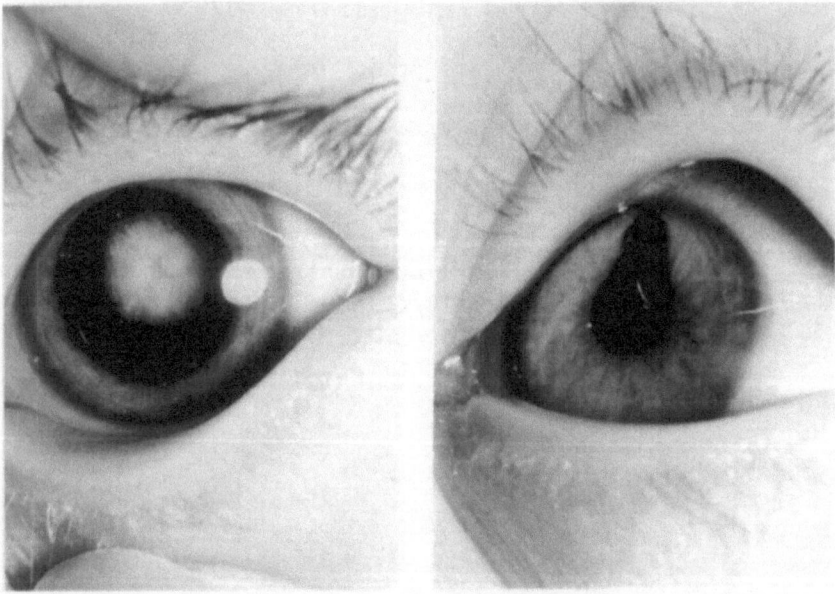

Fig. 22. Persistent hyperplastic primary vitreous 8 months old – (left): (right) post-operative appearance with inadvertent sector iridectomy.

hypertension and 2 secondary to branch vein occlusion. Diabetic unabsorbed vitreous hemorrhage, requiring only vitrectomy included 10 patients and
there were 24 additional diabetic cases of vitreous hemorrhage and cataract
requiring lensectomy and vitrectomy.

The next case illustrated is a diabetic, 30 years of age, who underwent an
unsuccesful vitrectomy in his right eye a year earlier which was subsequently enucleated because of hemorrhage and glaucoma. His left eye had
organized vitreous hemorrhage with good light projection in all quadrants. A
vitrectomy was performed and several layers of dense fibrous membranes
cut and removed. The smooth, blunt probe tip was then used to deflect the
fibrous tissue aside to visualize the underlying retinal attachments. Two
fibrous retinal attachments were noted and the fibrous band cut between
the two to isolate them. An attachment to the disc was then severed leaving
a 'Morning Glory' stalk emanating from the disc. Post-op result one year
later was 20/25. Fig. 23 shows the persistant fibrovascular stalk remnant
post-vitrectomy when visual acuity was 20/25.

Small vessels within fibrous retinitis proliferans can be severed and will
not bleed significantly. If bleeding occurs, it can be controlled by raising the
infusion pressure above the small capillary pressure so as to tamponade the
bleeder. That is the importance of the closed vitrectomy system, namely,
the ability to work in a pressurized eye. The goal in this type of surgery

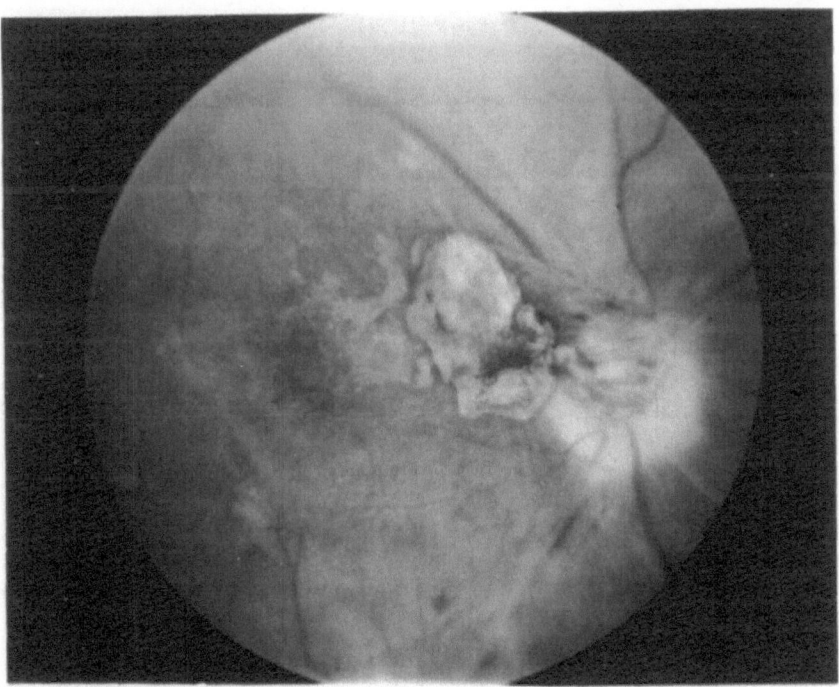

Fig. 23. Post-operative pars plana vitrectomy (20/25 visual acuity) with residual
fibrous retinitis proliferans stalk.

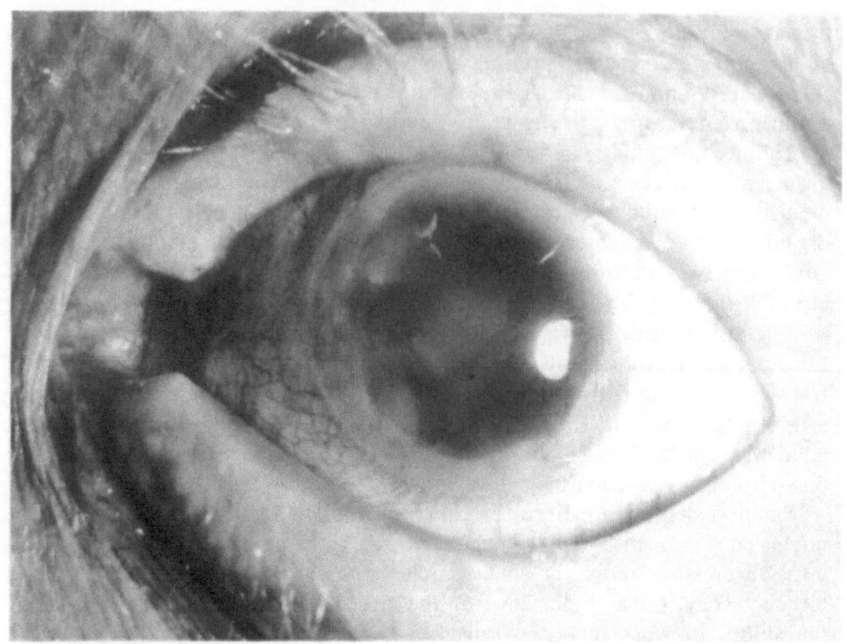

Fig. 24. Totally luxated 93 year old cataract with phacolytic glaucoma and early corneal decompensation with a posteriorly dislocated lens.

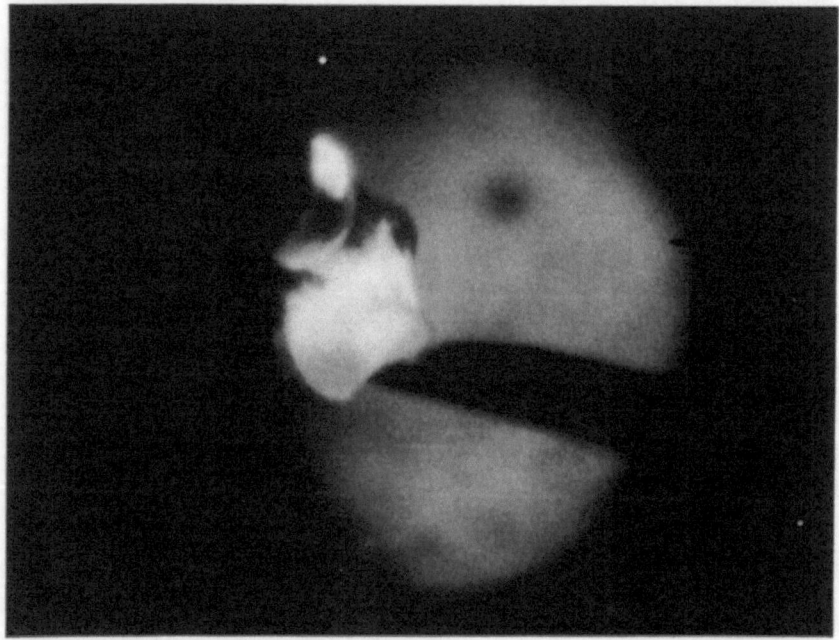

Fig. 25. Crushing luxated lens fragment within the mid-vitreous cavity between Roto-Extractor probe tip and a 21 gauge needle while packing lens into aspiration-cutting port.

where membranes are cut or peeled is to eliminate areas of two point traction that can give rise to subsequent shrinkage and detachment.

The next case is that of a 93 year old patient with a totally luxated lens following an attempted intracapsular cataract extraction with vitreous loss elsewhere. She had developed phacolytic glaucoma with a decompensated cornea (Fig. 24). A pars plana incision was made and cloudy opacified vitreous and lens cortex removed by the Roto-Extractor. An infusion Goldmann contact lens was then applied to the cornea to permit deeper visualization. Additional cortical material was removed down to the 93 year old rock hard nucleus, too hard to aspirate. A 21 gauge needle introduced through the opposite pars plana was used to crush the nucleus into the side cutter. Because of the long duty cycle and high speed cutting with minimal interruption of vacuum, we were able to retain this nucleus without dropping it in the mid-vitreous cavity. The crushed fragments were picked up from the retinal surface and packed into the aspiration opening where the cutter blade could engage them (Fig. 25). Ultimately, all lens material was removed from the eye. The decompensated cornea cleared, the glaucoma was cured and the vision was restored to this one-eyed patient. I have had occasion to utilize this crushing technique five times thus far. All have done well without complication except for one cutter which was ruined by sticking the needle tip into the cutter opening.

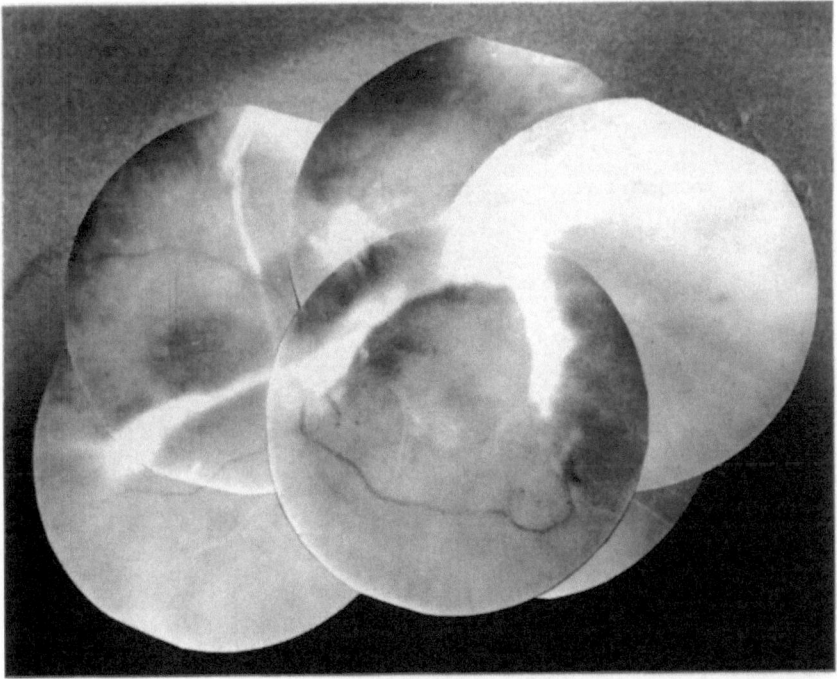

Fig. 26. Collage of a pre-operative diabetic retinitis proliferans with traction retinal detachment and a pre-retinal macular membrane or veil.

151

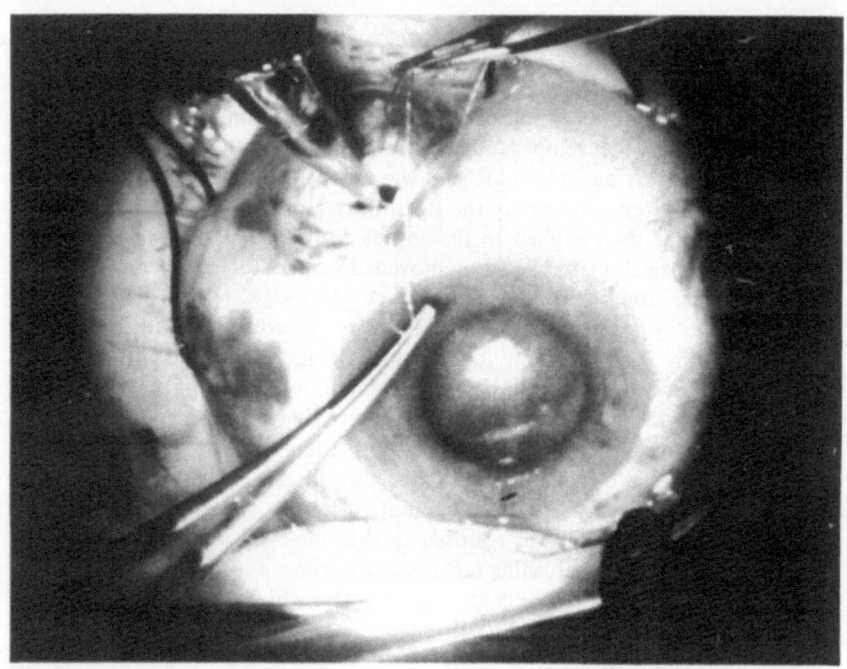

Fig. 27. Roto-Extractor trocar and cannula prepared for entry into sclerotomy wound everted by 7 '0' Vicryl safety suture loops.

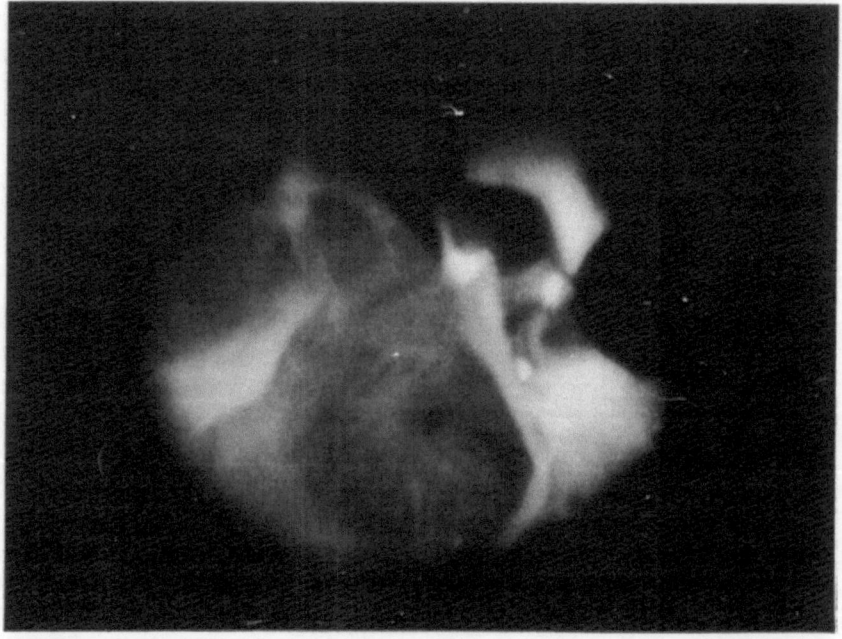

Fig. 28. Two instrument technique – 22 gauge hooked needle peeling pre-macular membrane or veil with Roto-Extractor feberoptic illumination.

The next case had a traction detachment due to a diabetic fibrous retinitis proliferans with pre-retinal membrane veiling the macula (Fig. 26). Two sclerotomy sites were prepared, one nasally and one temporally. The uvea within the sclerotomy was cauterized with a wet-field cautery to produce retraction and a Vanas scissors was used to enlarge and make certain the opening through the uvea was adequate. A dilating trocar and cannula (Fig. 27) prepared a pathway for the Roto-Extractor probe tip with the fiber-optic light pipe. The opacified vitreous was first removed anteriorly. A 22 gauge straight needle with a syringe on the barrel was then inserted through the superior-nasal pars plana to prepare a pathway for the hooked 22 gauge needle used for membrane peeling. The preretinal membrane was then hooked and peeled from the macula (Fig. 28) and the fibrous ring-like arcade fragmented and the material aspirated. This patient, ten days after surgery was able to read small newsprint with effort and the retina had flattened out (Fig. 29).

The visual results of these 100 cases are shown in Table II. These results show a fairly high success rate in diabetics. I should emphasize that I am very conservative and careful in case selection. Perhaps, I have been too conservative and should not have had this high success rate in this series.

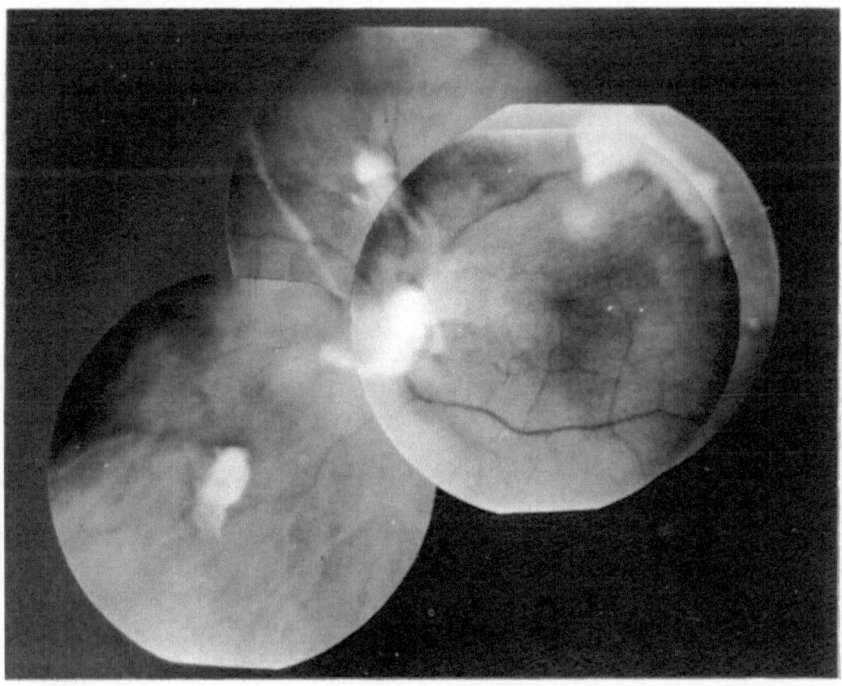

Fig. 29. Collage of a post-operative vitrectomy and membranectomy appearance (same patient as Fig. 25, 26 and 27).

TABLE II

VISUAL RESULTS
100 CONSECUTIVE ROTO-EXTRACTOR OPERATIONS WITH VITRECTOMY

		Improved	*Not-Improved*	*Worse*
1.	Congenital & Developmental Cataract	12	0	0
2.	Traumatic Cataract	14	3	0
3.	Cataracta Complicata – Uveitis	3	0	0
4.	Hyphema with Glaucoma	2	0	0
5.	Complications of Intracapsular Cataract	15	3	1
6.	Complications of Phaco-Emulsification	1	1	0
7.	P.H.P.V.	1	0	0
8.	Traumatic Massive Vitreous Hemorrhage	1	2	2
9.	Opaque Vitreous & Retinal Detachmant with Uveitis	2(1)*	0	0(1)*
10.	Vitreous Hemorrhage & Branch Vein Occlusion	2	0	0
11.	Hypertensive Vitreous Hemorrhage – P.P. Vit.	1	0	0
12.	Diabetic Vitreous Hemorrhage – P.P. Vit.	6	2	2
13.	Diabetic Vitreous Hemorrhage & Cataract	19	2	3

( )*	=	Late Failure
P.P.	=	pars plana
L.	=	lensectomy
V.	=	vitrectomy
P.H.P.V.	=	primary hyperplastic primary vitreous

REFERENCES

DOUVAS, N.G. Microsurgical Roto-Extractor instrument for vitrectomy. *Modern Problems in Ophthalmology* 15: *253-260* (1975). Karger Basel.
DOUVAS, N.G. The cataract Roto-Extractor. *Trans Am Acad Ophthalmol Otolargngol,* 77: *792-800* (1973).

Author's address:
Port Huron Eye clinic
1131 Erie Street at Pine Grove
Port Huron, Michigan. USA.

Note

The individual case examples and illustration presented in this paper were edited from movies shown at the conference. Those cases which seemed to best illustrate the Roto-Extractor techniques and results were selected.

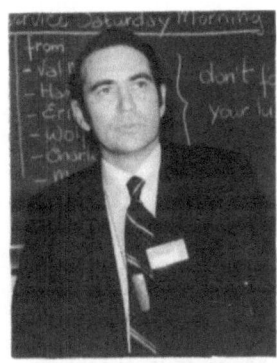

SOME OBSERVATIONS ON THE BLOOD-RETINAL BARRIERS IN HEALTH AND DISEASE

D.B. ARCHER

(Belfast, Northern Ireland)

ABSTRACT

The retinal pigment epithelium and the endothelial cells of the retinal vessels constitute two important cellular barriers which control the movement of substances and fluid into the retina. Both cellular layers may further influence the internal environment of the retina by actively transporting organic anions and fluid out of the retina. Functional failure of either layer results in intraretinal accumulation of fluid.

The retinal endothelial cells form a particularly resilient barrier, withstanding a wide variety of stresses without loss of integrity. They are, however, vulnerable to acute stretching or prolonged ischaemia. The retinal endothelial cells are also susceptible to inflammation, products of inflammation and certain chemicals, particularly in the presence of ischaemia. The barrier function also fails when the endothelial cells are the site of developmental abnormalities or degenerative processes.

The retinal pigment epithelium also provides an effective tissue barrier which can maintain its integrity despite significant alterations to its structure and function. Decompensation may, however, follow acute inflammation, oedema and necrosis of the pigment epithelium, or extensive choroidal ischaemia. Severe mechanical and metabolic compromise may also lead to loss of integrity, particularly in association with choroidal neovascularisation.

The active transport properties of the retinal pigment epithelium and retinal endothelial cells are ill-understood, but failure of such mechanisms could theoretically lead to the formation of retinal oedema in the presence of clinically normal barrier functions.

INTRODUCTION

The movement of fluid into and out of the retina appears to be controlled largely by two semipermeable membranes, the retinal pigment epithelium and the endothelium of the retinal vasculature (blood-retinal barrier). The contiguous cells of each membrane are fused together at specialised junctions (zonulae occludentes) which completely seal the intercellular spaces. Recent studies indicate that the endothelial cells of the retinal vessels may possess an additional regulatory mechanism with the ability to transport actively organic anions and fluid from the retinal parenchyma into the retinal vessels (CUNHA-VAZ & MAURICE, 1967). Thus the endothelial cells not only help to maintain optimum hydration of the retina, but probably provide a pathway for the removal of noxious and unwanted substances from the retina into the general circulation. A similar function has also been suggested for the retinal pigment epithelium, fluid being transported from the retina into the extravascular space of the choriocapillaris. Significant failure of either barrier results in intraretinal accumulation of fluid. In most instances of retinal oedema only one barrier is affected and the accumulation of fluid occurs at the site of decompensation; however, extensive or prolonged failure of either barrier may result in oedema of all layers. In certain clinical situations, particularly those characterised by severe ocular ischaemia, both barriers may be concurrently breached.

Mechanisms and proposed mechanisms of retinal oedema

I.   Retinal vascular endothelium malfunction − a barrier failure

The blood retinal barrier is remarkably resistent to changes in local environment (limited degrees of ischaemia-hypoxia) (CUNHA-VAZ 1966) and a wide variety of stresses (histamine, hypotonic and hypertonic solutions) (ASHTON & CUNHA-VAZ, 1965). However, five major sets of circumstances acting singly or in concert result in loss of vascular integrity. These are (a) acute distention of the vessel wall, (b) ischaemia, (c) certain chemical influences, (d) inflammation, and (e) defective endothelial cells.

(a) Acute distention and stretching of the vessel wall (acute retinal vein obstruction-occlusion): The retinal vessels can tolerate considerable traction and displacement without any observable ill effects on their barrier function. This is evident in severe preretinal macular fibrosis, where gross distortion of the normal vascular pattern may occur without any associated macular oedema or loss of endothelial integrity as judged by fluorescein angio-

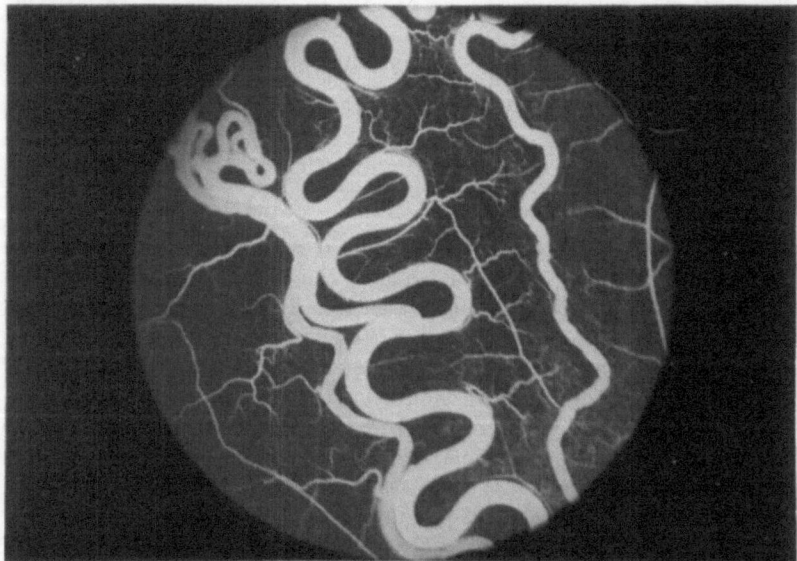

Fig. 1.   Late venous phase fluorescein angiogram of patient with large arteriovenous communication situated in the right superior fundus. The affected arteries, veins and intervening capillary network remain competent to dye despite gross alteration in calibre.

graphy. The retinal vasculature can also withstand moderate degrees of vaso-dilatation without observable alteration in barrier function, e.g., following paracentesis, or reactive hyperaemia induced by suction cup ophthalmo-dynamometry. Remarkable increases in vascular calibre can also occur without loss of integrity providing the changes occur slowly, permitting compensatory changes to occur in the endothelium. This is particularly striking in arteriovenous communications of the retina where arteries, veins and capillaries may reach alarming dimensions without producing any observable alteration in their barrier function (ARCHER et al, 1973) (Fig. 1).

Acute distention produced by sudden venous obstruction or occlusion, however, leads to immediate and widespread decompensation of the blood-retinal barrier with intraretinal oedema. Loss of integrity is most marked at the terminal venules which are particularly vulnerable to sudden rises in intraluminar pressure due to their relatively thin walls and large lumens (Fig. 2). The endothelial cells become attenuated and may demonstrate breaks in the internal plasma membrane. Plasma insudation into the vessel wall or beyond the capillary lumen may occur. In most instances the junctional complexes remain intact.

Two further factors also operate in acute vein obstruction or occlusion, namely, a high hydrostatic or intraluminar pressure and hypoxia consequent upon venous stasis. The contribution of either of these factors to the immediate decompensation of the blood-retinal barrier is probably less important than acute distension of the vessel wall. The retinal microvasculature and venous tributaries appear to tolerate and adjust to high levels of intraluminar pressure, e.g., the increase in venous pressure produced by suction

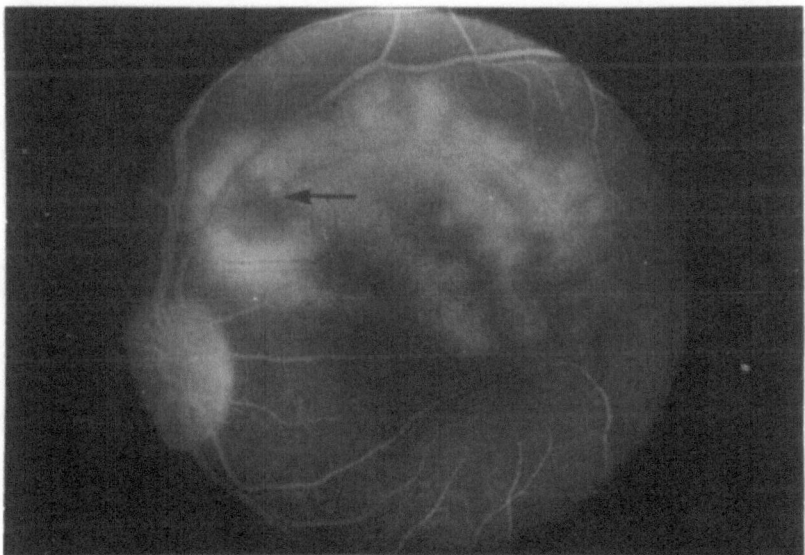

Fig. 2. Late phase fluorescein angiogram of Rhesus monkey fundus immediately following photocoagulation of the left supero-temporal macular vein (arrow). There is widespread extravasation of dye into the retina in the territory of the obstructed vein.

cup ophthalmodynamometry has little immediate effect on vascular competence. Similarly, direct arteriovenous shunts, where the venous circulation is subjected to arterial perfusion pressure, produce no observable loss of integrity.

The retinal endothelium is relatively insensitive (compared with nervous tissue) to *short periods* of anoxia or hypoxia. In various experimental animals the maintenance of endothelial structure and functions has been documented up to and beyond one hour of complete ischaemia; therefore, it would appear that in the acute vein obstruction the initial mechanism of macular oedema is due to sudden and marked stretching of the vessel walls. The endothelial changes that follow acute venous distention are reversible, and once the high intraluminar pressure has been relieved by the formation of collaterals, the microvasculature returns to normal or nearly normal calibre and regains its integrity (Fig. 3). The enlarged collateral vessels remain dilated for long periods of time, although they also retain their barrier competence due to the restructuring and rearrangement of their endothelial cells. Therefore, although acute distension of the retinal vasculature is of prime importance in the disturbance of endothelial function immediately following a venous occlusion it becomes less critical with the passage of time.

(b) Ischaemia – hypoxia, anoxia: Although the retinal vasculature can survive and recover from short periods of complete anoxia, ischaemia still remains the most potent cause of persistent failure of the blood-retinal barrier. The extensive oedema and haemorrhage commonly associated with

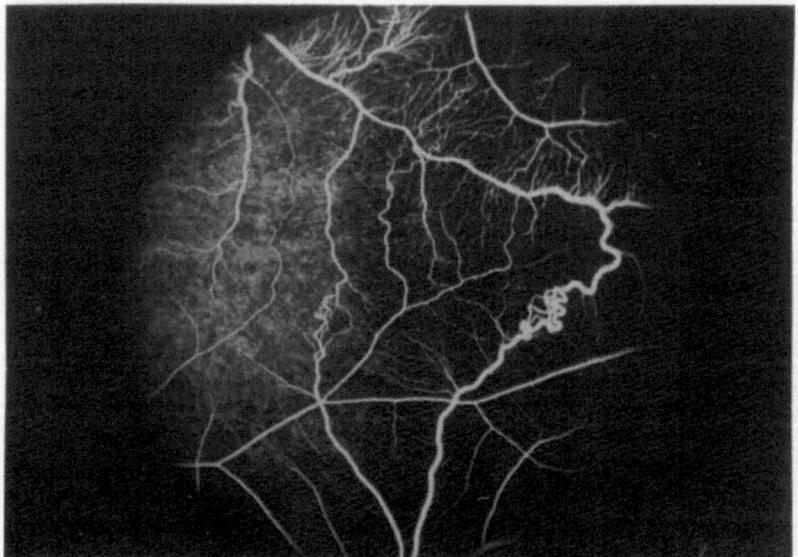

Fig. 3. Late phase fluorescein angiogram of Rhesus monkey fundus, several months following occlusion of a major branch retinal vein. Wellformed collaterals and capillaries within the distribution of the obstructed vein remain competent to dye.

a branch vein obstruction or occlusion probably represents the cumulative effects of hypoxia on the retinal endothelium, producing a complete breakdown in the blood retinal barrier. In the experimental animal these changes do not occur until 12-24 hours following the acute obstruction which is probably the length of time required for degenerative changes to occur in the endothelial cells (Fig. 4). Capillary collaterals are generally well developed within the first few hours following the acute obstruction so that it is unlikely that venous distension or high intraluminar pressure is a significant factor in the later breakdown of the blood retinal barrier.

Providing the degree of hypoxia is not excessive or prolonged the involved microvasculature has considerable powers of recuperation. Thus in many vein obstructions, particularly those of small order, the microvasculature demonstrates good recovery of function, even though the capillaries remain dilated and display structural abnormalities such as microaneurysms. Such recovery occurs in a significant number of branch retinal vein obstructions and should not be impeded by photocoagulation in the early stages of the disease. More intense ischaemia and prolonged hypoxia results in a permanent breakdown of the blood retinal barrier with persistent accumulation of fluid in the retina. Generally, once loss of capillary integrity has become established spontaneous recovery of function does not occur. Whether capillary function can be improved in such instances by reducing the amount of hypoxic retina using photocoagulation remains to be seen.

Acute retinal arterial obstruction produces a much more rapid breakdown in the blood-retinal barrier compared with chronic vein occlusion; however, because most arterial obstructions are incomplete the breakdown

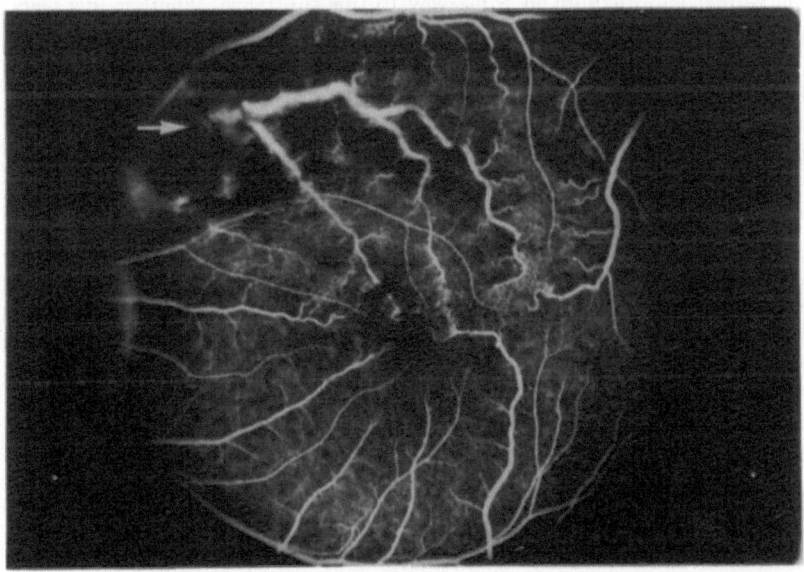

Fig. 4. Late phase fluorescein angiogram of Rhesus monkey fundus, several hours following occlusion of the supero-temporal macular vein by photocoagulation (arrow). There is extensive haemorrhage along the course of the obstructed vein.

159

is often delayed and mild. Severe ischaemia following an arterial occlusion precipitates an acute loss of integrity of the blood-retinal barrier, particularly on the arterial side of the circulation. Eventually all modalities of the retinal vasculature are implicated. The posterior pole of the eye, and particularly the macular area, are especially vulnerable.

(c) Chemically mediated influences: The retinal vascular endothelium in health can tolerate some remarkable chemical insults including hypertonic solutions and histamine. No biochemical substances elaborated by body tissues have thus far been shown to have a significant effect on the blood retinal barrier. Recently it has been shown that some of the prostaglandins have a significant action on certain ocular blood vessels, particularly in disrupting the blood aqueous barrier. Prostaglandins are also known to be present in most tissues in small amounts and in the fluids of chronic ocular inflammation. Therefore, it is not unreasonable to postulate that such a substance might be involved in or mediate some of the adverse reactions affecting the blood retinal barrier in disease. To explore this possibility the retinal vasculature of the Rhesus monkey was exposed to exogenous Prostaglandin E. (P.G.E.1) in varying concentrations via the carotid circulation. The results were negative, with high concentrations of P.G.E.1 in phosphate/alcohol buffer producing no untoward effect on the retinal vasculature as evaluated by fluorescein angiography. However, when P.G.E.1 was administered following an initial period of retinal ischaemia, there was a dramatic and extensive breakdown of the blood retinal barrier. Thus it would appear that although the retinal endothelial cells maintain their barrier function to prostaglandin in health, short periods of ischaemia sensitise the retinal endothelium in some way to this substance. Whether this reaction is specific for prostaglandin is not known.

(d) Inflammation: The blood retinal barrier is susceptible to a variety of inflammatory processes. The vessels may be affected by the actions of toxins or inflammatory products liberated from adjacent or remote foci of infection or inflammation, or by the implication of the vessel wall in the disease process itself (retinal vasculitis).

Active foci of toxoplasmosis retinitis may cause a remote retinal vasculitis due to the accumulation of inflammatory products about the vessel walls. The veins are predominantly affected although the arteries may also be involved. Fluorescein angiography in such instances demonstrates both staining of the endothelial cells and extravasation of dye into the adjoining retina. These changes are reversible following resolution of the inflammatory process. The peripheral retinal vessels may also be the site of acute inflammatory changes, particularly in pars planitis, where long segments of involved vessels become infiltrated with inflammatory cells. Fluorescein angiography indicates that these vessels are incompetent (PRUETT et al, 1974).

(e) Defective endothelial cells: The endothelial cells may be abnormal, either due to developmental defects such as Leber's miliary aneurysms and Coats's disease, or secondary to degenerative processes such as diabetes,

hypertension or sickle cell disease.

In some of the developmental disorders the retinal capillaries remain competent despite obvious structural changes until relatively late in the disease process. Eventually, however, decompensation occurs with the formation of retinal oedema, cystoid degenerative changes and, occasionally, retinal detachment. Of special interest in this group is the association of peripheral telangiectatic lesions with macular oedema and scarring despite the presence of clinically normal intervening retina. The mechanism of this remote effect is not known; however, ablation of the abnormal vessels often results in resolution of the macular oedema.

In severe diabetic retinopathy there is a generalised breakdown in the blood retinal barrier associated with numerous structural abnormalities of the microvasculature, including dilatation, fusion, collapse and closure of capillaries and the presence of multiple microaneurysms. These vessels are incompetent and profusely leak fluorescein during angiography. The aetiology of these capillary changes is not known; however, marked and consistent basement membrane changes have been demonstrated in the precapillary arterioles, and it may be that the abnormal vascular permeability is secondary to ischaemia (ASHTON, 1974). Such ischaemia would also render the vascular endothelium vulnerable to any coexisting metabolic abnormality.

II. Malfunction of the retinal vascular endothelium — pump failure

(a) Defective endothelial cells: CUNHA–VAZ & MAURICE (1967) have demonstrated that the retinal capillaries can actively transport organic anions out of the vitreous body into the retinal circulation. They also showed that when fluorescein was injected into the vitreous body it passed out across the entire retinal surface even against a high concentration gradient. Occluding the retinal vessels by diathermy or blocking endothelial activity by a variety of metabolic and competitive inhibitors abolished this unidirectional movement of fluorescein across the retina (CUNHA-VAZ & MAURICE, 1967). It is, therefore, possible that some varieties of macular oedema represent failure of this active transport mechanism by the endothelial cells. Prolonged elevation of the intraocular pressure in monkey eyes has been noted to produce macular oedema in the absence of significant decompensation of the blood retinal barrier as gauged by fluorescein angiography. Subtle macular oedema has also been noted in aphakic patients treated with epinephrine without any evidence of vascular decompensation (KOLKER & BECKER, 1968). The explanation for these findings is not yet immediately apparent. It may be that the pump mechanism of the endothelial cells of the retinal microvasculature is compromised whilst the barrier mechanism remains intact.

(b) Saturation of normal pump mechanism: Alternatively any condition that accelerates or facilitates the excessive movement of fluid into the retina, for example, from the vitreous or region of the optic nerve head, might also produce retinal oedema in the face of a normally functioning retinal vascular endothelium. Perhaps the macular oedema associated with

aphakia, pars planitis, pre-macular fibrosis or pits of the optic nerve head might be produced in part by such a mechanism.

III. Retinal pigment epithelium – barrier failure

The retinal pigment epithelium provides an effective tissue barrier against substances diffusing from the choroid via the fenestrated capillaries of that tissue. It has been demonstrated that the pigment epithelial cell and its tight junctions constitute a very selective semipermeable membrane resistant to even horseradish peroxidase (PEYMAN et al, 1971) and sodium fluorescein (GRAYSON & LATIES, 1971). Clinically, the extravasation of fluorescein in observable quantities does not occur from the choriocapillaris into the outer retina. Further evidence that the retinal pigment epithelium and its tight junctions constitute a rugged and persistent barrier is shown by the maintenance of its integrity in a number of pathological situations where considerable changes in its alignment, metabolism and structure occur.

(a) Lack of support – Discontinuity of Bruch's membrane (angioid streaks, choroidal tears, myopic lacquer cracks): The pigment epithelium can function adequately as a barrier despite the localised absence of Bruch's membrane. In angioid streaks, many of the large dehiscences in Bruch's membrane persist throughout life without any evidence of pigment epithelial incompetence or the accumulation of fluid in the subretinal space. The barrier generally fails only when the breaks are complicated by choroidal neovascularisation.

(b) Folds of retinal pigment epithelium: Alterations in the alignment of the retinal pigment epithelium, as occur in choroidal folds, rarely have any effect upon its competence. The alterations in fluorescent patterns merely reflect changes in alignment and density of pigment within the individual pigment epithelial cells. However, occasionally some degenerative changes may occur, observed as staining of the involved pigment epithelial cells during fluorescein angiography.

(c) Displacement (drusen) and detachment: Displacement of the pigment epithelium by drusen material or small serous detachments may also occur without appreciable disturbance in barrier function.

(d) Structural alterations: The pigment epithelium can withstand considerable structural insults without serious impairment of its barrier properties. Thus, in rubella and chloroquin retinopathies, despite marked alterations in pigment content and configuration and severe impairment of some physiological functions, there is little apparent effect on fluid transport at the outer retina.

(e) Accumulation of abnormal substances: The accumulation of abnormal substances within the retinal pigment epithelial cell as occurs in fundus flavimaculatus likewise seems to have little effect on the overall barrier integrity of the retinal pigment epithelium. In some instances, however,

degenerative changes do occur and staining of such cells is evident on fluo-rescein angiography.

Decompensation of the retinal pigment epithelial barrier does, however, occur in certain circumstances:
1. Extensive and severe choroidal ischaemia
2. Mechanical and metabolic compromise particularly when associated with choroidal neovascularisation
3. Acute inflammation, oedema or necrosis of the pigment epithelium.

1. Choroidal ischaemia: The retinal pigment epithelium and outer retina receive a high blood flow by means of an intricate and complex system of choroidal arteries. The blood is delivered to the choriocapillaris directly by means of large calibre arterioles, which maintain a high perfusion pressure down to a capillary level. The choroidal vasculature is also characterised by intervenular anastomoses which can circumvent most small choroidal artery obstructions. Thus it is not surprising that the retinal pigment epithelium functions exceptionally well despite considerable disease of the choroidal vasculature. In most clinical situations where segmental choroidal stasis is identified by fluorescein angiography it is unusual to detect any significant malfunction of the retinal pigment epithelium barrier or extravasation of dye into the sub-retinal space.

In the experimental animal severe choroidal stasis can be produced by occlusion of a major short posterior ciliary artery. When the lateral short posterior ciliary vessel is ligated, the choroidal circulation to the temporal

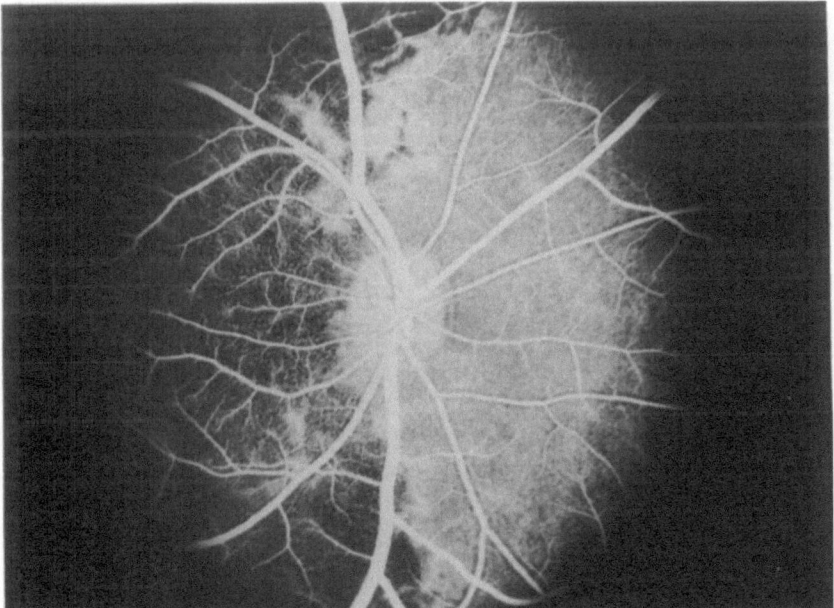

Fig. 5. Late venous phase fluorescein angiogram of Rhesus monkey fundus, taken 6 hours after ligation of right lateral posterior ciliary artery. There is marked delay in filling of the choriocapillaris temporal to the optic disc.

fundus is grossly impaired, although some flow is maintained by various communicating channels from the episcleral venous plexuses, the peripapillary vessels and venae vorticosae (HAYREH & BAINES, 1972) (Figs. 5 & 6). Nevertheless, despite this gross stasis the pigment epithelium maintains its barrier function as determined by angiography, at least for several hours. ERNEST and co-workers used an oxygen microelectrode, advanced some 200 microns into the retina to determine oxygen tension in the choroidal circulation of the macula. They found that following occlusion of the lateral short posterior ciliary artery, there was an immediate reduction in oxygen tension at the macula to about 1/3 of that measured in the normal nasal choroidal circulation (ERNEST et al, 1976). This finding further emphasises the resilience of the retinal pigment epithelium and its ability to withstand substantial hypoxia, at least for limited periods of time with the maintenance of a functional barrier.

When choroidal ischaemia is prolonged, areas of acute pigment epithelial necrosis develop, particularly at threshold zones of the collateral circulation. This is appreciated as discrete areas of retinal pigment epithelial oedema, and fluorescein angiography demonstrates complete breaching of the pigment epithelial barrier with extravasation of dye into the outer retina (Fig. 7). Histological sections of such areas demonstrate marked swelling and the formation of vacuoles in the pigment epithelium and accumulation of fluid in the sub-retinal space.

Individual units of the choriocapillaris can be obstructed by injecting small plastic microspheres into the choroidal circulation (STERN & ER-

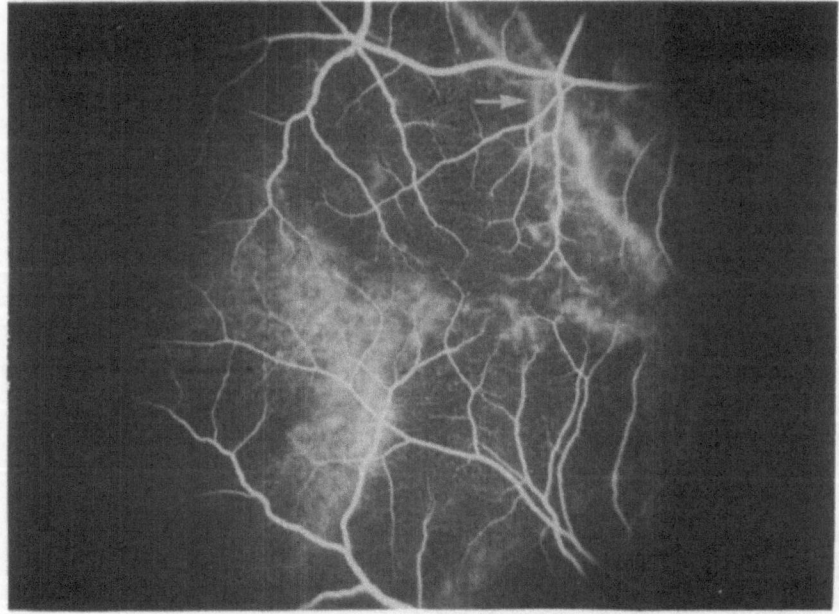

Fig. 6.   Late venous phase angiogram of temporal fundus of Rhesus monkey, following ligation of right lateral posterior ciliary artery. Large venous collaterals (arrow) divert blood to the ischaemic choriocapillaris.

NEST, 1974). This produces a similar acute ischaemia of the retinal pigment epithelium with loss of integrity of the retinal pigment epithelial barrier. Fluorescein angiography in such cases demonstrates extravasation of dye into the outer retina at sites of occlusions.

Acute ischaemia of the retinal pigment epithelium can be also observed in a number of clinical situations, e.g., acute disseminated intravascular coagulopathy and advanced temporal arteritis. Acute disseminated intravascular coagulopathy is characterised by widespread deposition of fibrin and platelet clots in small blood vessels. The choriocapillaris may be implicated with vacuolisation and disruption of the overlying pigment epithelium, leading to a localised serous detachment of the retina. The macula is particularly susceptible in this condition due to the sudden deceleration in flow that occurs as the posterior ciliary vessels rapidly unload their blood into the choriocapillary vasculature. This sudden stasis favours the local precipitation of clots in this hypercoaguable circulatory system (COGAN, 1975).

In advanced temporal arteritis, focal areas of choriocapillaris closure may be identified with necrosis of the overlying pigment epithelium (Fig. 8). Fluorescein angiography demonstrates extravasation of dye across the retinal pigment epithelium into the sub-retinal space.

2. Mechanical and metabolic compromise: Persistent detachment of the retinal pigment epithelium or the development of choroidal neovascularisation frequently breaches the retinal pigment epithelial barrier and leads to

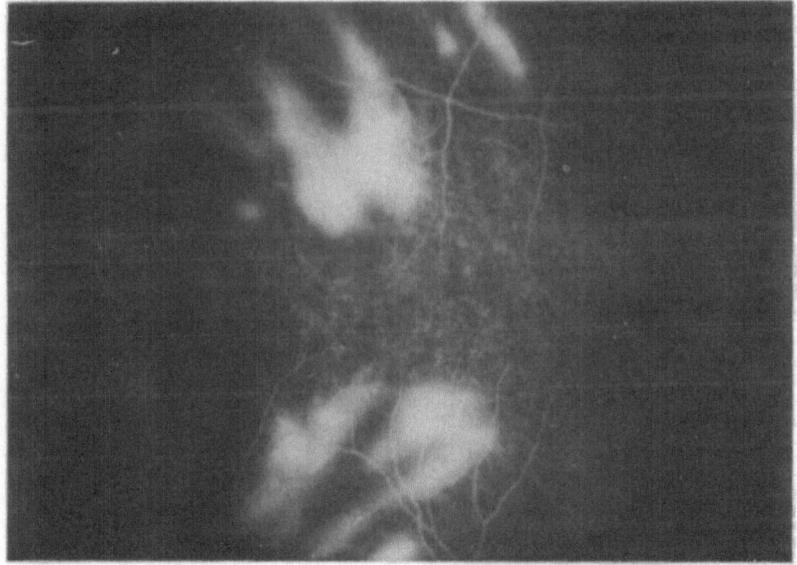

Fig. 7. Late phase angiogram of temporal fundus of Rhesus monkey, several days following ligation of lateral short posterior ciliary artery. Hyperfluorescent areas demonstrate sites of retinal pigment epithelial degeneration, with extravasation of dye into the outer retina.

the accumulation of fluid in the sub-retinal space. The precise factors which cause separation of the retinal pigment epithelium from Bruch's membrane or stimulate the ingrowth of choroidal vessels into the sub-pigment epithelial region are not known. It is probably a combination of mechanical factors such as microruptures of Bruch's membrane, metabolic factors resulting from the accumulation of substances within the sub-pigment epithelial space and some degree of local hypoxia.

3. Acute inflammation, oedema or necrosis of the pigment epithelium: The retinal pigment epithelial barrier may be breached by a number of conditions which lead to acute oedema, inflammation or necrosis of the retinal pigment epithelium, e.g., acute posterior multifocal placoid pigment epitheliopathy. Whether such acute oedema is the result of inflammation, virus infiltration, or a vasculitis of the choriocapillaris is not known. In any event, the pigment epithelium becomes acutely oedematous and loses its ability to function as a barrier to some degree. This loss of barrier integrity is usually only for a short time and complete recovery is the rule. Persistent defects of pigmentation, however, produce a hyperfluorescent pattern on fluorescein angiography.

4. Retinal pigment epithelium – pump failure: There is some evidence to indicate that the retinal pigment epithelium is capable of removing fluid and certain organic anions from the retina against a concentration gradient

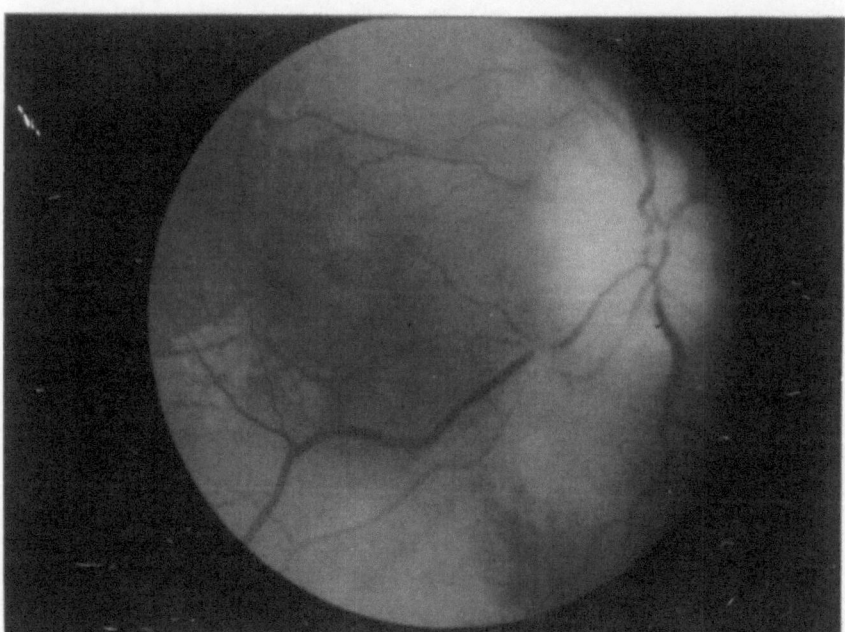

Fig. 8. Fundus photograph of patient with advanced temporal arteritis. Discrete areas of acute pigment epithelial necrosis are present inferotemporal to the right macula. The right optic disc demonstrates an acute ischaemic optic neuropathy.

(CUNHA-VAZ & MAURICE 1967). The part that such a mechanism plays in the formation of macular oedema is not known at this time. It is significant, however, that the inhibition of this pump mechanism of the retinal vasculature and pigment epithelium in the experimental animal results in detachment of the retina (CUNHA-VAZ & MAURICE, 1967).

REFERENCES

ARCHER, D.B., DEUTMAN, A.F., ERNEST, J.T. & KRILL, A.E. Arteriovenous communications of the retina. *Amer. J. Ophthal.* 75: *224-241* (1973).

ASHTON, N. Vascular basement membrane in diabetic retinopathy. *Brit. J. Ophthal.* 58: *344-366* (1974).

ASHTON, N. & CUNHA-VAZ, J.G. Effect of histamine on the permeability of the ocular vessels. *Arch. Ophthal.* 73: *211-223* (1965).

COGAN, D.G. Ocular involvement in disseminated intravascular coagulopathy. *Arch. Ophthal.* 93: *1-8* (1975).

CUNHA-VAZ, J.G. Studies of the permeability of the blood retinal barrier. III. Breakdown of the blood retinal barrier by circulatory disturbances. *Brit. J. Ophthal.* 50: *505-516* (1966).

CUNHA-VAZ, J.G. & MAURICE, D.M. The active transport of fluorescein by the retinal vessels and the retina. *J. Physiol.* 191: *467-486* (1967).

ERNEST, J.T., STERN, W.H. & ARCHER, D.B. Submacular choroidal circulation. *Amer. J. Ophthal.* (in press).

GRAYSON, M.C. & LATIES, A.M. Ocular localization of sodium fluorescein. *Arch. Ophthal.* 85: *600-609* (1971).

HAYREH, S.S. & BAINES, J.A.B. Occlusion of the posterior ciliary artery. I. Effects on choroidal circulation. *Brit. J. Ophthal.* 56: *719-735* (1972).

KOLKER, A.E. & BECKER, B. Epinephrine maculopathy. *Arch. Ophthal.* 79: *552-562* (1968).

PEYMAN, G.A., SPITZNAS, M. & STRAATSMA, B.R. Peroxidase diffusion in the normal and photocoagulated retina. *Invest. Ophthal.* 10: *181-189* (1971).

PRUETT, R.C., BROCKHURST, R.J. & LETTS, N.F. Fluorescein angiography of peripheral uveitis. *Amer. J. Ophthal.* 77: *448-453* (1974).

STERN, W.H. & ERNEST, J.T. Microsphere occlusion of the choriocapillaris in Rhesus monkeys. *Amer. J. Ophthal.* 78: *438-448* (1974).

Author's address:
Department of Ophthalmology
Eye and Ear Clinic
Royal Victoria Hospital
Belfast, Northern Ireland

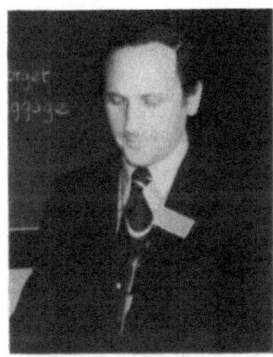

THE MANAGEMENT OF THE VASCULAR RETINOPATHIES

R.K. BLACH

(London, England)

The first classification of the vascular retinopathies was given by DESMAR-RES in 1858. He described the retinopathy of Glycosuria, Albuminuria and Spermatorrhoea. Today we include:
1) Retrolental fibroplasia,
2) Sickle cell retinopathy,
3) Venous retinopathy,
4) The retinopathies associated with hyperviscosity,
5) Diabetic retinopathy,
6) Hypertensive retinopathy and the collagenoses,
7) The predominantly ischaemic retinopathies.

It has been suggested that the common factor in all these retinopathies is vascular occlusion (BLACH, 1974). Certainly, they all share clinical features in common although the distribution and development of these features are characteristic of each individual retinopathy.

There are two basic types of response to vascular occlusion in the retina; (1) abnormal vascular permeability and, (2) ischaemia.

The abnormal vascular permeability response is seen on fluorescein angiography as leaking dilated capillaries (Fig. 1) and gives rise, ophthalmoscopically, to retinal haemorrhages, hard exudates and retinal oedema.

The ischaemic response is represented on fluorescein angiography by areas of capillary nonperfusion (Fig. 2). Under these circumstances, the retina is ischaemic but not anoxic, because the retina still receives a part of its blood supply from the choroid and the vascular occlusion is seldom complete. As a response to the retinal ischaemia, especially if it is peripheral, neovascularization occurs and this in turn can give rise to haemorrhage, fibrosis, vitreous detachment and retinal traction, the so called ischaemic response.

The picture of any individual retinopathy depends, by and large, on the balance of the abnormal permeability response and the ischaemic response (Fig. 3).

A wide variety of therapies are available for the vascular retinopathies. Some have proved their worth, others are under trial and yet others are merely speculative. We may broadly classify the therapies into those concerned with:
1) prophylaxis,
2) treatment of the cause,

3) treatment of the condition,
4) the management of complications.

We shall choose examples of the various retinopathies under these headings to illustrate practical clinical problems, but special emphasis will be given to photocoagulation.

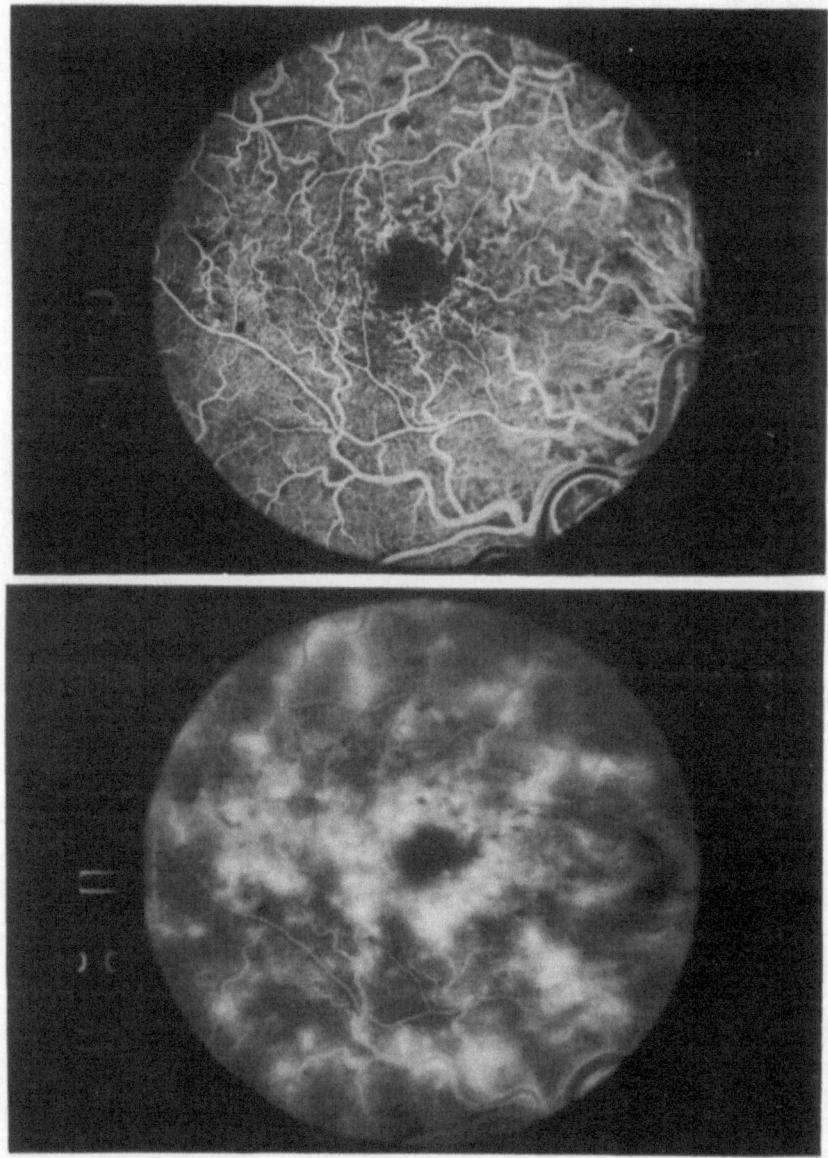

Fig. 1. a & b. Fluorescein angiograms showing capillary dilatation giving rise to the abnormal permeability response in a case of retinal vein occlusion.

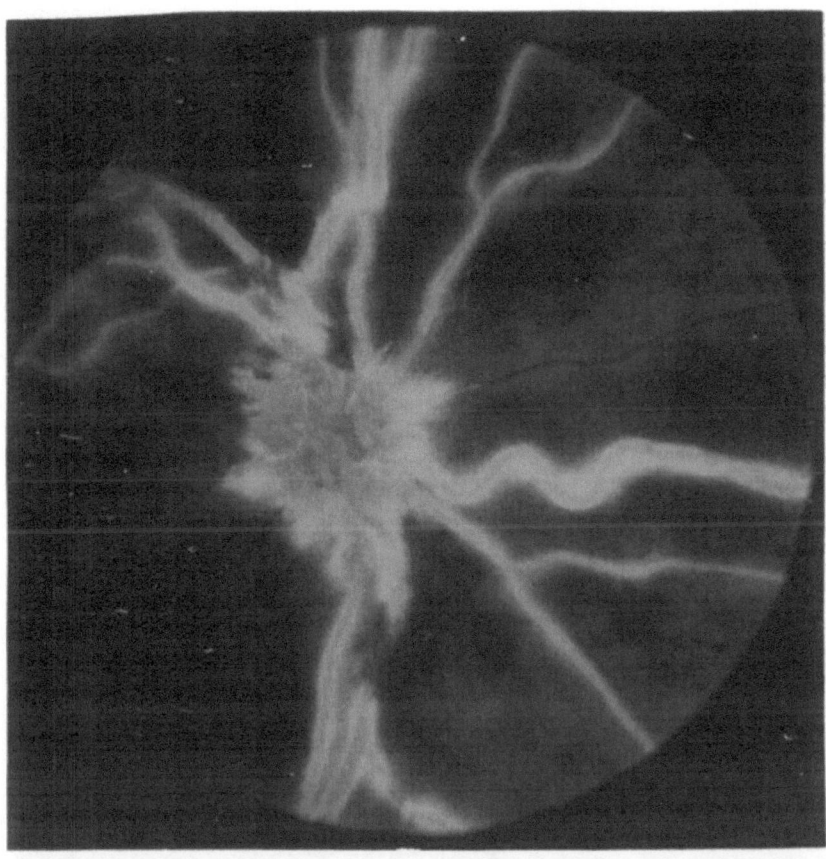

Fig. 2. Fluorescein angiogram showing capillary non-perfusion giving rise to the ischaemic response in a case of retinal vein occlusion.

1. PROPHYLAXIS

Prophylaxis is important in a number of retinopathies such as radiation retinopathy. However, the most controversial aspect of prophylaxis, as far as the ophthalmologist goes, concerns retrolental fibroplasia (TIZARD, 1971). The development of retrolental fibroplasia is stimulated not by the high environmental oxygen concentration of the baby, but by a high arterial oxygen tension. Certainly, premature babies do not need oxygen routinely and the oxygen that is given for birth asphyxia is so transient as to be unimportant. However, in babies that have the respiratory distress syndrome (hyaline membrane disease) and that suffer from recurrent apnoeic attacks, oxygen may be required. Arterial blood pO2 (from the umbilical artery) should be monitored, aiming to have the arterial oxygen tension between 60 and 90 mmHg, never above 160 mmHg. It is not known what is a safe level of arterial oxygen for the premature infant. This depends upon the degree of immaturity of the retinal vessels and on the duration of exposure to these

171

levels. The intra-uterine arterial pO2 of the foetus is only between 30 and 40 mmHg and this may be raised to 75 mmHg when he breathes air. Forty per cent ambient oxygen in the air may therefore not be safe, but under other circumstances a 100% oxygen in the environment may fail to raise the arterial oxygen tension in the baby to reasonable levels. The danger of very high environmental oxygen is the sudden recovery of the baby such as occurs in recurrent apnoeic attacks, and therefore continuous monitoring of pO2 would be ideal. Giving oxygen therapy, therefore, to premature babies always involves a calculated risk between the effects of giving the baby too much oxygen and too little. Ophthalmological changes cannot be observed until some time after the cessation of oxygen therapy so that the role of the ophthalmologist in the premature baby unit is limited. Nevertheless, he should be in a position to give informed advice to the paediatrician (MUSHIN, 1974).

2. TREATMENT OF THE CAUSE

The second method of treating a vascular retinopathy is treating its cause. The hypertensive retinopathies are the least controversial of this group. However, we shall briefly consider the problem of the retinopathy associated with central retinal vein occlusion as a great deal has been written on this. Three forms of treatment have been considered for retinal vein occlusion in terms of its cause:
1) anticoagulants
2) drugs that interfere with the fibrin of the blood
3) drugs that affect the blood viscosity.

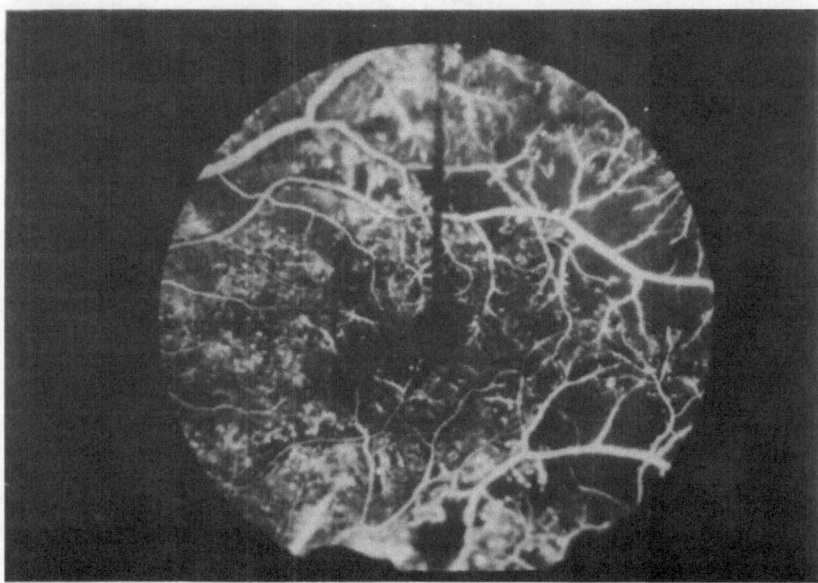

Fig. 3. Fluorescein angiogram in a case of diabetic retinopathy showing areas of abnormal capillary permeability and areas of capillary closure.

Although there are many conditions associated with retinal vein occlusion, the actual cause is seldom established. It is unlikely that a thrombus is the primary event in retinal vein occlusion (WISE et al, 1971) since fluorescein angiography suggests that blood flow through the retinal vein continues. However, the development of collaterals suggests that secondary occlusion may occur. Anticoagulants, which act by preventing clots forming in the first place, would not be a logical form for therapy since the formation of a clot is probably only rarely the cause of retinal vein occlusion. The same argument might therefore be applied against the fibrinolysins, such as streptolysin, which can dissolve a blood clot in its early days, and also against defibrinating agents such as Arvin. One great problem with both these groups of drugs is that, if it is felt that they are useful in preventing secondary thrombosis, then how long should they be continued?

Whether hyperviscosity is a factor in retinal vein occlusion is difficult to establish although central vein occlusion is not an uncommon complication of hyperviscosity states and may indeed be a consequence of reduced flow or stasis. This may occur when external pressure is put on the retinal vein for example in arterial disease and glaucoma. Under these circumstances it might appear logical to use an agent which will reduce hyperviscosity, such as low molecular weight dextrans (Rheomacrodex). This has, in fact, been used in a number of cases, although the results have not been especially encouraging (RADNOT & FOLLMAN, 1969).

There is a large literature on the use of drugs that affect blood clotting in central retinal vein occlusion but the great mass of this literature can be criticised on the grounds that there have been no controlled studies (WISE et al., 1971). It has, however, been an incidental observation that acute vitreous haemorrhages are more common in patients who receive these drugs and that the incidence of thrombotic glaucoma might be reduced by these therapies (KOHNER et al., 1974).

3 TREATMENT OF THE CONDITION

The most popular way of treating the vascular retinopathies directly is by means of photocoagulation The rationale of photocoagulation is threefold:
1) It can be used to destroy the abnormally permeable blood vessels so as to prevent leakage from the capillaries which give rise to the abnormal permeability response
2) It can be used to destroy new vessels directly.
3) It can be used to destroy areas of ischaemic retina, thereby destroying the stimulus for further neovascularization.

While the application of this form of therapy to various retinopathies can therefore be defended on these grounds, the assessment of the effect of this form of treatment is complex

In the evolution of any form of therapy a number of stages should be considered:
1) The definition of the condition to be treated.
2) The study of the natural history of the condition.
3) The idea of therapy.
4) A pilot feasibility study of therapy.

173

5) A direct comparison of the effects of treatment with the natural history of the condition (a clinical trial).
6) A general recommendation of therapy.
7) The application of this knowledge to medicine generally.

In photocoagulation, the first three or four steps in the evolution of therapy have already been passed. It is tempting to add 2 and 4 and suggest that that is the same as a clinical trial, but medical statisticians have repeatedly shown that this is not valid. We have passed the pioneering days and reached the age of accountability in photocoagulation and we may illustrate our problems by taking the example of three retinopathies — diabetic retinopathy, the retinopathy associated with branch vein occlusion, and sickle cell retinopathy.

Diabetic Retinopathy

Broadly speaking, there are two types of diabetic retinopathy; background retinopathy, which is the manifestation of the abnormal permeability response, and proliferative retinopathy, which is the manifestation of the ischaemic response. However, in diabetes this simple classification does not hold true entirely as abnormal permaebility and vascular occlusion often

TABLE I

RANDOMISED CONTROLLED CLINICAL TRIALS FOR
THE TREATMENT OF DIABETIC MACULOPATHY

AUTHOR	YEAR	NUMBER	VISUAL RESULT		
			B	S	W
Irvine	1971	C 10	13%	10%	80%
		T 10	20%	30%	50%
Patz	1973	C 63	10%	27%	63%
		T 63	27%	66%	7%
B.D.A.	1 yr 1975	C 76	24%	32%	48%
		T 76	38%	32%	30%
	2 yrs	C 44	23%	16%	61%
		T 44	34%	25%	41%
	3 yrs	C 25	32%	24%	44%
		T 25	54%	24%	24%

B = better
S = same
W = worse
C = control
T = treatment

174

coexist (Fig. 3). Thus, in the maculopathies, especially those with the worst prognosis, large areas of posterior capillary closure occur, and in the severest of the proliferative retinopathies, that is florid retinopathy, a mass of leaking dilated capillaries or new vessels are apparent. Nevertheless, all cases of new vessels do have peripheral closure.

The large literature on the benefits of photocoagulation in diabetic retinopathy gives hope to the clinician, but often the fate of individual patients makes him despair of the literature. EDERER & HILLER (1975) re-analysed five controlled studies of photocoagulation in a kind but critical way, pointing out the value of properly controlled trials and the weaknesses of studies that did not obey the basic statistical rules. Fortunately a number of randomised controlled clinical trials have been published.

The results of the maculopathy and background retinopathy trials are indicated in Table I. The results of PATZ (1973) and those of the British Diabetic Association (1975), which are only preliminary, suggest that there is a statistically significant bias in favour of treatment although it is impor-

TABLE II

CONTROLLED TRIALS FOR PROLIFERATIVE DIABETIC RETINOGRAPHY

AUTHOR	YEAR	NUMBER	VISUAL ACUITY		
			B	S	W
Okun	1968	C 52	10%	54%	36%
		T 52	36%	54%	10%
Beetham	1970	C 144	11%	59%	30%
		T 144	24%	61%	15%
Irvine	1971	C 24	13%	21%	67%
		T 24	17%	25%	58%
B.D.A.	1 yr 1975	C 68	15%	47%	38%
		T 68	19%	49%	32%
	2 yrs	C 23	13%	35%	52%
		T 23	30%	26%	43%
	3 yrs	C 16	13%	31%	56%
		T 16	25%	38%	38%

B = better
S = same
W = worse
C = control
T = treatment

tant that these trials be continued for a sufficient period of time to assess the long term effects.

The published results of the randomised controlled clinical trials of proliferative retinopathy have so far been more disappointing (Table II). There is no statistical evidence in favour of treatment. The most favourable trial is that of OKUN (1969), although many of the control patients were withdrawn for treatment. It may well be that in the photocoagulation trials now being undertaken by the British Diabetic Association, and more recently in America, will suggest subgroups which are responsive to photocoagulation but it is still important that proliferative patients be treated at centres where the information on the results of treatment can be of some value to the medical profession. We have not yet reached the stage where isolated physicians can legitimately be advised to treat proliferative retinopathy by photocoagulation since we have yet to learn what subgroups are most susceptible to treatment and what methods of treatment are most effective.

Branch Retinal Vein Occlusion

Branch retinal vein occlusion may present as a pure retinopathy either showing the abnormal permeability response or the ischaemic response. Cases with the predominantly abnormal permeability response lose their vision as the result of macular oedema, whereas those with the predominantly ischaemic response lose their vision as a result of vitreous haemorrhage or foveal atrophy. Only a few of the published studies differentiate between the two mechanisms and it is therefore not surprising that the published results on the visual prognosis for retinal vein occlusion are variable (Table III). It will be seen, however that, in spite of this variation, nearly half the cases improve their vision.

TABLE III

NATURAL HISTORY OF BRANCH VEIN OCCLUSION

AUTHOR	YEAR	NUMBER	VISUAL RESULTS		
			B	S	W
Duff	1951	71	42%	27%	31%
Hill	1970	44	41%	50%	11%
Blankenship	1973	48 (M)	27%	46%	27%
		18 (V)	28%	56%	16%
Cairns	1974	26	35%	42%	23%
Michels	1974	43	53%	14%	30%

B = better
S = same
W = worse
M = Maculopathy
V = Vitreous haemorrhage

Applying the rationale of photocoagulation, it would be logical to treat the abnormal permeability response by photocoagulating leaking capillaries. Where the ischaemic response is predominant then new vessels can be treated either directly or, especially where new vessels are present on the optic disc, the whole drainage area of the vein may be treated so as to reduce the stimulus for neovascularization. Collateral vessels should not be treated. However, the results of treatment in published cases are rather disappointing when compared with the natural history, especially bearing in mind that these are uncontrolled studies (Table IV). This is the more so as treatment itself carries a certain morbidity in terms of field loss, haemorrhage and retinal detachment. Therefore in the present state of our knowledge, it would be irresponsible to recommend the general ophthalmologist to treat retinal branch vein occlusion until we have objective evidence as to its efficacy. This can only be obtained by careful randomised clinical trials, both for the patient with the abnormal permeability response and those with the ischaemic response. Such a trial is in fact under way at Moorfields Eye Hospital but the preliminary results are not in favour of treatment. However, we await the full results of this trial with interest.

Sickle Cell Retinopathy

Lastly we may consider sickle cell retinopathy. We do not have the figures of the morbidity of this disease but its natural history has been beautifully documented by GOLDBERG (1971) and CONDON (1974). GOLDBERG compares the results of photocoagulation with a group of 25 cases previ-

TABLE IV

TREATMENT OF BRANCH VEIN OCCLUSION

AUTHOR	YEAR	NUMBER	VISUAL RESULTS		
			B	S	W
Campbell	1973	20 (M)	75%	15%	10%
Blankenship	1973	13 (M)	38%	54%	8%
		23 (V)	13%	70%	17%
Cleasby	1974	52 (M)	73%	14%	14%
		18 (V)	67%	28%	5%
Cairns	1974	12	58%	42%	0
Gitter	1975	51	60%	24%	16%

B = better
S = same
W = worse
M = maculopathy
V = vitreous haemorrhage

177

ously observed untreated. In this group of 25 cases not a single sea fan was observed to occlude spontaneously and yet we have noticed this on a number of occasions. The feasibility of treatment has therefore been established but we have only got to stage 2 or 3 along our evolution of therapy and it would be too soon to recommend therapy generally until the results of a randomised controlled clinical trial, comparing the natural history with treatment, have been published. We do not know yet whether occlusion of the fans without peripheral retinal ablation of the ischaemic retina encourages further neovascularization in the future. As this is often a symmetrical disease, it is very suitable for a randomised clinical trial and, incidentally, there is no better way of studying the natural history of a condition.

4. THE COMPLICATIONS OF THE RETINOPATHIES

The major complications of the retinopathies are – (1) vitreous organisation and traction, (2) retinal detachment, and (3) thrombotic glaucoma. Vitreous traction and membrance formation are the subject of separate communications of this congress and will not be considered further. Retinal detachments may either be serous or traction detachments. Serous detachments usually follow an acute hypertensive type of retinopathy, in which case they settle when the underlying condition is treated. Traction detachments occur in association with vitreous pathology, when they present problems in therapy beyond the subject of this paper.

Thrombotic glaucoma is perhaps the most dreaded complication of some of the vascular retinopathies. Filtering operations have been universally unsuccessful in practice. This condition has now become the subject of a number of randomised controlled clinical trials at Moorfields Eye Hospital in order to assess -- (1) the effect of peripheral retinal ablation (a) as a prophylactic measure and (b) as a treatment for rubeosis of the iris and, (2) cyclocryotherapy as a pain relieving procedure in established neovascular glaucoma. It was suggested many years ago (SMITH, 1961) that peripheral retinal ablation might reduce neovascularization in the anterior segment and, although there is much anecdotal evidence in favour of this, no proper trial has yet been undertaken. We are now in the process of doing this and it is hoped that the results will be available late next year.

In conclusion, therefore, we are at an interesting stage in the development of treatment of the vascular retinopathies. Prophylaxis of the vascular retinopathies has obvious implications in radiation retinopathy and complex factors affect the ophthalmologist in retrolental fibroplasia. In treating the cause of the retinopathies, the hypertensive retinopathies are outside the ophthalmologist's field of work, but the problems of retinopathy associated with central retinal vein occlusion have shown that his studies are not up to the scientific acumen expected of physicians in the testing of new drugs. In treating the actual retinopathy, photocoagulation plays an important part. We have passed the pioneering stages and have come to the stage of accountability, less dramatic for us but more important for the patient. Here our social responsibility towards our patients as a group often outweighs the individual therapeutic enthusiasm that we might

like to apply to individual patients. Lastly the complications of the retinopathies are the subject of new and exciting surgical techniques.

REFERENCES

ARCHER, D.B. Natural Course of Branch Retinal Obstruction. *Trans. Ophthalmol.
Soc. U.K.* 94: *623* (1974).
BEETHAM, M.P., AIELLO, L.A., BALODIMOS, M.R. & KONEZ, L. Ruby Laser Photo-
coagulation of early Diabetic Neovascular Retinopathy. *Arch. Ophthalmol.* 83: *261*
(1970).
BLACH, R.K. Vascular Occlusion, the Key to the Retinopathies. Trans. Asia-Pacific
Congress Ophthalmol. 1974, in press.
BLANKENSHIP, G.W. & OKUN, E. Retinal Tributary Vein Occlusion. *Arch. Ophthal-
mol.* 89: *363* (1973).
BOWELL, R.E., MARMION, U.J. & MCCARTHY, C.F. Treatment of Central Retinal
Vein Thrombosis with Ancrod. *Lancet* i: *173* (1970).
British Diabetic Association Trial: Xenon Arc Photocoagulation in the Treatment of
Diabetic Retinopathy. Lancet 1110, 2, C 1975.
CAIRNS, J.D. Photocoagulation in the Treatment of Retinal Branch Vein Occlusion.
Austral. J. Ophthalmol. 2: *5* (1974).
CAMPBELL, J.G. & WISE, G.N. Photocoagulation Therapy of Branch Vein Obstruc-
tions. *Am. J. Ophthalmol.* 75: *28* (1973).
CLEASBY, G.W., HALL, D.O., FUNG, W.E. & WEBSTER, R.G. Retinal Branch Vein
Occlusion Treatment by Photocoagulation. *Mod. Probl. Ophthalmol.* 12: *275*
(1974).
CLEMETT, R.S., KOHNER, E.M. & HAMILTON, A.M. The Visual Prognosis in Reti-
nal Branch Vein Occlusion. *Trans. Ophthalmol. Soc. U.K.* 93: *523* (1973).
CONDON, P.I. & SERGEANT, G.R. Photocoagulation and Diathermy in the Treat-
ment of Proliferative Sickle Retinopathy. *Brit. J. Ophthalmol.* 58: *650* (1974).
DESMARRES, L.A. Maladies des Yeux. Vol. III, 2nd ed. p. 523, Paris 1858, Gernier
Baillier.
DUFF, I.F., FALLS, H.F. & LIMMAN, J.W. Anticoagulant Therapy in Occlusive Vas-
cular Disease of the Retina. *Arch. Ophthalmol.* 46: *601* (1951).
EDERER, E. & HILLER, R. Clinical Trials, Diabetic, Retinopathy and Photocoagula-
tion. *Survey of Ophthalmol.* 19: *267* (1975).
GITTER, A.K., COHEN, G. & BABER, B.W. Photocoagulation in Venous Occlusive
Disease. *Am. J. Ophthalmol.* 79: *578* (1975).
GOLDBERG, M.F., Treatment of Proliferative Sickle Retinopathy. *Trans. amer. Acad.
Ophthalmol. Otolarving.* 75: *532* (1971).
HILL, D.W. & GRIFFITHS, J.D. The Prognosis of Retinal Vein Thrombosis. *Trans
ophthalmol., Soc. U.K.* 96: *309* (1970).
IRVINE, A.R. & NORTON, E.W. Photocoagulation for Diabetic Retinopathy. *Am. J.
Ophthalmol.* 71: *423* (1971).
KOHNER, E.M., HAMILTON, A.M., BULPITT, C.J. & DOLLERY, C.T.. Streptokinase
in the Treatment of Central Retinal Vein Occlusion. *Trans. ophthalmol. Soc. U.K.*
94: *599* (1974).
MICHELS, R.G. & GASS, J.D.M. Natural Course of Retinal Branch Vein Obstruction.
Trans. amer. Acad. Ophthalmol. 78: *166* (1974).
MUSHIN, A.C. Retinopathy of Prematurity · A Disease of Increasing Incidence?
Trans. ophthalmol. Soc. U.K. 94: *251* (1974).
OKUN, F. & JOHNSTON, G.P. Role of Photocoagulation in the Treatment of Prolifer-
ative Diabetic Retinopathy, in The Treatment of Diabetic Retinopathy. Eds. Gold-
berg, M.F. & Fine. S.L. U.S. Public Health Service Publication No. 1890, p. 523,
Washington, 1969.
PATZ, A., SCHATZ, H., BERKOW, T.W., GITTELSON, A.M. & TICHO, U. Macular-
Oedema, and overlooked Complication of Diabetic Retinopathy. *Trans. amer.
Acad. Ophthalmol Otolarygol.* 77: *34* (1973).

179

RADNOT, M. & FOLLMAN, P. Rheomacrodex (Dextran) in the Treatment of the Occlusion of the Central Retinal Vein. *Ann. Ophthalmol.* 1: *58* (1969).
SMITH, R.S. Neovascularization in Ocular Disease. *Trans. Ophthalmol. Soc. U.K.* 81: *125* (1961).
TIZARD, J.P.M. Retinopathy of Prematurity. *Pro. roy. Soc. Med.* 64: *771* (1971).
WISE, G.N. ,DOLLERY, C.T. & HENKIND, P. The Retinal Circulation. Harper Row. New York, 1971, p. 127.
WISE, G.N., DOLLERY, C.T. & HENKIND, P. The Retinal Circulations Harper & Row. New York, 1971, p. 363.

Author's address:
Moorfields Eye Hospital
City Road
London
England

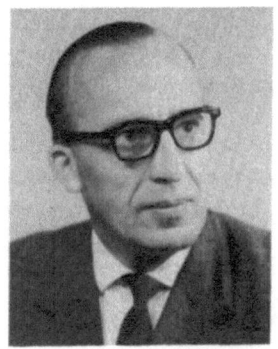

ADVANCES IN ELECTRO-OPHTHALMOLOGY
ITS USE IN RETINAL VASCULAR DISEASES

HAROLD E. HENKES

(Rotterdam, The Netherlands)

Since KARPE (1946) published his thesis 'Basis of clinical electroretino-graphy' the field of electro-ophthalmology has much expanded.

Although the basic ERG procedures have not changed essentially in the last 30 years — we still use contactlens electrodes, a stimulus light source, amplifiers and recording systems — the quality of the apparatus has greatly improved.

In the early 50ties we published cases of central retinal vein obstruction some of which demonstrated a recovery of the scotopic b-wave, while in others an attenuation, even a complete loss of b-wave amplitude was observed.

At that time we suggested that the height of the b-wave might be of value in the prognosis of venous occlusive diseases (HENKES 1953).

At present, we know that loss of b-wave amplitude, subsequent change in b/a-ratio and loss of oscillatory potentials (OP's) in retinal vascular occlusive

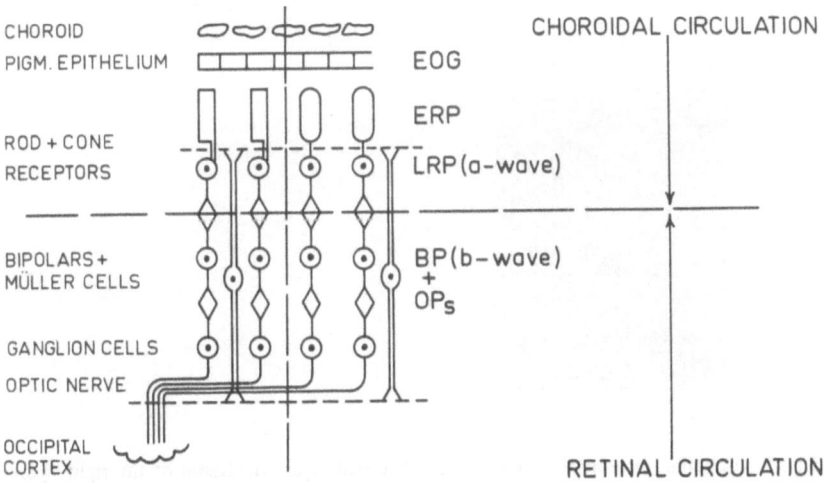

Fig. 1   Retinal section in relation to origin of EOG and ERG components.

181

disease, are prominent features serving as sensitive indicators for inner retinal layer viability (FRANÇOIS et al., 1973). The study of separate components of the ERG has deepened our understanding as to the localization of a given retinal process.

Figure 1 illustrates schematically the structures from which the EOG and the various components of the ERG derive. Disorders confined to the deep

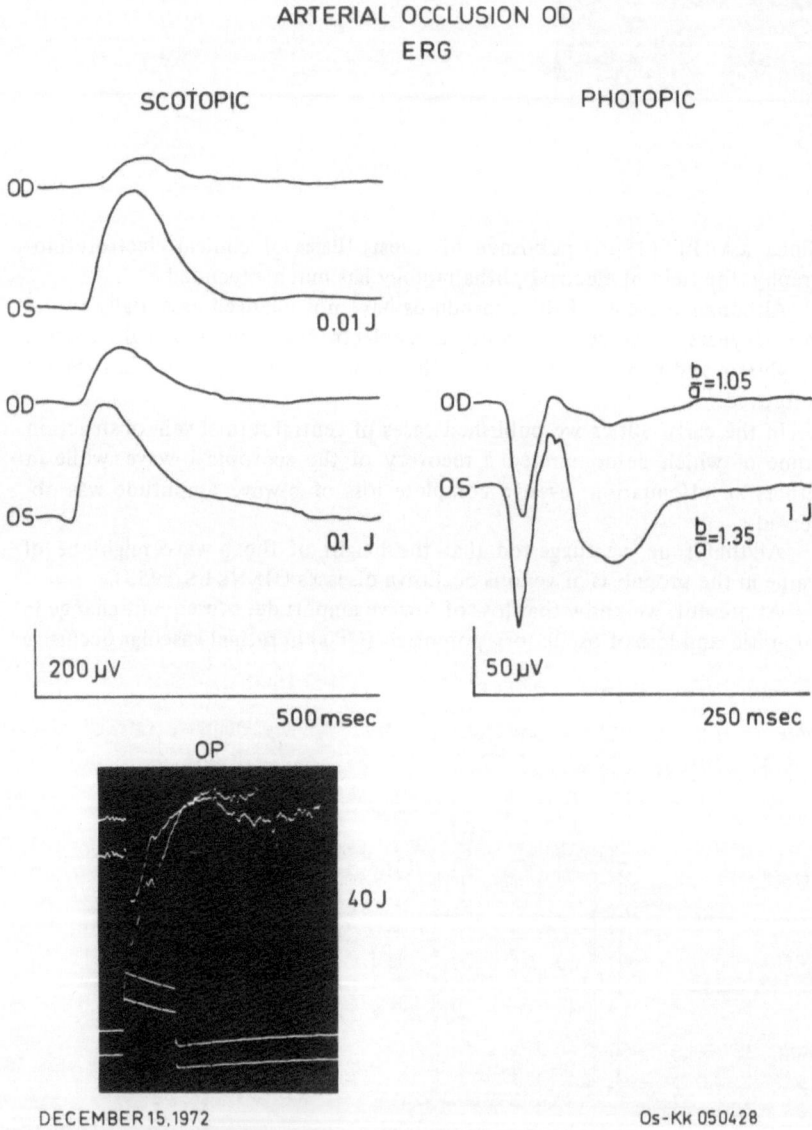

Fig. 2. Ischemic retinopathy due to central retinal artery occlusion of the right eye. Significant loss of b-wave and OP's. Markedly reduced b/a-ratio, of the 'normal' eye as well.

182

retinal layers may produce an abnormal EOG lightrise and changes in the early receptor potential (ERP), as well as in the late receptor potentials (scotopic and photopic a-waves).

Dysfunctions of the superifcial layers of the retina will be reflected in changes of the b-waves and the oscillatory potentials (OP's).

Attenuation of the circulation in the ophthalmic artery will lead to a reduction, or a complete loss of retinal electric activity.

A disturbance in the choroidal circulation will influence the EOG and the early ERG components, leaving the electric activity of the superficial

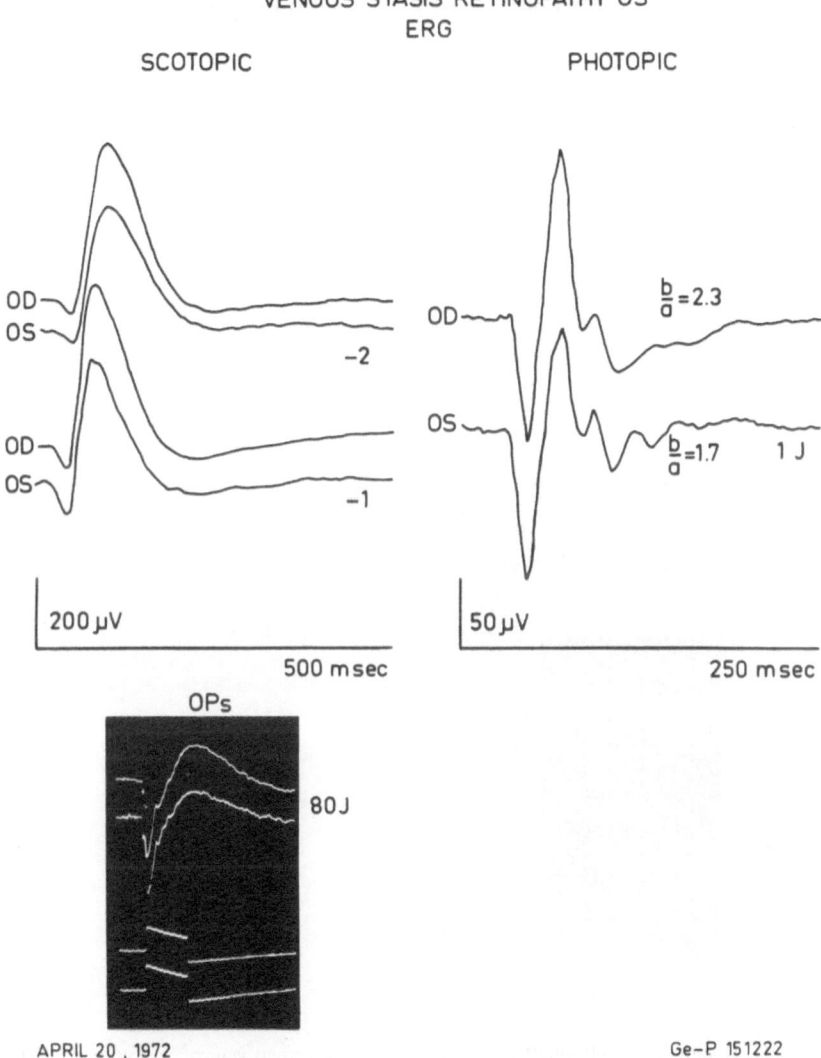

Fig. 3. Venous stasis retinopathy of the left eye. Normal b-wave and OP's. The b/a-ratio is reduced.

183

layers intact. A disturbance in the retinal vasculature will result in changes in the late ERG components, viz. the b-waves and the OP's.

Thus in central retinal artery occlusion, a normal ERP and normal a-waves are to be expected, whereas the b-waves and OP's will be markedly reduced or absent due to ischemia of the inner retinal layers (Fig. 2).

Strangely enough, the EOG lightrise is greatly reduced too, but NEU-MANN (1962) demonstrated a concomitant oedema of the choroid over the area of the ischemic retina. This may explain the local loss of function of the pigment-epithelium, from which the EOG lightrise is said to derive.

Retinal venous obstructions are to be divided into cases of venous stasis

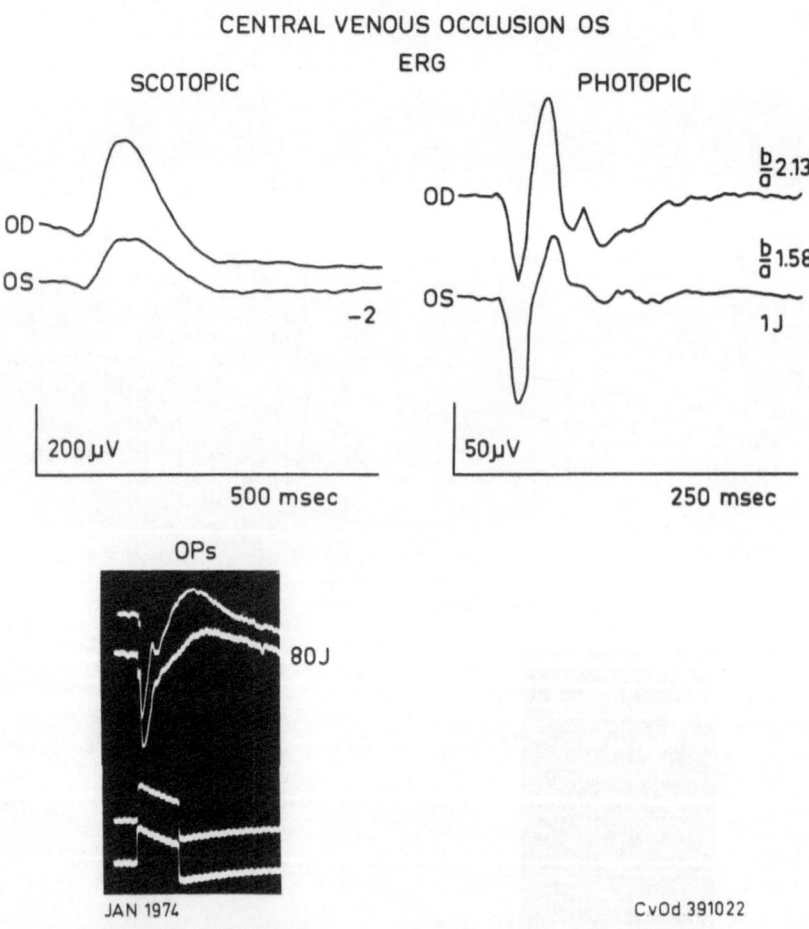

Fig. 4. Hemorrhagic retinopathy in a case of central retinal vein occlusion of the left eye.
A: Markedly reduction of scotopic b-wave and of b/a-ratio. Complete loss of OP's. The socalled 'normal' right eye shows reduction of OP's as a sign of diminished retinal viability.

retinopathy in which the circulatory disturbance is restricted to the venous system, and hemorrhagic retinopathy in which at the same time the arterial circulatory system is involved.

In venous stasis retinopathy (Fig. 3) the ERG may be either normal, or a slight reduction in b/a-ratio may be present. The OP's may be reduced too. Recovery of electric activity is the rule. The prognosis is favourable.

A hemorrhagic retinopathy may demonstrate more extensive loss of retinal activity due to inherent retinal inschemia (Fig. 4A). The prognosis is uncertain. Recovery of electric activity may occur (Fig. 4B). This development however, is more questionable than in venous stasis retinopathy. In cases, in which a complete loss of electric activity occurs, the development of a neovascular glaucoma is to be feared.

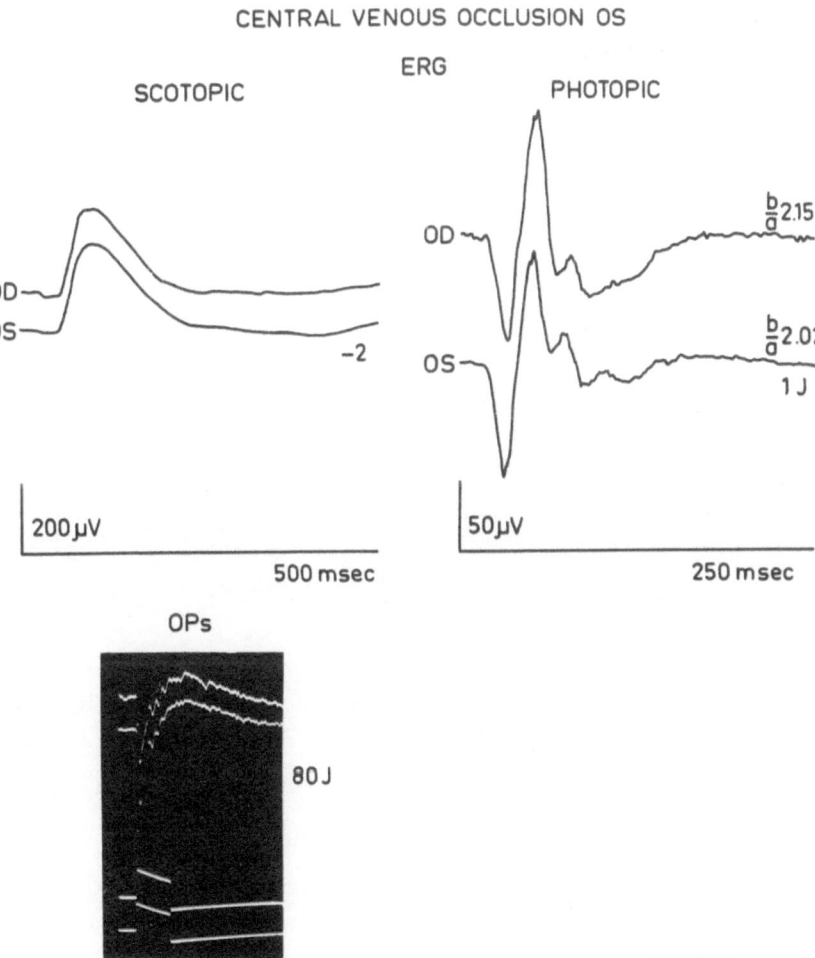

B: One year later, recovery of electric activity of the left eye is obvious. Recovery of OP's of the right eye points towards improvement of the general circulation.

References

FRANÇOIS, J., ROUCK, A. DE., CAMBIE, E. & ZANEN, A., L'électro-diagnostic des affections rétiniennes. *Bull. Soc. Belge d'Ophtal.* 166: *1-494* (1973).

HENKES, H.E. Electroretinography in circulatory disturbances of the retina. I. Electroretinogram in cases of occlusion of central retinal vein or of one of its branches. *Arch. Ophthal.* 49: *190-201* (1953).

KARPE, G. The basic of clinical electroretinography. *Acta Ophthal., Suppl.* 24, (1946).

NEUMANN, E. Histology of choroid and retina after multiple recent occlusions of the retinal arteries as revealed by coronal serial sections of the globe. *Brit. J. Ophthal.* 46: *357-364* (1962).

Author's address:
Eye Hospital
Erasmus University
Rotterdam, The Netherlands

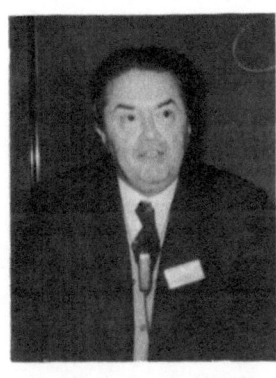

QUELQUES IDEES NOUVELLES CONCERNANT LA CIRCULATION CHOROÏDIENNE

PIERRE AMALRIC

(Albi, France)

La lecture de tous les traités d'ophtalmologie ne nous permet guère de penser que nos connaissances sur la choroïde se soient quelque peu transformées depuis 20 ans. Il n'y est encore question que de 'big vessels' sans aucune étude topographique précise.

Et cependant, lorsque l'on retrace l'historique des publications de ces dernières années, on est obligé de remarquer que nos connaissances sur cet ensemble vasculaire ont beaucoup progressé.

Nous voudrions dans cette brève présentation rappeler quelques uns des derniers travaux concernant la circulation choroïdienne artérielle, capillaire ou veineuse. Nous verrons ensuite sur le plan topographique comment cette circulation s'organise dans une zone privilégiée de l'oeil, la région maculaire.

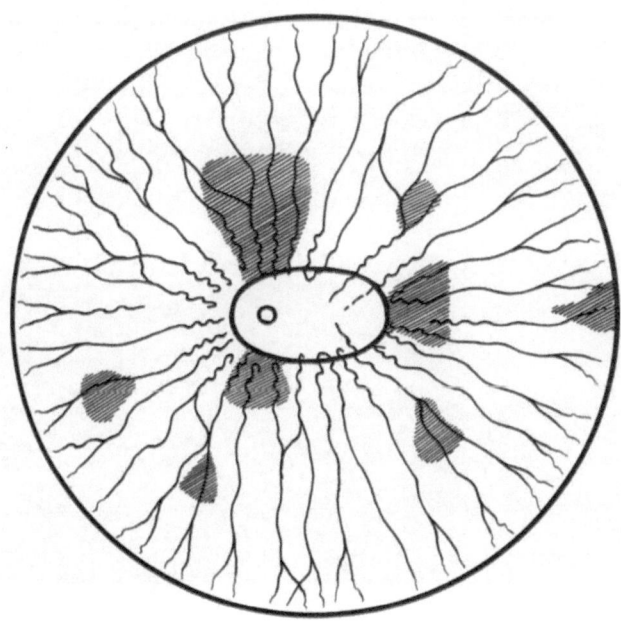

Fig. 1. Schéma des artères ciliaires courtes et longues. Quelques types de triangle.

187

1 LES ARTERES CILIAIRES

En 1963, ayant eu l'occasion de constater chez un malade une image triangulaire périphérique centrée sur l'artère ciliaire longue postérieure, nous
avons pensé à l'existence d'un syndrome ischémique choroïdien, provoqué
par l'oblitération de cette artère. A partir de ce fait d'observation, nous
avons avec REMKY constaté une concordance de notre vision ophtal-
moscopique de l'artère avec ce que l'examen histologique nous révélait. En
1964, à Heidelberg, les variations physiologiques du paquet vasculo nerveux
ciliaire long postérieur, ont fait l'objet d'une première exposition scienti-
fique. Dans les années suivantes, nous avons consacré à ce problème de
nombreuses publications. Nous n'avions à l'époque pour examiner nos malades que l'ophtalmoscopie, directe ou indirecte, et la diaphanoscopie trans-
sclérale qui nous permettait de visualiser chez tous nos malades les branches
périphériques des artères ciliaires.

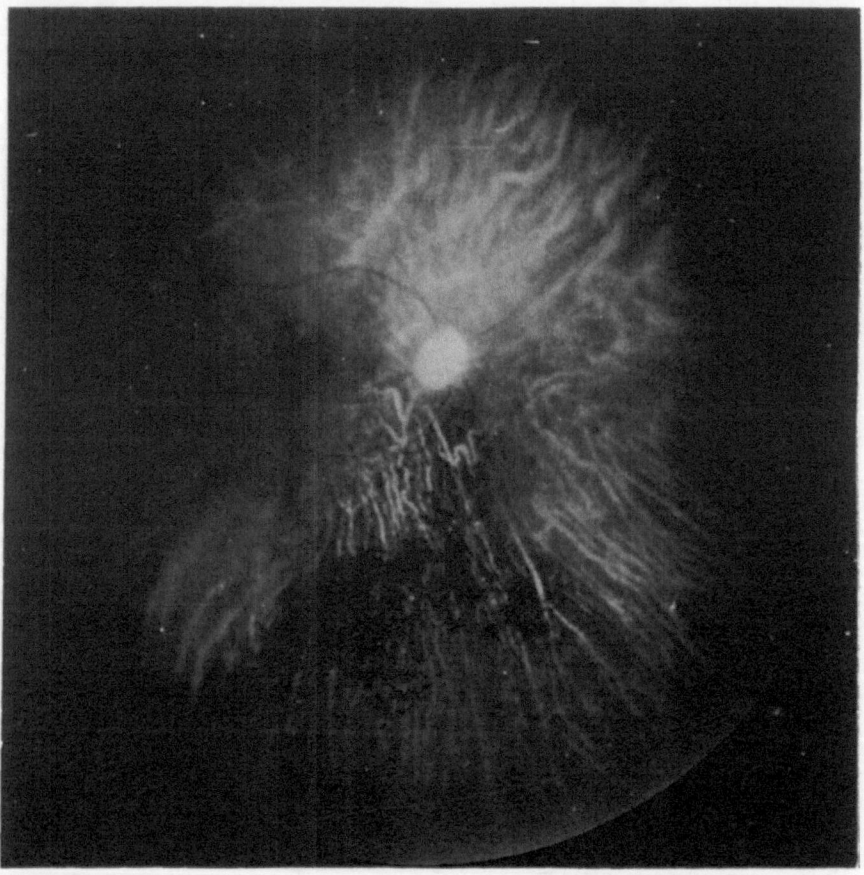

Fig. 4. Visualisation au rétinographe grand angle (avec filtre rouge) d'un très large
triangle sous papillaire.

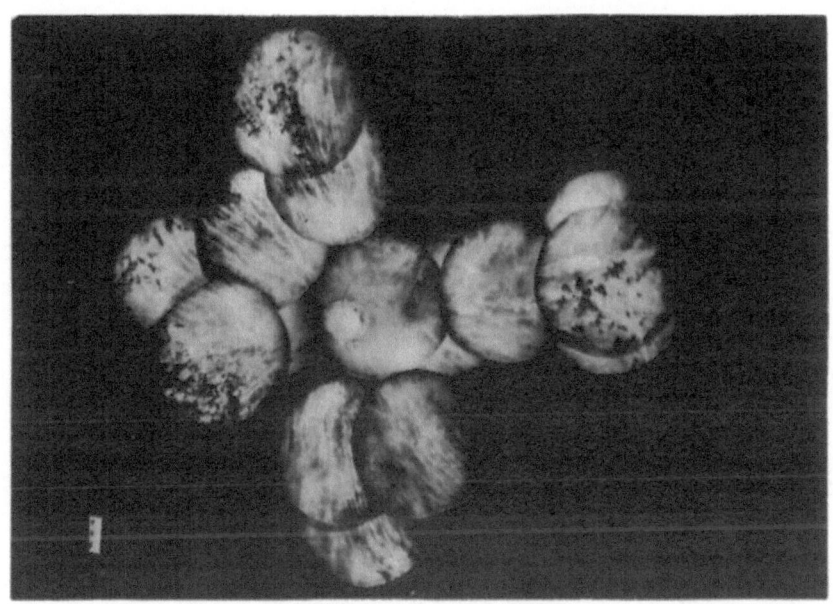

Fig. 2. Triangles ischémiques choroïdiens au cours d'une maladie de Raynaud grave. Aspect en infra rouge.

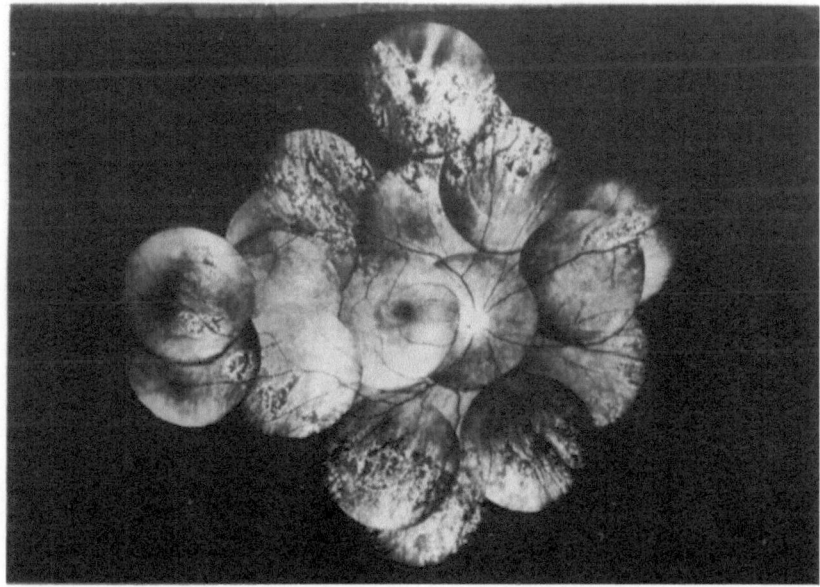

Fig. 3. Triangles périphériques dans un cas d'ischémie choroïdienne aiguë au cours d'un accident gravidique. Aspect en lumière anérythre.

Vers 1966 à partir de rétinographies en rouge et en infrarouge, chez des malades atteints de sclérose choroïdienne, nous avons pu préciser la topographies des réseaux ciliaires courts postérieurs et réunir aussi de nombreuses observations de plusieurs types de syndromes triangulaires siégeant en des points très variés du fond d'oeil.

A la même époque, l'angiographie fluorescéinique a permis d'apporter à cette étude des 'éléments précieux, morphologiques et dynamiques; et cela surtout dans certaines circonstances pathologiques le réseau vasculaire ciliaire étant rendu visible par l'atrophie pigmentaire sus jacente.

Les artères se dirigent en rayons de roue vers la périphérie. L'origine sinueuse initiale de ces grosses artères ciliaires s'associe à une direction en spirale à partir de l'émergence intraoculaire. Ce premier chapitre de nos recherches concernant les artères ciliaires longues et courtes avec la traduction pathologique de leur oblitération par un syndrome d'atrophie triangulaire parait aujourd'hui admise par tous, surtout depuis que cette vue anatomoclinique a été confirmée par l'expérimentation animale.

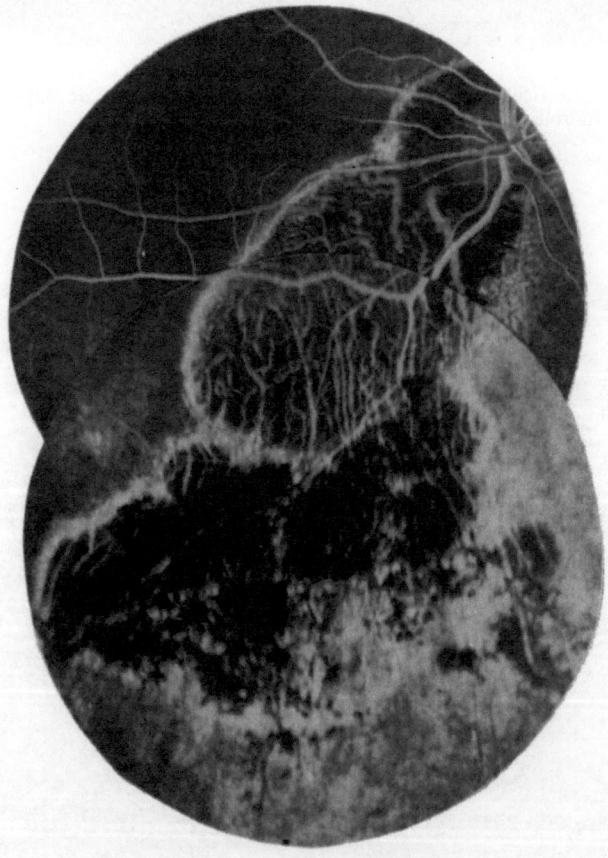

Fig. 4.bis   Le même cas en angiographie avec le rétinographe 30° se revèle formé par plusieurs 'cercles'

HAYREH a montré en effet chez le singe que l'oblitération des artères ciliaires provoquait des ischémies triangulaires adoptant le même aspect avec un apex central et une base périphérique.

2 LES CAPILLAIRES

Il est cependant un autre type d'image que l'on remarque très souvent au niveau du fond d'oeil: c'est l'image choroïdienne circulaire atrophique à bords nettement limités et à pigmentation plus ou moins accusée. Les études de micro circulation entreprises à Pavie par OTTAVIANT, MORONE et leur equipe, à Chicago par ERNEST & KRILL, ont confirmé que la choroïde sur *le plan capillaire* se terminait par des unités arrondies de taille plus ou moins grande suivant que l'on allait du centre vers la périphérie et cela permettait d'expliquer non seulement des images atrophiques de l'atrophie gyrée, mais

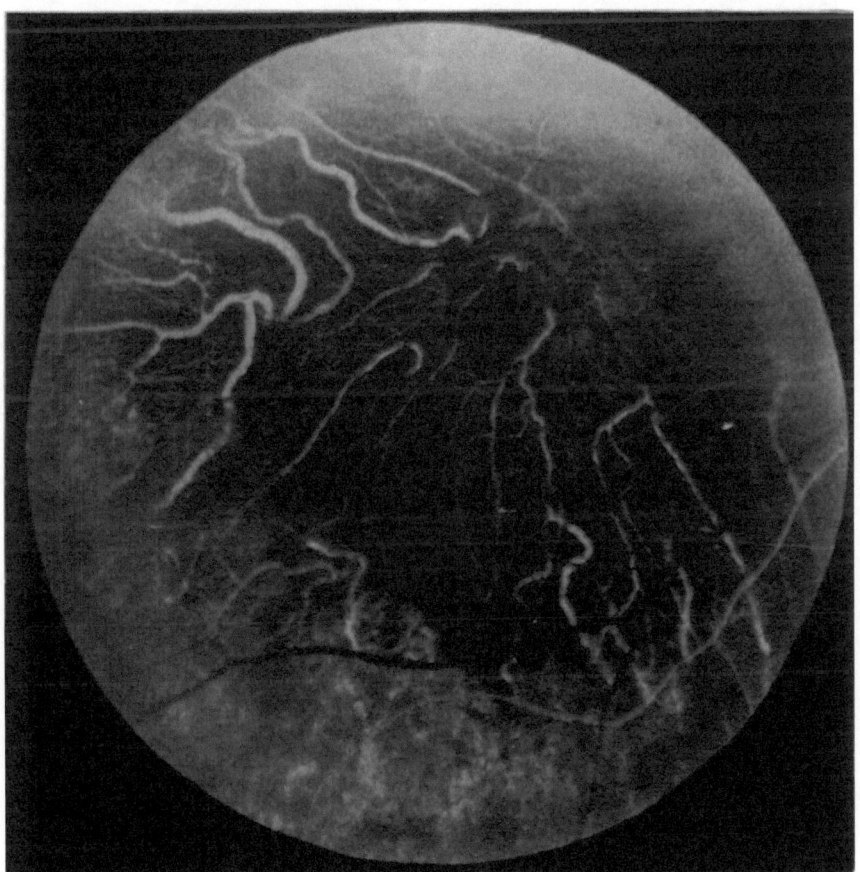

Fig. 5. Origine sinueuse en tourbillons des artères ciliaires dans leur émergence péri-maculaire.

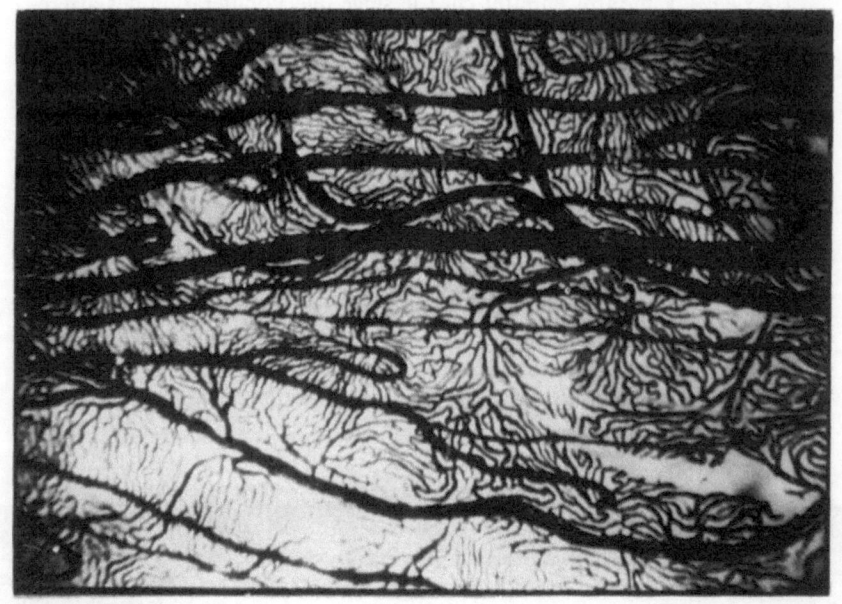

Fig. 6. Unités circulatoires capillaires centrées par une artériole (OTTAVIANI, MORONE et collaborateurs).

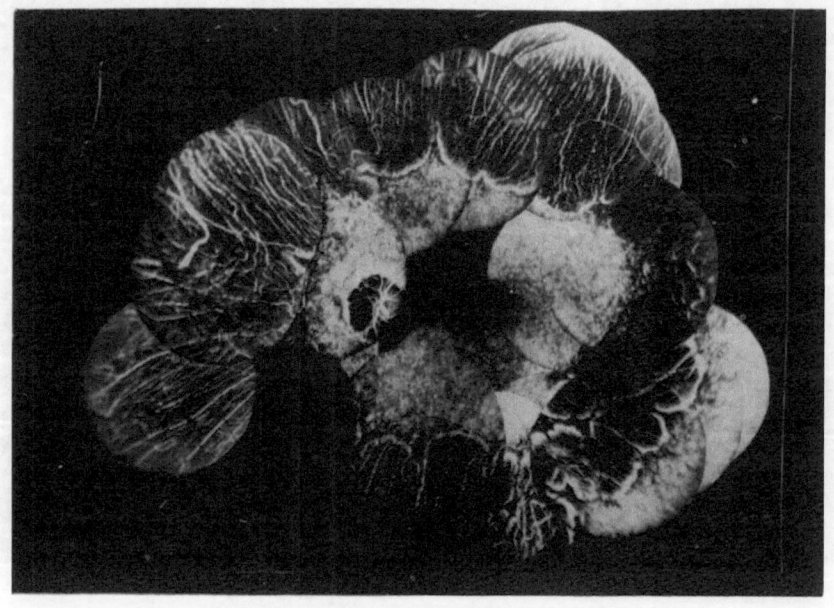

Fig. 7. Unités choroïdiennes rondes dans l'atrophie gyrée.

aussi certains foyers inflammatoires isolés correspondant à une artériole terminale.

La conjonction d'images arrondies et d'images triangulaires est également possible comme cela peut se voir au cours de certains syndromes triangulaires dont l'angiographie révèle la formation à partir de plusieurs cercles de plus en plus étendus du centre vers la périphérie.

3 LES VEINES

L'ensemble de ces formations géométriques au niveau de la choroïde laisse supposer une systématique vasculaire nettement définie. Cela est devenu encore plus évident depuis la vision panoramique réalisée avec des rétinographes grand angle: on a alors sur un seul cliché une vision globale de la plus grande partie du réseau vasculaire choroïdien. Ainsi se trouvent évités de fastidieux montages plus ou moins éronnés lorsqu'ils couvrent une surface très grande.

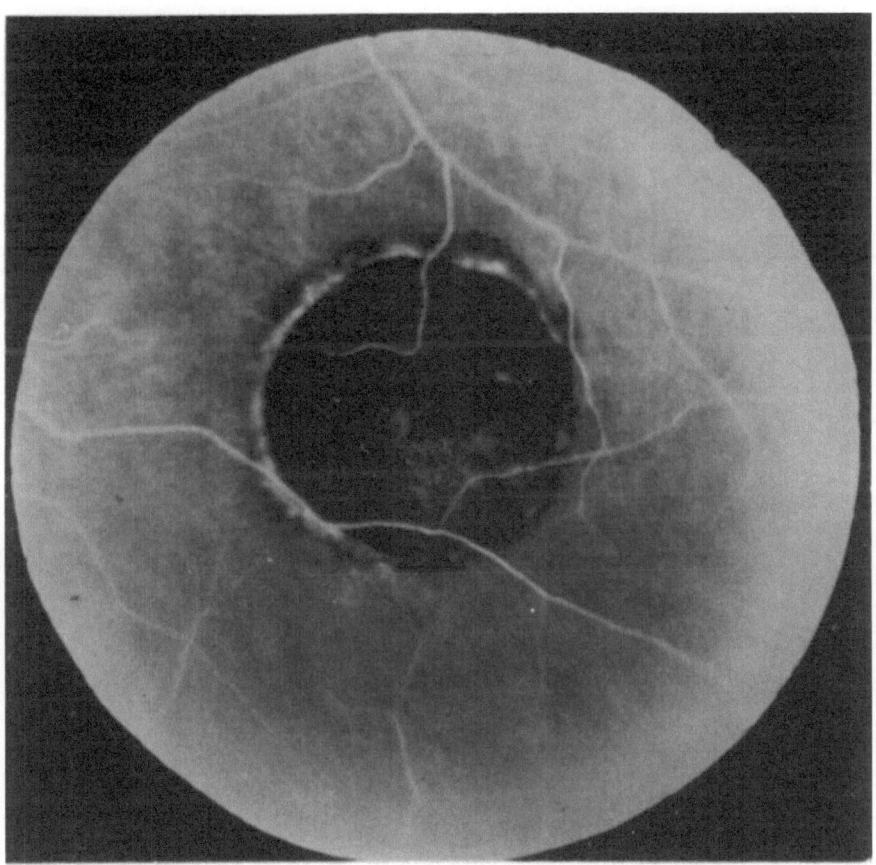

Fig. 8. Foyer inflammatoire très pigmenté simulant un naevus.

L'adjonction de filtres colorés, l'infra-rouge surtout, a été à l'origine d'une meilleure connaissance du *réseau veineux vortiqueux*. L'étude du réseau veineux choroïdien en est encore à son début. Les extrêmes variations que nous avons pu constater dans la forme, la direction et le nombre de réseaux vortiqueux, expliquent que l'on hésite à rapporter à leurs altérations certains tableaux pathologiques choroïdiens. Cependant en perfectionnant les méthodes d'examen et en pensant plus particulierement aux veines vortiqueuses il arrive souvent que l'on puisse évoquer cette pathogénie devant des altérations choroïdiennes profondes siégeant au niveau de ces zones de sortie veineuse. Cela est surtout vrai en ce qui concerne les vortiqueuses temporales supérieure et inférieure, dont les veines émissaires proviennent pour une grande part de la région maculaire.

Dans des circonstances étiologiques très diverses vont apparaitre des signes de souffrance veineuse se traduisant par des réactions hémorragiques ou exsudatives profondes soulevant la rétine, gagner secondairement à partir de la périphérie, les parties centrales du fond d'oeil; parfois un décollement

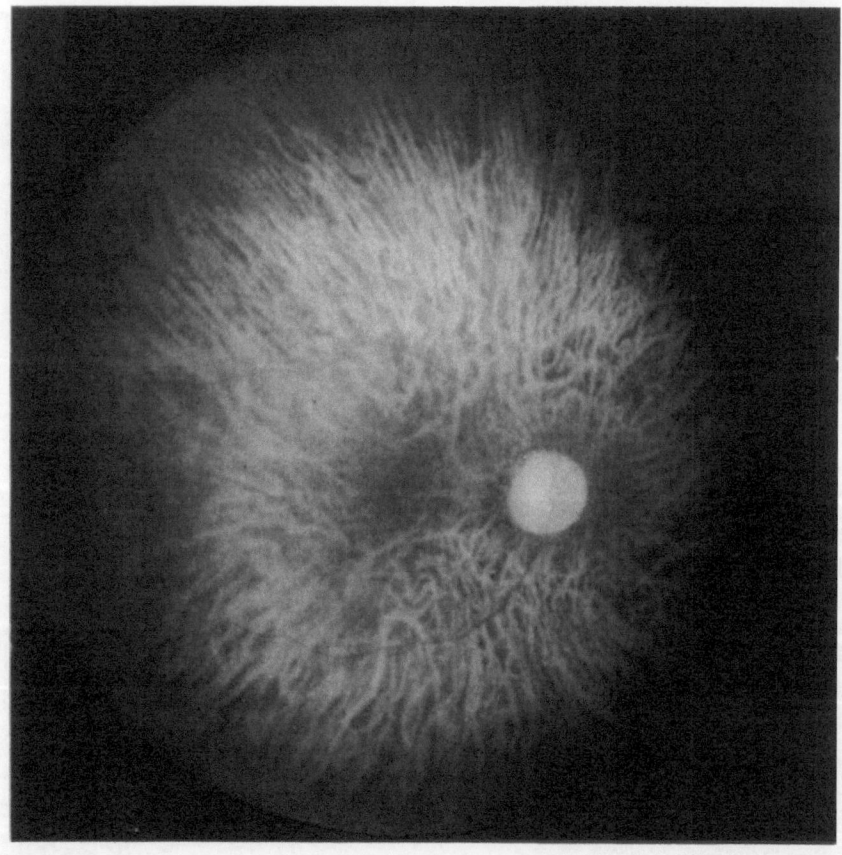

Fig. 9. Systématisation des vaisseaux choroïdiens. Rétinographie grand angle. Vision en infra rouge.

194

choroïdien surajoute ou une réaction pigmentaire importante rendent plus complexe encore le diagnostic.

Dans ce bref aperçu, nous ne pouvons envisager tous les problèmes; mais nous voudrions surtout que devant tout syndrome choroïdien, hémorragique, exsudatif ou transudatif, siégeant dans les régions périphériques, on évoque en premier lieu une altération du réseau veineux vortiqueux que l'étiologie en soit traumatique, vasculaire, infectieuse, dégénérative et parfois même pseudo-tumorale.

LA REGION MACULAIRE

Enfin, pour terminer, la région maculaire reste de tout le fond d'oeil, celle où les problèmes choroïdiens sont les plus complexes. Elle le doit non seulement à l'importance de son réseau, en raison de l'extrême délicatesse

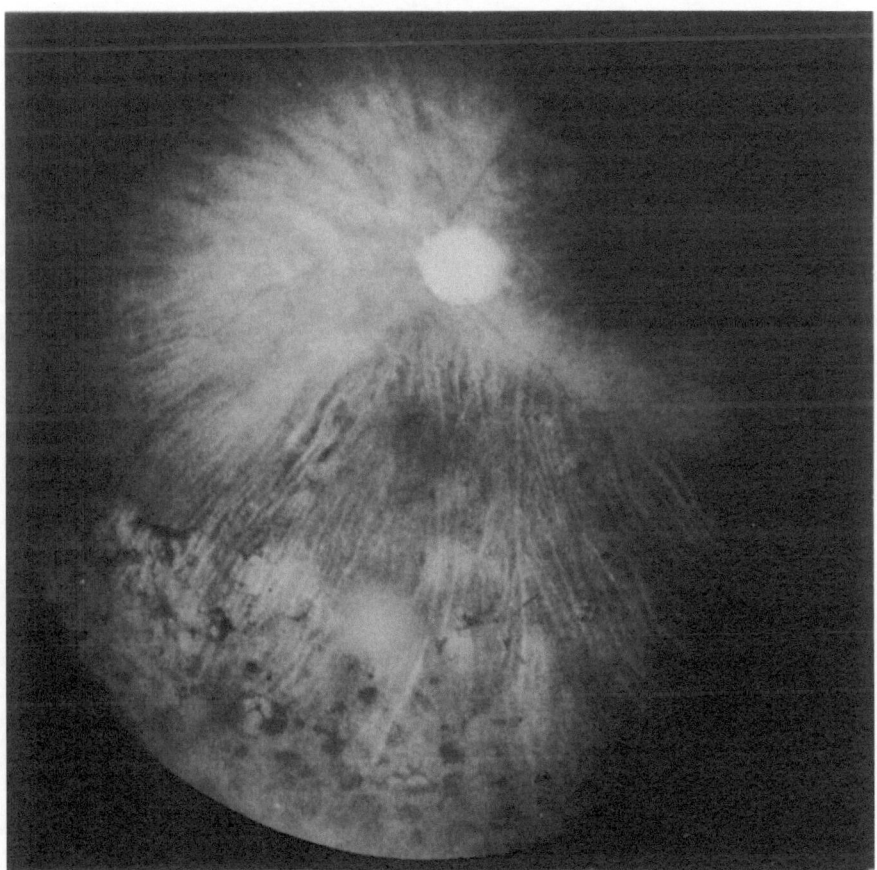

Fig. 10. Larges triangles inférieurs au rétinographe grand angle. Il faut remarquer aussi qu'autour du golfe vortiqueux nasal inférieur, s'organise un large éventail atrophique. (vision en infra rouge).

195

des structures qu'il irrigue mais aussi à la rapidité du courant sanguin à son niveau. Rendu invisible par l'écran pigmentaire rétinien, elle ne peut en clinique être explorée qu'avec difficulté. Seul dans quelques cas pathologiques privilégiés ou chez certains sujets dont le réseau pigmentaire est très peu dense, on a pu mettre en évidence les réseaux qui l'irriguent.

Les artères maculaires nous paraissent provenir des branches des artères ciliaires courtes faisant émergence sous la macula; elles sont de diamètre plus ou moins important mais aboutissent en fait en dernière analyse à des petites artérioles irriguant des unités circulatoires entourant la zone centrale sous fovéale. S'il est fréquent de voir l'origine sinueuse des gros troncs artériels périmaculaires, il est rare de pouvoir observer les petites artères maculaires qui leur font suite.

Sur le plan embryologique, HEIMANN a bien montré cependant leur individualité, celle ci n'est contestée maintenant par personne et récemment

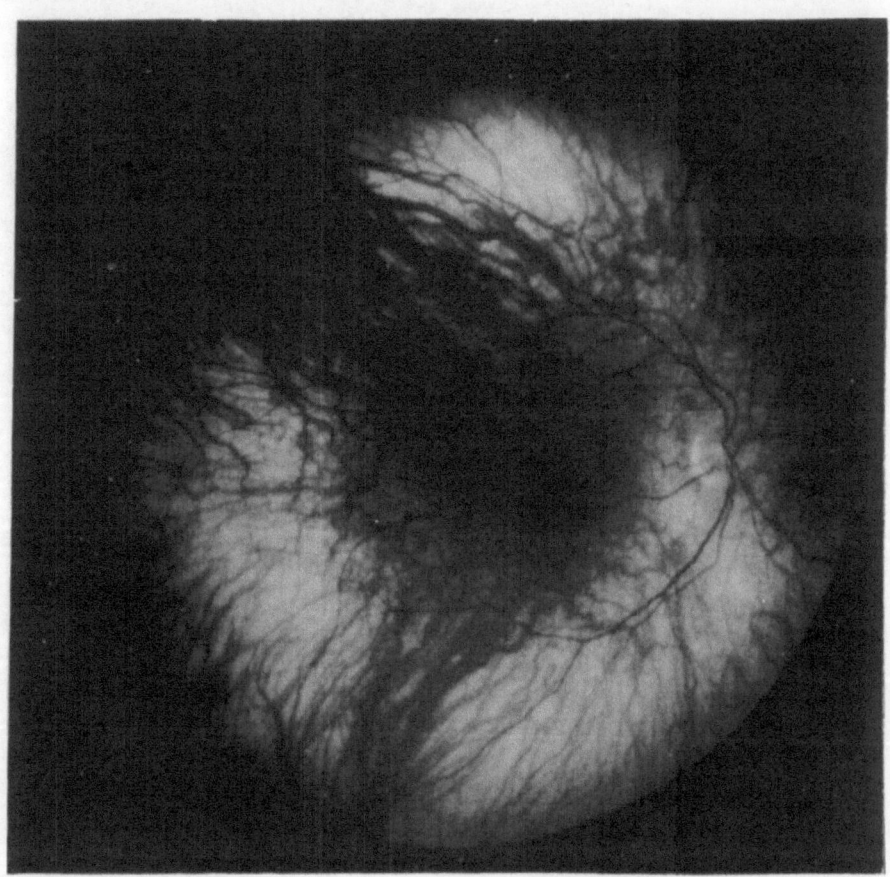

Fig. 11. Circulation veineuse de la macula se dirigeant vers le réseau vortiqueux. Rétinographie grand angle.

ERNEST a observé aussi certaines branches à destination proprement maculaire.

Enfin, OTTAVIANI distingue des artères de trois types; les plus petites se terminent dans un réseau capillaire de forme arrondie. Elles forment en somme le centre d'un cercle capillaire très dense qui se continue à la périphérie par un réseau veineux. Cette image en nénuphar correspond à la formation la plus parfaite pour obtenir l'équilibre d'un flux sanguin très rapide. Cela évoque la répartition d'un jet en parapluie dans toutes les directions.

Nous avons sur le plan clinique de nombreux exemples qui appuient cette conception de la choroïde maculaire. Nous savons par exemple que dans la choroïderémie, il persiste souvent une très bonne acuité visuelle lorsque toute la choroïde périphérique est atrophiée. Comment expliquer cela s'il n'y avait encore dans ces cas la persistance d'une circulation propre-

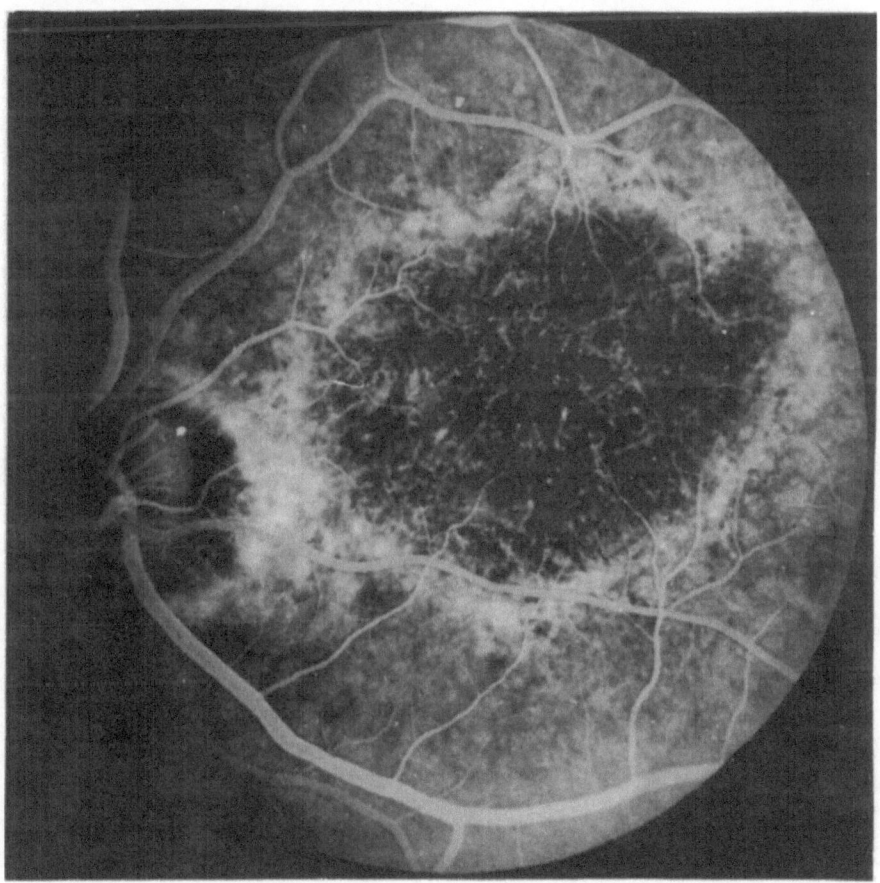

Fig. 12. Petites artèrioles prenant leur émergence autour de la macula dans une maladie de Stargardt.

ment maculaire. Nous avons aussi un ensemble de tableaux cliniques où la disposition des artères maculaires explique les images qui succédent à l'embolisation des plus fines artérioles terminales. C'est le cas en particulier de l'image en rosette de FRANÇOIS dans la toxoplasmose.

Dans tous les processus scléreux ou atrophiques, on voit souvent certaines unités circulatoires qui disparaissent en formant des plages plus ou moins rondes avoisinant la fovea. L'angiographie permet de bien en préciser les limites dans de nombreux cas de maladie de Stargardt ou de dégénérescence maculaire survenant dans le fundus flavimaculatus. Ce qui est frappant dans ces cas c'est de constater la persistance d'une circulation centrale foveale alors que la circulation péri-fovéale est totalement atrophique. Ces malades conservent longtemps une acuité visuelle chiffrable.

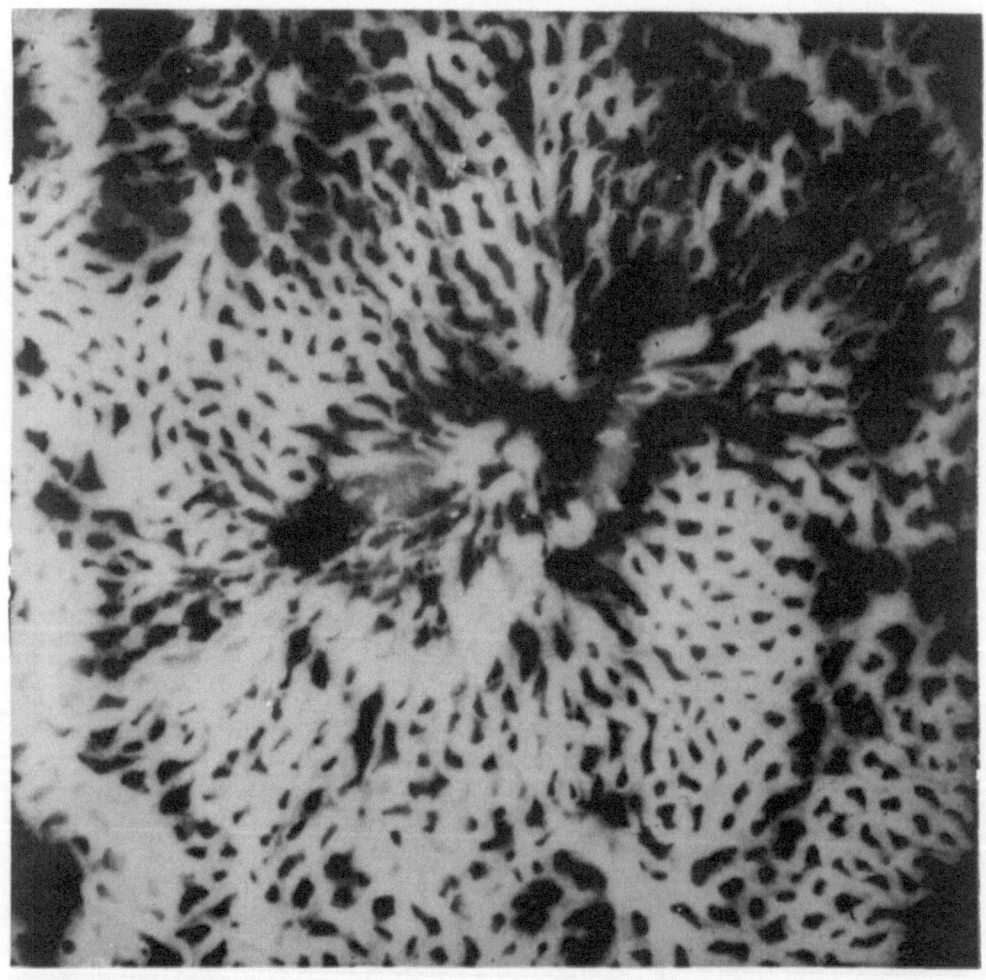

Fig. 13. Schéma d'une unité circulatoire centrée par l'artère avec son réseau veineux périphérique (OTTAVIANI).

Nous pensons que cette interprétation de la choroïde maculaire nous permet de mieux comprendre tout un ensemble de faits pathologiques survenant au voisinage même de la fovea. En particulier tout le processus de néovascularisation prenant son origine non pas au centre mais dans son voisinage immédiat, semble être en rapport avec des altérations d'unités maculaires distinctes du réseau foveal. Il est possible dans certains cas avec une photocoagulation bien appliquée de supprimer tout danger d'aggravation du processus hémorragique.

Si nous voulons donc résumer notre conception de la circulation choroïdienne maculaire, nous dirons qu'il existe des unités capillaires arrondies (7 à 8 en moyenne) autour d'une zone capillaire centrale correspondant à la fovea.

Certes, les anastomoses entre ces unités sont nombreuses mais elles conservent cependant une certaine autonomie comme cela peutse voir dans les scléroses progressives.

Le réseau veineux maculaire très dense aboutit surtout par des voies de large diamètre et à grand débit aux golfes vortiqueux.

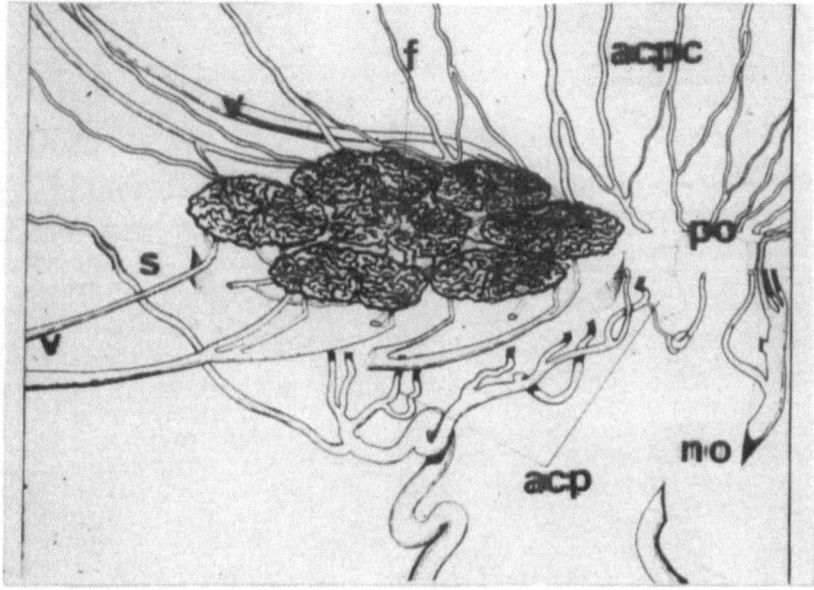

Fig. 14. Notre schéma   de la circulation capillaire de la zone maculaire. (Dessin de Savojni).
A.C.P. = artère ciliaire postérieure
A.C.P.C. = artère ciliaire courte postérieure
F = Fovea
N.O. = Nerf optique
P.O. = Papille optique
S = sclérotique
V = veines choroïdiennes

Il faut cependant ajouter qu'au delà de ce schéma normal, il existe souvent, en particulier chez le myope ou au cours d'anomalies congénitales, des veines vortiqueuses anormales sortant du globe au niveau de la macula ou au niveau de la papille. Tous ces cas sont importants car ils peuvent expliquer des complications circulatoires qui se produisent souvent, en particulier pensons nous pour les taches de Fuchs.

Nous voyons chaque jour par l'accumulation de documents que nous pouvons à partir de nos observations cliniques ou rétinographiques, dessiner une pathologie vasculaire choroïdienne nouvelle. La systématisation que nous donnons aujourd'hui ne constitue qu'un point de départ.

Author's address:
6, rue Saint-Clair
Albi, France

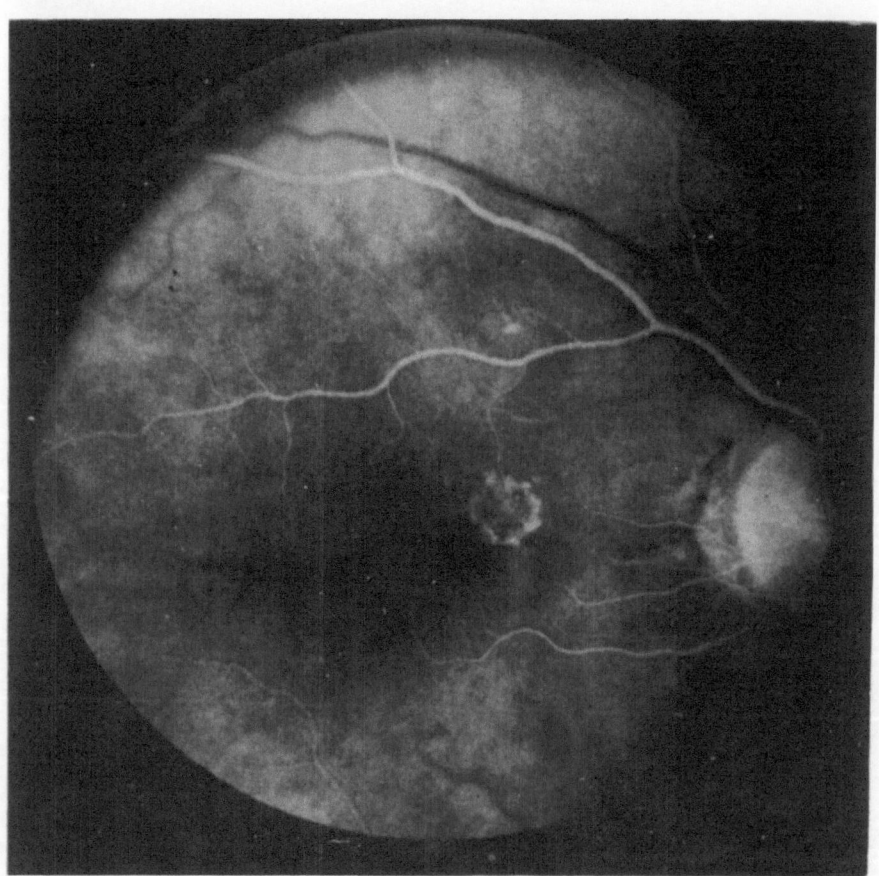

Fig. 15. Visualisation du réseau capillaire d'une unité circulatoire péri-maculaire.

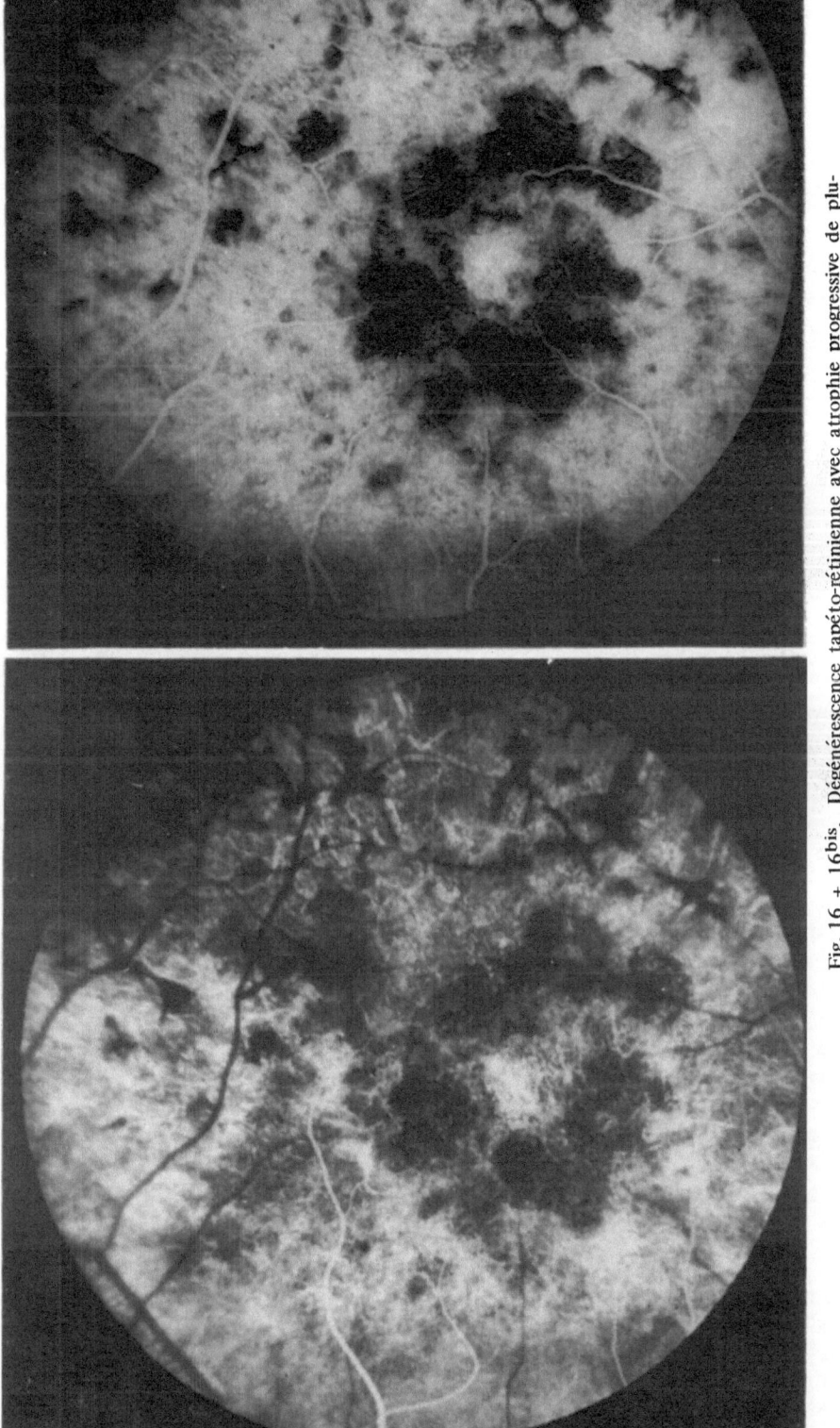

Fig. 16 + 16bis. Dégénérescence tapéto-rétinienne avec atrophie progressive de plusieurs unités circulatoires choroïdiennes péri-fovéales. Il persiste une circulation centrale. Ceci explique la conservation de l'acuité visuelle. Large scotome annulaire autour du point de fixation.

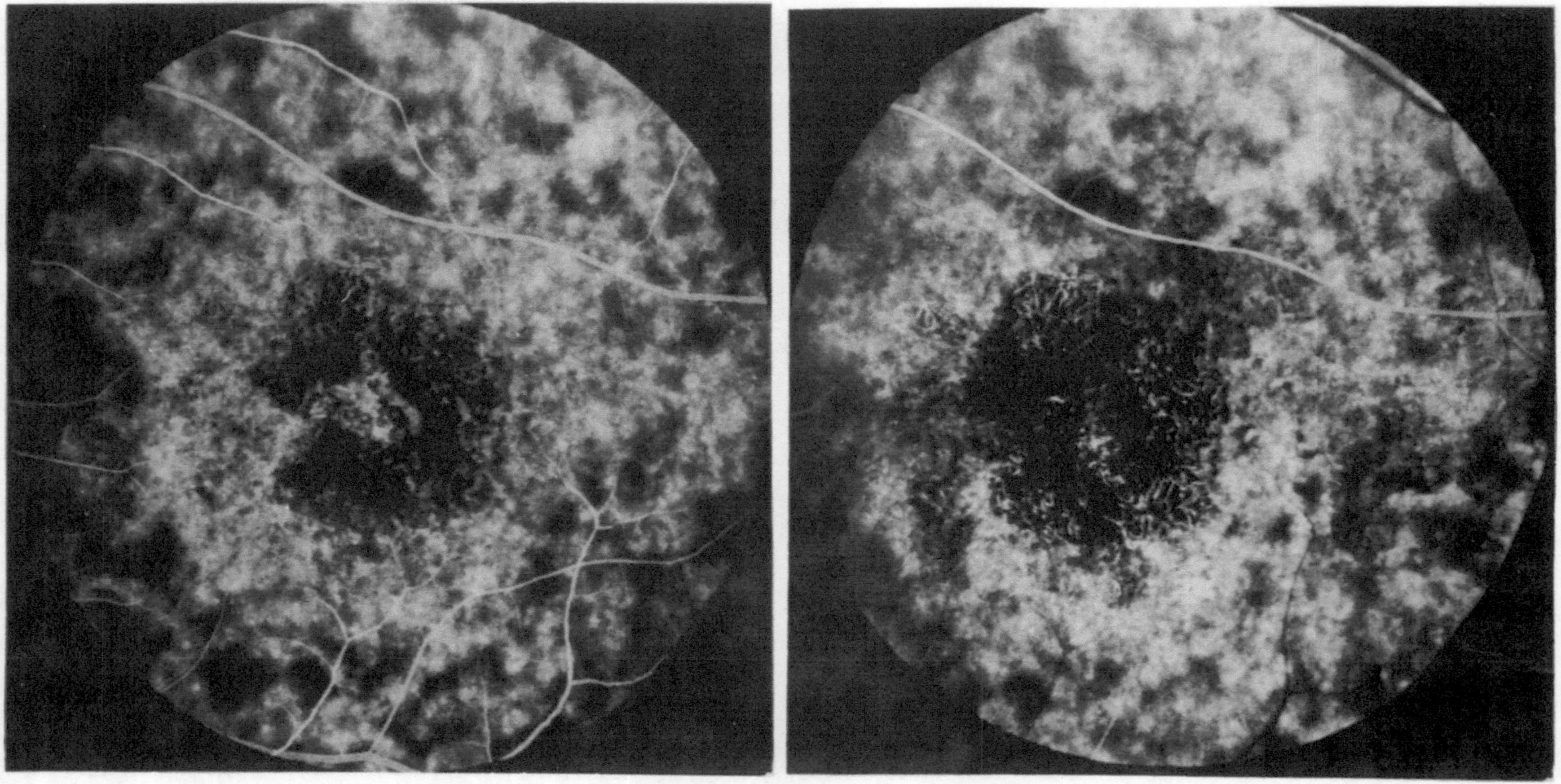

Fig. 17 + 17bis. Autre cas, absolument comparable au précédent.

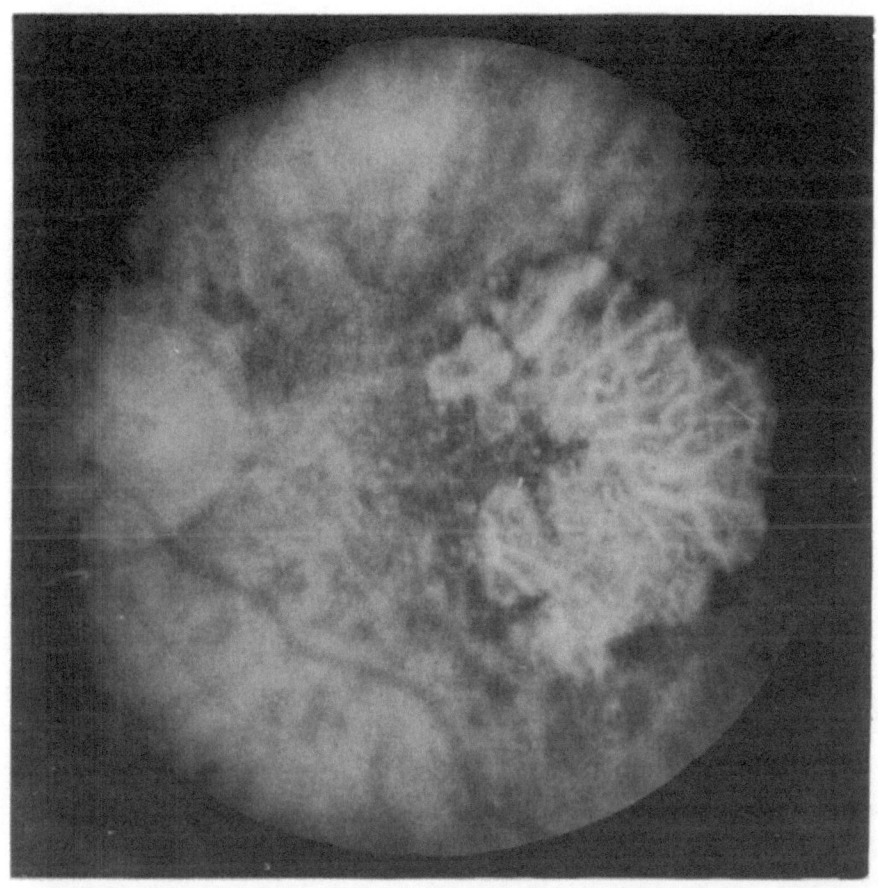

Fig. 18. Atrophie capillaire de plusieurs unités maculaires périfovéales. L'aspect se maintient semblable depuis 8 ans. Conservation d'une bonne acuité visuelle.

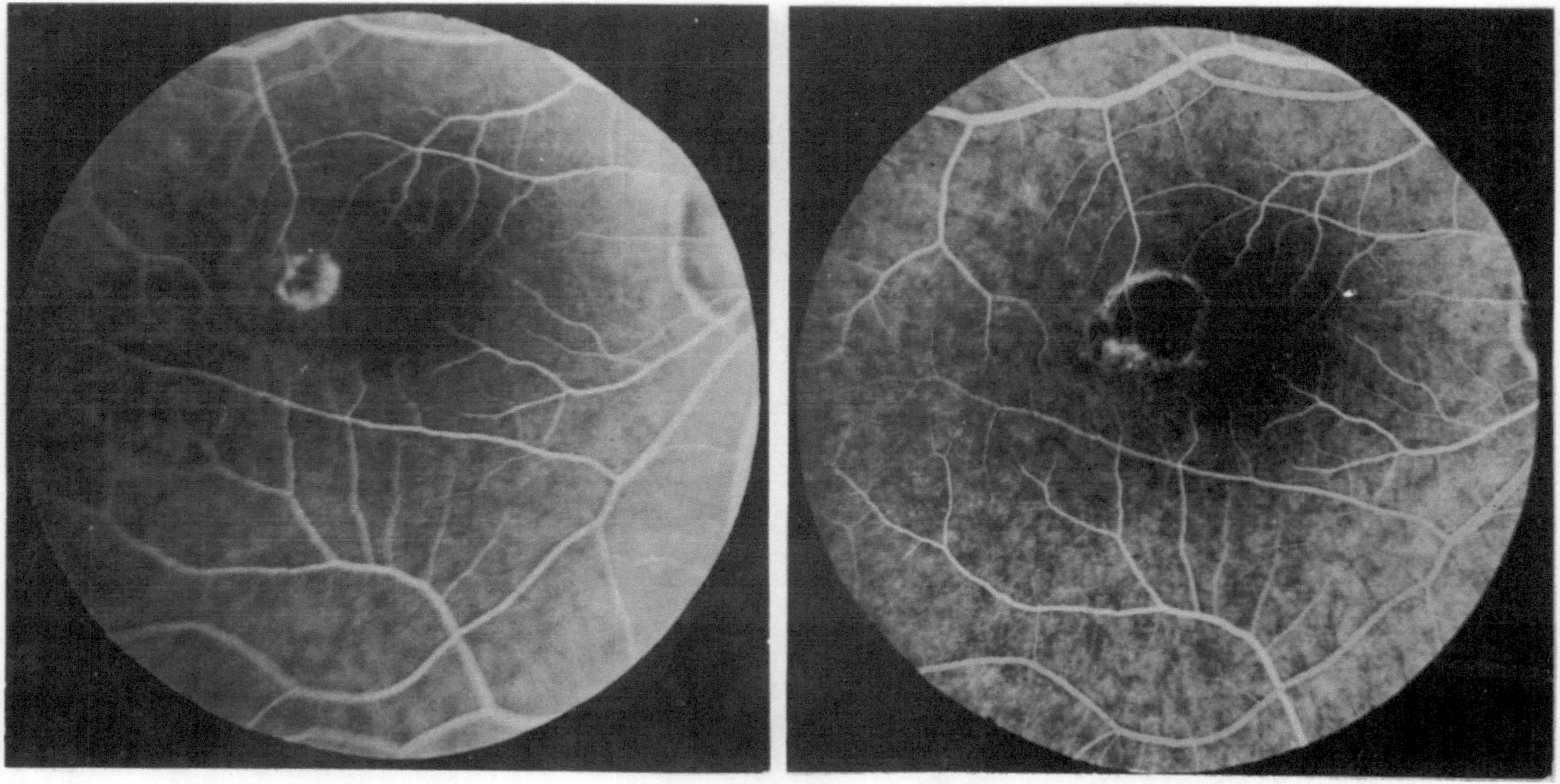

Fig. 19 + 19bis. Néovascularisation péri-fovéale stoppée par une photocoagulation correspondant uniquement à la lésion.

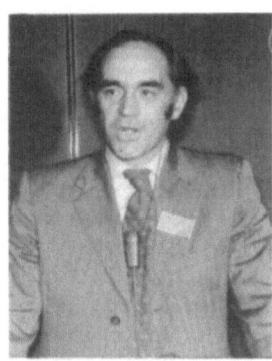

THE MACULAR DISCIFORM RESPONSE AND LASER TREATMENT

ALAN C. BIRD

(London, England)

In disciform macular degeneration the retina and pigment epithelium are detached from the underlying choroid by serous fluid, and the subpigment epithelial space is occupied by blood vessels originating from the choroid. Recent interest in the disease is due to the realisation that disciform degeneration in the elderly is the commonest cause of registerable blindness in England and Wales (SORSBY, 1966), to fluorescein fundus angiography which allows the study of the morphology of the disease during life (GASS, 1967) and to photocoagulation which provides a means of treating the lesion.

Disciform lesions represent the response of the tissues in the posterior fundus to pre-existing disease affecting the posterior choroid and retina, such as trauma (FULLER & GITTER, 1973), granulomatous chorioretinitis, (WOODS & WAHLEN, 1960; KRILL & ARCHER, 1970), Myopia (SALZMANN, 1902; SATTLER, 1907) and angioid streaks (GASS, 1967). However, in the vast majority of cases the predisposing disease is characterised by drusen and pigment epithelial changes which may be genetically determined or the result of age alone (GASS, 1973). It has been shown histopathologically that there is progressive accumulation of abnormal material in Bruch's membrane, degeneration of the fibres within Bruch's membrane, and closure of choroidal capillaries with age (HOGAN, 1967; HOGAN, ALVARADO & WEDDELL, 1971; SARKS, 1974). The pathogenesis of these changes and their relationship to disciform response are as yet not understood, so that as yet there is no rational basis for treatment of the basic disease.

It is likely that the behaviour of the established disciform lesion is determined by the behaviour of the subretinal blood vessels; early in the disease the blood vessels grow causing the lesion to become larger, whilst in old lesions there is capillary closure and the retina may flatten (TEETERS & BIRD 1973a, b). Successful treatment of the disciform lesions depends upon destruction of the subretinal neovascular system. The results of treatment have been reported by many authors (WATZKE & SNYDER, 1968; WISE, CAMPBELL, WENDLER & RITTLER, 1968; ZWENG, LITTLE & PEABODY, 1968; JIPSON & WETZIG 1969; LITTLE, ZWENG & PEABODY, 1970; SNEIDER, 1970; CLEASBY, FUNG & FIORE, 1971; L'ESPERANCE, 1971. PATZ, MAUMENEE & RYAN, 1971a, b; GASS, 1971, 1973; SCHATZ & PATZ, 1973a b; BIRD, 1974). The results in early reports were disappointing, but in more recent series, better therapeutic results have been obtained due to more careful selection of cases for treatment and to the availability of the argon laser with slit lamp delivery system which allows more accurate placement of destructive energy. However, ignorance of the natural history of disciform lesion and of its visual prognosis make it difficult to assess the significance of these results.

The status of pigment epithelial detachments without evidence of subretinal neovascularisation in patients over 50 years old with diffuse disease of Bruch's membrane and the pigment epithelium is in doubt; GASS (1967) termed these avascular disciform lesions. TEETERS & BIRD (1973) recorded that 67% developed a vascular disciform lesion within a year in a small series of such patients. In view of SARK's findings (1973) it is likely that some of these patients have undetectable subretinal neovascularisation, and it is undeniable that others may have had variants of central serous choroidopathy with its attendent good visual prognosis. The outcome suggests that few of the latter group were included in the study of TEETERS & BIRD (1973).

It is the purpose of this paper to report the results of treatment of 172 vascular disciform lesions and to compare them with 41 disciform lesions which were deemed treatable but were not treated. An additional 53 'avascular disciform lesions' were treated.

VASCULAR DISCIFORM LESIONS

Patients

172 disciform lesions in 161 patients over the age of 50 years have been treated in the retinal unit, Moorfields Eye Hospital, and have been followed for at least six months. The average age of these patients was 64 years (range 50 to 83). In 88 of these cases there was a pre-existing disciform lesion in the other eye, and in 84 the other eye had drusen and pigment epithelial changes. In all patients the subretinal neovascular system was adequately visualised by fluorescein angiography. The lesions were treated by high intensity burns giving rise to contiguous lesions over the whole of the area of neovascularisation. The patients were then reviewed every two weeks, until the retina was flat or the lesion no longer treatable, the lesion being retreated as required. At the time of review the distance of the foveola from the edge of the neovascular tissue was assessed using a grid superimposed upon the most suitable negative on the initial fluorescein fundus angiogram. The patients were sub-divided according to the distance of the subretinal neovascular tissue from the foveola: more than 400 microns, 400 to 200 microns, 200 to 50 microns or underlying the foveola. The measurement of 200 and 400 microns were relatively accurate but at 50 microns was somewhat arbitary; the last was estimated by identifying a discernable gap between the subretinal blood vessels and foveola of about the diameter of a large retinal arteriole. Measurement was hampered, in a few cases, by difficulty in locating the fovea accurately.

The results were assessed using the maximum likelihood ratio test.

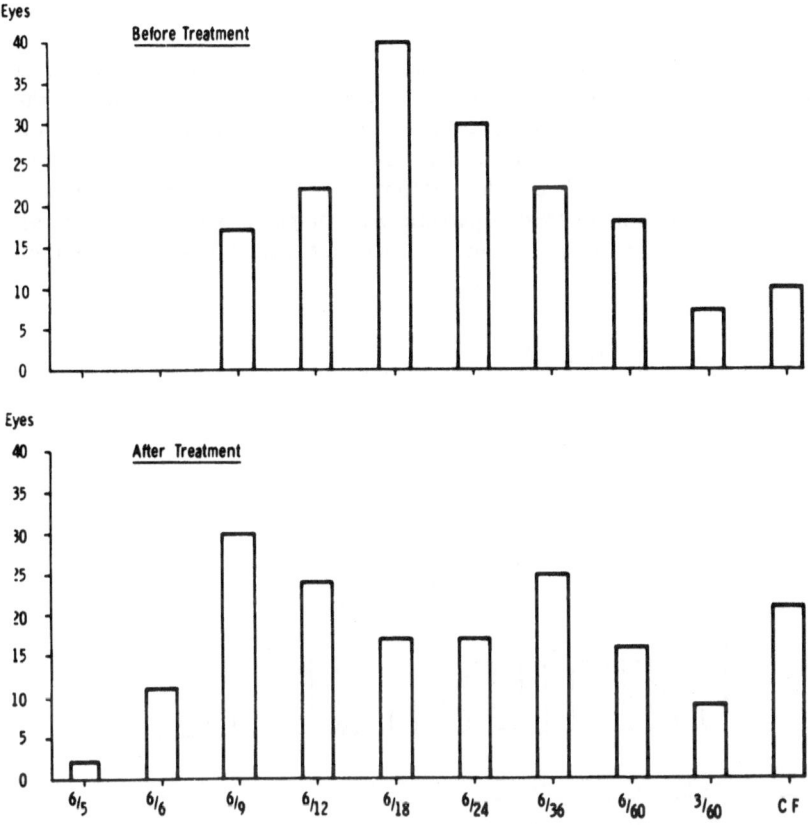

Fig. 1. The visual acuity of eyes prior to treatment compared with the visual acuity 6 months or more after treatment of vascular disciform lesions by argon laser photocoagulation.

	COMPARISON GROUP	TREATED PATIENTS		
distance of blood vessels from fovea	4	retina flat	disciform lesion	total
400 + microns	4	31	0	31
400 – 200 microns	18	46	12	58
200 -- 50 microns	19	28	13	41
less than 50 microns	0	6	36	42
	41	111	61	172

Table: This shows the distance between the subretinal new blood vessels and the fovea in the treated patients and the comparison group. It also shows the morphological outcome 6 months after treatment of the disciform lesion by argon laser photocoagulation.

Results

In 111 of the 172 lesions the retina was flattened by treatment and remained flat for six months after treatment. The success rate correlated well with the distance of the neovascular tissue from the foveola (Table). The visual outcome is shown in Fig. 1. The average visual acuity improved from 6/24 to between 6/18 and 6/24, but the difference was not statistically significant. The visual outcome of treated patients was compared with that of a group of patients deemed treatable but who were not treated, either because they

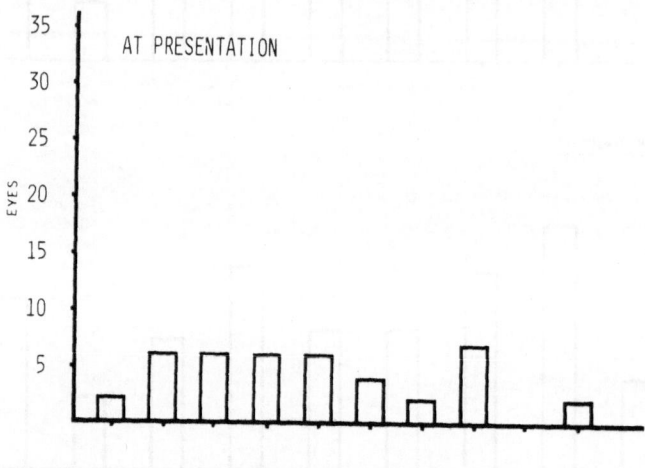

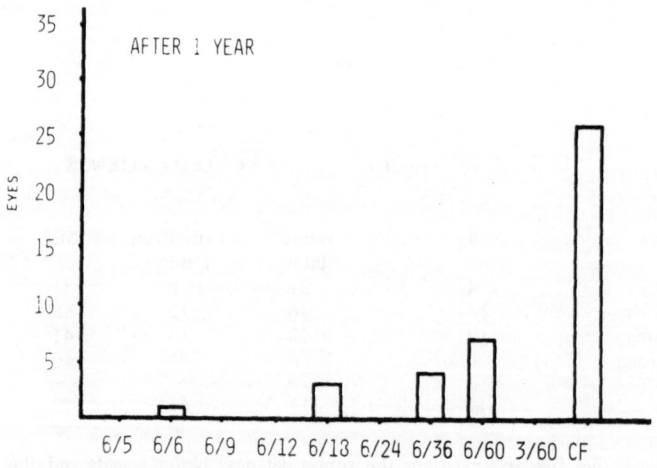

Fig. 2. The visual acuity of eyes with disciform macular lesions when initially seen and one year later which were deemed treatable at the beginning of the follow-up period but which were not treated.

were seen before the argon laser was available or because the referring ophthalmologist elected that they should not be treated. The non-treated patients were comparable in terms of age (average 65 years, range 50-82) and in terms of initial visual acuity. No patient with blood vessels nearer than 50 microns was included in the comparison group (Table). The visual outcome in the comparison group (Fig. 2) shows that the visual prognosis is poor for the disease but that some patients maintained good vision for one year.

There was a highly statistically significant difference between visual outcome of the treated against the nontreated patients (probability less than 0.001). The patients with a distance of less than 50 microns between the edge of the neovascular tissue and the foveola fared no better than the nontreated patients.

Of the 111 patients whose retina was flattened for six months, 68 have been followed for a further year and 11 (16%) developed another disciform lesion in this period. 17 have been followed for a second year and 3 (16.5%) have developed another lesion.

Comment

These results indicate that treatment of disciform degeneration by photocoagulation may be justified in well selected cases. The lack of success in treating lesions near the fovea is due, in part, to the reluctance to place intense burns near the fovea. There is also evidence that intraretinal absorption of argon laser energy occurs in the sensory retina at the fovea (MARSHALL, HAMILTON & BIRD, 1974, 1975), so that centrally it is difficult to deliver sufficient energy to the subretinal tissues.

A comparative study of this type cannot replace a stratified controlled trial, but it indicates that such a trial is justified and that the patients should be stratified on the basis of distance of the neovascular tissues from the fovea.

The recurrence rate of 16% for the first year and 16.5% for the second year differ little from the 12-15% per year occurrence of second eye involvement in patients with unilateral disciform macular degeneration.

AVASCULAR DISCIFORM LESIONS

Patients

53 avascular pigment epithelial detachments in 47 patients over the age of 50 years have been treated by argon laser photocoagulation. The average age of these patients was 61 years (range 50-74). In 16 patients there was a vascular disciform lesion in the other eye, and in six an avascular disciform lesion. In the remaining 31 there were drusen and pigment epithelial changes only, in the fellow eye. In all lesions there was even accumulation of dye in the subpigment epithelial space on fluorescein fundus angiography without evidence of subretinal neovascularisation.

The lesions were treated by an even grid of lesions over the surface of the pigment epithelial detachment avoiding the foveal area. The patients were then followed every two weeks until the lesion was flat or was untreatable, with further treatment as required.

Results

Of the 53 lesions, 48 became flat after treatment and remained flat for six months. In three it was evident soon after the initial treatment that there was subretinal neovascularisation beneath the fovea so that the lesions could not be treated further; in two of the cases the neovascular tissue was identified two weeks after treatment. In two cases there was a small pigment epithelial detachment at the fovea; in each case four burns on the edge of the lesions failed to flatten the lesion and attempts to retreat the lesion were thought unwise.

The visual outcome is shown in Fig. 3. There was an improvement in vision in the group during the period following treatment and the improvement was shown to be statistically significant (probability = 0.024).

Of the 53 lesions in which the retina was flat for six months after treatment, 36 were followed for a further year and 5 of these developed a

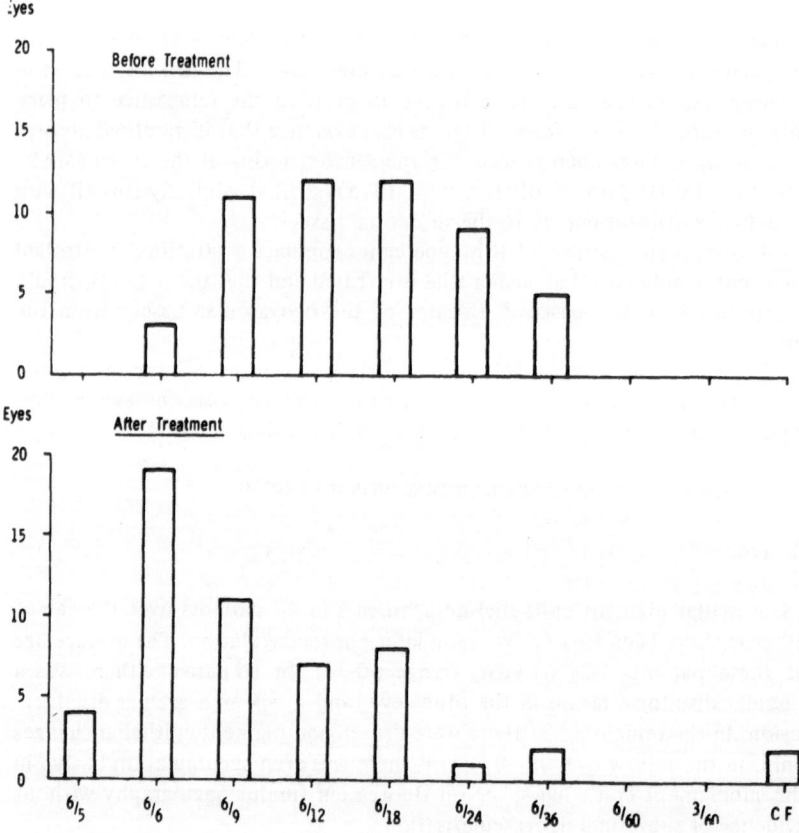

Fig. 3. The visual acuity of eyes before treatment and 6 months or more after treatment of pigment epithelial detachments by argon laser photocoagulation.

210

disciform in the eye (14%). 14 were followed for a second year and 7 for a third year and recurrence occured in one of each group (10% per year over the two years).

Comment

The results of treatment in this group compare favourably with those in vascular disciform lesions. In two of the three patients who developed a vascular disciform lesion within two weeks it seems likely that the neovascular tissue was present at the time of initial treatment but was not recognised. These results indicate that is is probably justified to treat older patients with avascular pigment epithelial detachments, but this justification would be much stronger if it were shown that such lesions were likely to develop into vascular desciform lesions with its attendent poor visual prognosis. The average age of this group is only slightly less than that for patients with vascular disciform lesions. One third of the patients had a vascular disciform lesion in the other eye, though this figure is less than in the first group. The recurrence rate is close to that which may be expected in patients with ocular disease which predisposes to vascular disciform lesions. Therefore, it may be concluded that most, if not all the patients in this group could be included within the spectrum of disciform macular disease with its relatively poor visual prognosis, and that the treatment of pigment epithelial detachments in patients over 50 years with diffuse changes in Bruch's membrane and the pigment epithelium is justified.

REFERENCES

BIRD, A.C. Treatment of senile disciform macular degeneration by photocoagulation. *Brit. J. Ophthal.* 58: *367* (1974).
CLEASBY, G.W., FUNG, W.E. & FIORE, J.V. Photocoagulation of exudative senile maculopathy. *Arch. Ophthal. (Chicago)* 85: *18* (1971).
FULLER, B. & GITTER, K.A. Traumatic choroidal rupture with late serous detachment of macula. Report of a successful argon laser treatment. *Arch. Ophthalmol.* 89: *354* (1973).
GASS, J.D.M. Pathogenesis of disciform detachment of the neuro-epithelium. General concepts and classification. *Amer. J. Ophthal.* 63: *573* (1967).
GASS, J.D.M. Photocoagulation of macular lesions. *Trans. Amer. Acad. Ophthal. Otolaryng.* 75: *580* (1971).
GASS, J.D.M. Drusen and disciform macular detachment and degeneration. *Arch. Ophthal.* 90: *206* (1973).
HOGAN, M.J. Bruch's membrane and disease of the macula. Role of elastic tissue and collagen. *Trans. Ophthal. Soc. U.K.* 87: *113* (1967).
HOGAN, M.J., ALVARADO, J. & WEDDELL, J.E. Histology of the human eye; An atlas and textbook, p. 344. Saunders, Philadelphia, 1971.
JEPSON, C.N. & WETZIG, P.C. Photocoagulation in disciform macular degeneration. *Amer. J. Ophthal.* 67: *920* (1969).
KRILL, A.E. & ARCHER, D. Choroidal neovascularisation in multifocal (premused histoplasmin) choroiditis, 84: *595* (1970).
L'ESPERANCE, F.A. Argon and ruby laser photocoagulation of disciform macular disease. *Trans. Amer. Acad. Ophthal. Otolaryng.* 75: *609* (1971).
LITTLE, H.K., ZWENG, H.C. & PEABODY, R.R. Argon laser slit lamp retinal photocoagulation. *Trans. Amer. Acad. Ophthal. Otolaryng.* 74: *85* (1970).

MARSHALL, J., HAMILTON, A.M. & BIRD, A.C. Intraretinal absorption of argon laser irradiation in human and monkey. *Experimentia* 30: *1335* (1974).

MARSHALL, J., HAMILTON, A.M. & BIRD, A.C. Histopathology of ruby and argon laser lesions in monkeys and human retina: a comparative study. *Brit. J. Ophthal.* (1975) in press.

PATZ, A., MAUMENEE. A.E. & RYAN, S.J. Argon laser photocoagulation. Advantages limitations. *Trans. Amer. Acad. Ophtal. Otolaryng.* 75: *569* (1971a).

PATZ, A., MAUMENEE, A.E. & RYAN, S.J. Argon laser photocoagulation in macular diseases. *Trans. Amer. Ophthal. Soc.* 69: *71* (1971b).

SALZMANN, M. Die atrophie der adherhaut im Kursichtigen Auge. *v. Graefe Arch. Ophthal.* 54: *337* (1902).

SARKS, S.H. New vessel formation beneath the retinal pigment epithelium in senile eyes. *Brit. J. Ophthal.* 57: *951* (1973).

SATTLER, H. The pathology and treatment of myopia. *Trans. Ophthal. Soc. U.K.* 27: *1* (1907).

SCHATZ, H. & PATZ. A. Exudative snile maculopathy. I. Results of argon laser treatment. *Arch. Ophthal. (Chicago)* 90: *183* (1973a).

SCHATZ, H. & PATZ, A. Exudative senile maculopathy. II. Complication of argon laser treatment. *Arch. Ophthal. (Chicago)* 90: *197* (1973b).

SNEIDER, R.J. Serous detachment of the macula. *Canad. J. Ophthal.* 5: *117* (1970).

SORSBY, A. The Incidence and Causes of Blindness in England and Wales, 1948-62, p. 14. Reports on Public Health and Medical Subjects, No. 114, H.M.S.O., London, 1966.

TEETERS, V.W. & BIRD, A.C. A clinical study of the vascularity of senile disciform macular degeneration. *Amer. J. Ophthal.* 75: *53* (1973a).

TEETERS, V.W. & BIRD, A.C. The development of neovascularisation of senile disciform macular degeneration. *Amer. J. Ophthal.* 76: *1* (1973b).

WATZKE, R.C. & SNYDER, W.B. Light coagulation for haemorrhagic disciform degeneration of the macula. *Trans. Amer. Acad. Ophthal. Otolaryng.* 72: *389* (1968).

WISE, G.N.. CAMPBELL. C.J., WENDLER. P.F. & RITTLER, M.C. Photocoagulation of vascular lesions of the macula. *Amer. J. Ophthal.* 66: *542* (1968).

WOODS, A.C. & WAHLEN, H.E. The probable role of benign histoplasmosis in the etiology of granulomatous uveitis. *Trans. Amer. Ophthal. Soc.* 57: *318* (1959).

ZWENG, H.C.. LITTLE, H.L. & PEABODY, R.R. Laser photocoagulation of macular lesions. *Trans. Amer. Acad. Ophthal. Otolaryng.* 72: *377* (1968).

Key words: Disciform macular degeneration, Argon laser photocoagulation.

Author's address:
Department of Clinical Ophthalmology
Institute of Ophthalmology
Moorfields Eye Hospital
City Road
London EC1V 2PD. England

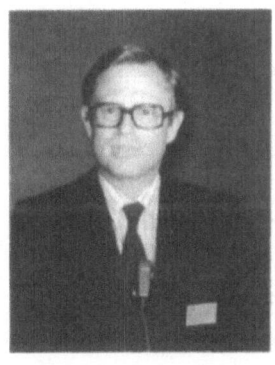

THE VALUE OF DIAGNOSTIC TESTS IN NAEVUS, MELANOMA AND HAEMANGIOMA OF THE CHOROID*

JENDO A. OOSTERHUIS, R.A. VAN DIJK & E.K.J. PAUWELS

(Leyden, The Netherlands)

Diagnostic assessment of choroidal melanoma can be extremely difficult; on histologic examination of eyes enucleated under the clinical diagnosis of a melanoma diagnostic errors have been found in the past in up to 20% of large series of eyes (FERRY, 1964; SHIELDS et al., 1973).

Nowadays quite a few diagnostic tests are available, which are a great help in establishing the proper diagnosis. Comparative evaluation of their usefulness as diagnostic tool is the subject of this study in 61 patients with the clinical diagnosis of choroidal melanoma which after enucleation was confirmed by histologic examination. Results of the following examination methods are given: ophthalmoscopy, fluorescence angiography, perimetry, diaphanoscopy, isotope uptake of phosphor ^{32} and technetium $^{99\,m}$, echography, and general examination for detection of metastatic disease and melaninuria.

1. OPHTHALMOSCOPY

Differences in ophthalmoscopic appearance between naevus, melanoma and haemangioma of the choroid are summarized in Table I.

Table I confirms the clinical findings that the ophthalmoscopic diagnosis is relatively easy in large, prominent tumours but that slightly elevated choroidal melanomas may show a great similarity in appearance with choroidal naevi which have developed secondary lesions of Bruch's membrane and retinal pigment epithelium (GASS, 1974). In these cases other examination methods are required for assessment of the diagnosis.

2. FLUORESCENCE ANGIOGRAPHY

Fluorescein-angiographic examination is a great help in establishing malignancy of pigmented choroidal tumours (OOSTERHUIS & VAN WAVEREN, 1968; GASS, 1974). Its value is discussed elsewhere in this issue (DE LAEY, p. 95).

---

* This study was part of the research programme of the Dutch Interuniversity Institute, Amsterdam.

TABLE I

OPHTHALMOSCOPIC ASPECT OF NAEVUS, MELANOMA AND HAEMANGIOMA OF THE CHOROID

Size		NEAVUS	MELANOMA	HAEMANGIOMA
	elevation	flat − 2 dioptres	any number of dioptres	variable (retinal detachment)
	diameter	up to 6 disc φ average 1.5 disc φ	variable	variable
Aspect	pigmentation	hyper/hypopigmentation	hyper/hypo-pigmentation	no or slight pigmentation; typical: orange-rose colour
	lipofuscin	-	+ (47%)ᐃ	−
	secondary lesions:			
	drusen	+ (51%)*	+	−
	dystrophy) RPE detachment	rare (6%)*	+	−
	neovascularization	rare	+	−
	retinal detachment	−	+	50%
	shape	flat	flat mushroom dome-shaped	flat
	margin	merging into normal choroidal pigm. pattern	sharp demarcation	

+ : regularly observed
− : absent or very rare
ᐃ : according to Smith and Irvine (1973)
* : according to Naumann et al. (1971)

TABLE II

VISUAL FIELD DEFECTS IN CHOROIDAL NAEVUS AND MELANOMA

Visual field defects	45 choroidal melanoma	21 choroidal melanoma with elevation up to 2 dioptres	84 choroidal naevus*
relative scotoma	13% (6)	15% (3)	23% (20)**
absolute scotoma	87% (39)	85% (18)	0

* according to Naumann et al. (1971)
** all 20 naevi were elevated; in all but one drusen and pigment-epithelial changes were present

214

3. PERIMETRY

Perimetric examination has been performed in 46 melanoma patients, with the aid of the Goldmann perimeter and the Friedmann visual field analyzer. Patients with large tumours protruding into the vitreous, in whom visual field loss could easily be assessed by hand movements and − in most of the cases − central vision was lost, were left out of the evaluation. The results are summarized in Table II.

The great diagnostic value of perimetry appears from the fact that we found an absolute scotoma in 87% of 45 melanoma patients, which contrasts highly with the absence of an absolute scotoma in choroidal naevi (NAUMANN et al., 1971). Thus, the presence of an absolute scotoma is a bad omen.

It is remarkable that in the whole group of melanomas as well as in those tumours with only a slight elevation up to 2 dioptres, the presence of an absolute scotoma was about equally frequent. As Table II shows, when a relative scotoma is found the lesion may equally ewll be a melanoma or a naevus with secondary lesions simulating a melanoma (NAUMANN et al., 1971).

The overall incidence of visual field defects in choroidal naevi in the literature up to 1967 was quoted by KARICKHOFF (1967) to be 21%; NAUMANN et al. (1971) found a figure of 23%. However, using the very sensitive Tübinger static and kinetic perimeter, FLINDALL & DRANCE (1969) found 85% relative scotomas corresponding with the site of the naevi.

4. DIAPHANOSCOPY

As a rule, transconjunctival diaphanoscopy was performed.

For diaphanoscopy of lesions at the posterior pole of the eye a fibre optics transilluminator of own design was used, which was introduced via a conjunctival incision and which at the same time was used for locating the tumour prior to the measurement of the P^{32} activity. Of the 35 patients examined, transillumination was normal in 2, diminished in 12 and extinct in 21 eyes.

Both in naevus and melanoma the light absorption greatly depended on the degree of pigmentation and, to a lesser extent, on the thickness of the tumour layer. Thus, diaphanoscopy, although useful for establishing the degree of pigmentation in tumours, is not of great value in the differentiation between naevus and melanoma. However, it has its value in special cases, e.g. for location of a pigmented tumour in a non-rhegmatogenous retinal detachment. It has a distinct diagnostic value in the choroidal haemangioma, since in these cases the light passing through the tumour has a remarkable, bright red colour and is not or only insignificantly absorbed by pigment.

5. ISOTOPE UPTAKE TESTS

Beta-ray emission was measured approximately 48 hours after intravenous

215

injection of phosphor ^{32} according to the method of HAGLER et al. (1970, 1972). Scintigraphic measurement of gammaray emission was performed after intravenous injection of technetium ^{99m} ; the technique has been described previously (VAN DIJK & OOSTERHUIS, 1974). The results of both tests are summarized in Table III.

TABLE III

RESULTS OF ISOTOPE UPTAKE TESTS IN EYES WITH CHOROIDAL MELANOMA

	Phosphor ^{32} β-emission	Technetium ^{99m} γ-emission
Number of patients	61	49
positive	96% (59)	56% (28)
negative	4% (2)	38% (18)
dubious		6% (3)

Of the 61 eyes with choroidal melanoma, confirmed on histologic examination, the P^{32} test was negative in only 2 eyes; in one eye the tumour was largely necrotic, which explains the negative outcome, the other negative result was due to incorrect localization of the tumour since a positive result was obtained when the test was repeated on the eye directly after enucleation.

The technetium ^{99m} scanning examination proved to be less reliable than the phosphor ^{32} test. This is at least partly due to the low resolution of the collimator which does not allow reliable measurements of tumours with a diameter of less than 5 millimeters. Fortunately, the prospects for a higher resolution to about 1.5 millimeters diameter of the tumour seem to be favourable.

6. ECHOGRAPHY

Our experience in this field is too limited for evaluation of this method. In very experienced hands correct echographic diagnoses in verified cases of melanomas of choroid and ciliary body rated 93.5% (VANÝSEK et al., 1971) or even 96% (OSSOINIG et al., 1975). Tumours with a prominence from the sclera of more than 1.5 mm may be differentiated by echography. On the other hand, in the clinically suspected or diagnosed melanomas the rate of 13.2% echographic borderline cases was relatively high (OSSOINING et al., 1975).

7. GENERAL EXAMINATION: METASTATIC DISEASE, MELANINURIA

A thorough general examination was carried out in all patients, especially directed to the detection of metastatic disease and the presence of melaninuria. In none of the patients abnormalities were encountered.

The results indicate that no method of examination in itself is sufficiently reliable for establishing the diagnosis of choroidal melanoma. But when the results of various methods of examination, especially ophthalmoscopy, fluorescence angiography, perimetry and phosphor [32] uptake, and also echography, are evaluated, they often fit in well together. The diagnosis of choroidal melanoma can then almost certainly be assessed or ruled out, so that the decision whether or not to perform enucleation can be taken without delay.

Haemangioma of the choroid differs from choroidal melanoma in ophthalmoscopic and fluorescein-angiographic aspect. Haemangiomas are round or oval, slightly elevated, orange-red with yellow spots on the surface. They have an indistinct margin, measure two to ten disc diameters in size and have a preference for the paramacular area. Half of the haemangiomas is associated with a serous retinal detachment (GASS, 1974). The fluorescein-angiographic aspect, which is very characteristic, will be discussed elsewhere in this issue (DE LAEY, p. 95).

On diaphanoscopy the haemangioma shows a remarkable, bright red transillumination. Isotopic examination is also a useful diagnostic aid (see Table IV).

TABLE IV

RESULTS OF ISOTOPE UPTAKE TESTS IN
7 PATIENTS WITH PRESUMED CHOROIDAL
HAEMANGIOMA

	Phosphor [32] β-emission	Technetium [99 m] γ-emission
positive	1	4
negative	6	3

Only in 1 patient with choroidal haemangioma the phosphor [32] test was positive. One year previously it was negative, but since on fluorescence angiography, performed at regular intervals, the size of the tumour appeared to increase and the pattern suggested the presence of a choroidal melanoma, the phosphor [32] test was repeated: this time it was positive and thus, unfortunately, the eye was removed. It is very probable that a technical failure, due to improper functioning of the probes, is responsible for the false positive result at the second isotope uptake examination.

In 4 of the 7 choroidal haemangiomas the technetium [99 m] scintigram was positive; the number might have been greater, had measurement at higher resolution been possible. The combination of positive scintigram and negative phosphor [32] test as found in 4 of the haemangioma patients, has not been observed in our melanoma patients, but other conditions, especially those of inflammatory origin, may give a similar result.

The diagnosis of choroidal haemangioma can further be supported by subtraction angiography of the skull, as the vascular tumour may show as a thickening of the choroid (Fig. 1) but incidentally also a choroidal melanoma may give a slight contrast on the subtraction angiogram (LOEWER-SIEGER & OOSTERHUIS, 1971; ZIEDSES DES PLANTES, 1975).

As in melanoma, also in choroidal haemangioma the results of various examinations, such as ophthalmoscopy, fluorescence angiography, isotope uptake and subtraction angiography, often fit in well together. This is of great importance, not only because thus enucleation of the eye can be avoided but also because photocoagulation treatment is indicated when a secondary retinal detachment spreads into the macular area. Fig. 2 shows a cavernous haemangioma of the choroid immediately after photocoagulation. Afterwards the retinal detachment in the macular area disappeared but visual acuity improved only from 0.4 to 0.6 owing to pigmentary dystrophy in the macular area.

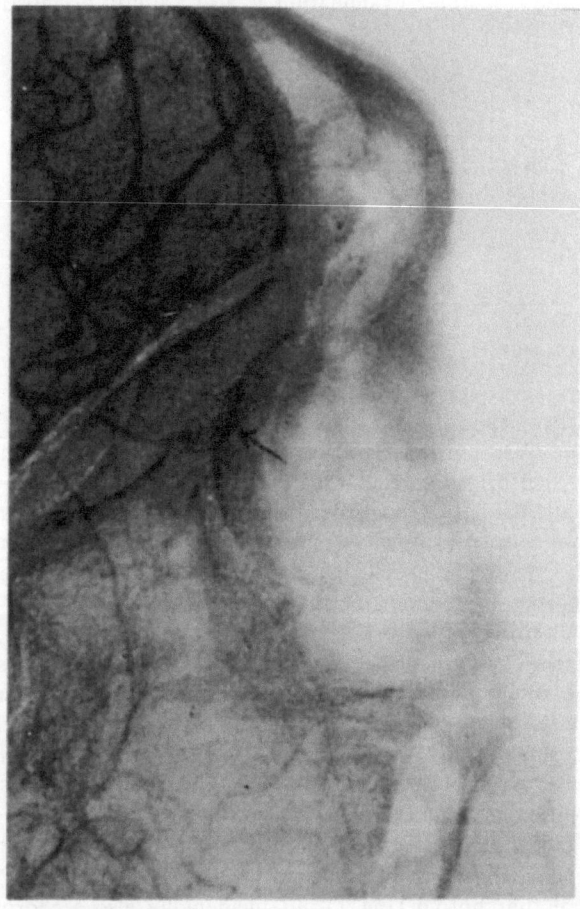

Fig. 1. Choroidal haemangioma in subtraction angiography.

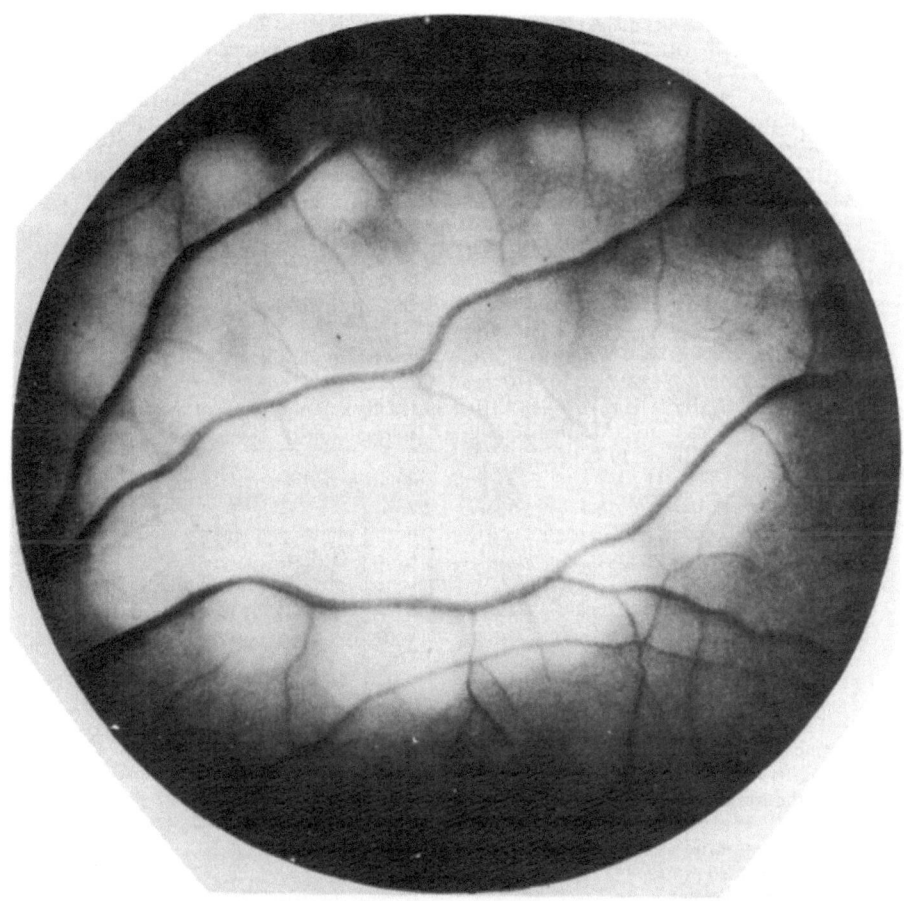

Fig. 2. Haemangioma of the choroid after photocoagulation.

SUMMARY

The value of various diagnostic tests for the differential diagnosis of naevus, melanoma and haemangioma of the choroid is discussed. Most important are: ophthalmoscopy, fluorescence angiography, perimetry, isotope uptake examination and, possibly, echography. Comparison of the results of the various tests is the best guide to the treatment required.

REFERENCES

VAN DIJK, R.A. & OOSTERHUIS, J.A. The diagnosis of intraocular tumours with the aid of radioactive phosphor. Netherl. Ophthal. Soc., 169th Meeting, Enschede, 1974, to be published in *Ophthalmologica*.

FERRY, A.P. Lesions mistaken for malignant melanoma of the posterior uvea. *Arch. Ophthal.* 72: *463-469* (1964).

FLINDALL, R.J. & DRANCE, S.M. Visual field studies of benign choroidal melanomata. *Arch. Ophthal.* 81: *41-44* (1969).

GASS, J.D.M. Differential diagnosis of intraocular tumors. Mosby, St. Louis, 1974.

HAGLER, W.S., JARRETT, W.H. & HUMPHREY, W.T. The radioactive phosphorus uptake test in diagnosis of uveal melanoma. *Arch. Ophthal.* 83: *548-557* (1970).

HAGLER, W.S., JARRETT, W.H., SCHNAUSS, R.H., LA ROSE, J.H., PALMS, J.M. & WOOD, R.E. The diagnosis of malignant melanoma of the ciliary body or choroid: use of the radio-active fosforus uptake test. *Southern Med. J.* 65: *49-59* (1972).

KARICKHOFF, J.R. Loss of visual function and visual cells in 600 cases of malignant melanoma. *Amer. J. Ophthal,* 64: *268-273* (1967).

LOEWER-SIEGER, D.H. & OOSTERHUIS, J.A. Melanoma or haemangioma of the choroid? *Ophthalmologica* 163: *32-35* (1971).

NAUMANN, G.O.H., HELLNER, K. & NAUMANN, L.R. Pigmented nevi of the choroid. Clinical study of secondary changes in the overlying tissues. *Trans. Amer. Acad. Ophthal. & Otolaryngol.* 75: *110-123* (1971).

OOSTERHUIS, J.A. & VAN WAVEREN, Ch.W. Fluorescein photography in malignant melanoma. *Ophthalmologica* 156: *101-116* (1968).

OSSOINING, K.C., BIGAR, F. & KAEFRING, S.L. Malignant melanoma of the choroid and ciliary body. In: Ultrasonography in Ophthalmology. *Bibl. ophthal.* 83: *141-154.* Karger, Basel, 1975.

SHIELDS, J.A. & ZIMMERMAN, L.E. Lesions simulating malignant melanoma of the posterior uvea. *Arch. Ophthal.* 89: *466-471* (1973).

SMITH, L.T. & IRVINE, A.R. Diagnostic significance of orange pigment accumulation over choroidal tumors. *Amer. J. Ophthal.* 76: *212-216* (1973).

VANÝSEK, J., PREISOVÁ, J. & OBRAZ, J. Ultrasonography in ophthalmology. Butterworths, London, and Czechoslovak Medical Press, Prague, 1971, p. 262.

ZIEDSES DES PLANTES, B.G. Subtraction angiography of the orbit. In: Modern Problems of Ophthalmology. Karger, Basel, 1975, pp. 74-82.

Author's address:
Departments of Ophthalmology and Radiology
University Hospital
Leyden, the Netherlands

Requests for reprints:
Prof. Dr. J.A. Oosterhuis,
Oogheelkundige Kliniek
Academisch Ziekenhuis
Leyden, The Netherlands

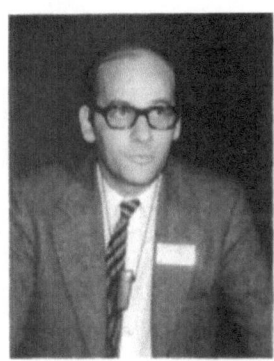

FLUORESCEIN ANGIOGRAPHIC ASPECTS
OF CHOROIDAL MELANOMAS

J.J. DE LAEY

(Ghent, Belgium)

Since MC LEAN & MAUMENEE described in 1960 the staining of choroidal haemangiomas by intravenously injected fluorescein, fluorescein angioscopy and angiography have become an essential step in the diagnosis of suspected fundus lesions. Fluorescein angiography as well as echography and the radio-active phosphorus uptake test account for a decreased incidence of eyes enucleated for lesions simulating malignant melanomas. The most important factor, however, is still careful clinical observation (SHIELDS & MC DONALD, 1974). Fluorescein angiography is perhaps of greatest value in cases of small tumours of the posterior pole when echography is useless and radioactive phosphorus uptake tests cannot be done without a surgical procedure. Even if the P 32 test is done carefully, the method is not without danger, and hemorrhages or ruptures of Bruch's membrane after the test have been reported (BURTON, 1975).

I. CHOROIDAL NAEVI

According to NAUMANN (1970) naevi are found in 11% of autopsy eyes in the choroid or in the ciliary body. Two thirds of them are situated in the posterior pole. They are probably congenital but appear only at the age of 6 to 10 when the fundus has become sufficiently pigmented. They are flat or slightly elevated, greyish with usually well defined borders (Fig. 1). Their size is variable, usually one to two disc diameter, and more than one may be found in the same eye.

Some naevi are surrounded by a halo of depigmentation (Fig. 2) but the most common associated change is the presence of drusen. In a survey of 62 choroidal naevi we found drusen in 22 cases; this correlates fairly well with the observations of HAYREH (1974). Naevi may also be associated with serous and even haemorrhagic detachment of pigment epithelium and sensory retina (GASS, 1974) (Fig. 3).

Unless an associated serous detachment involves the macular region, the patient is unaware of the lesion (Fig. 3). Naevi, however, may be the cause of relative and even absolute scotomas (NAUMANN et al., 1966). According to FLINDALL & DRANCE (1969) relative scotomas are found in 85% of cases of naevi by static perimetry.

The pigmented lesion blocks the underlying fluorescence and the lesion appears darker than the surrounding retina. If drusen are present some early

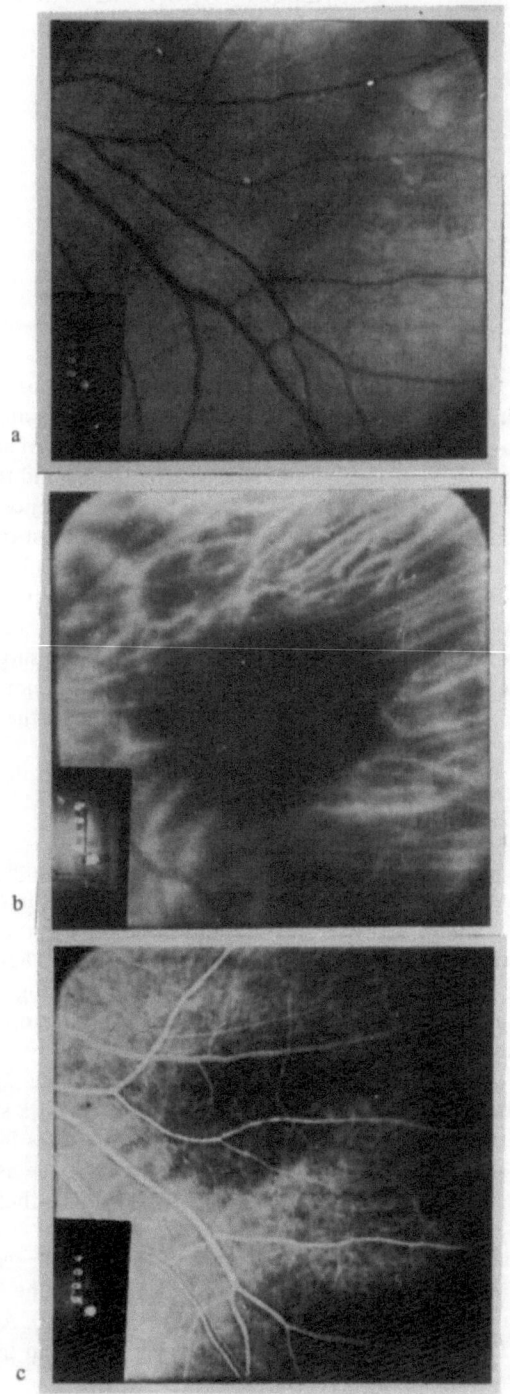

Fig. 1. Choroidal naevus. a. aspect in red-free light. b. aspect in red light. c. fluoroan-giographic aspect.

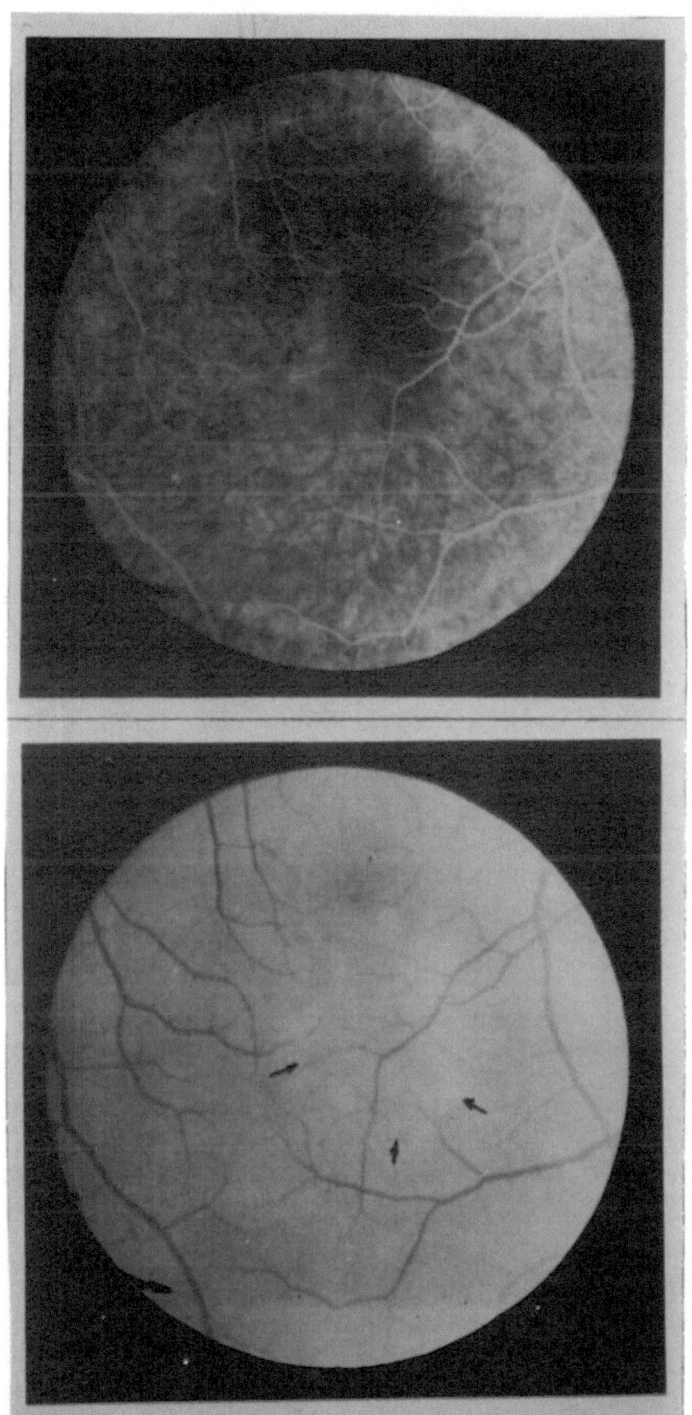

Fig. 2.   Naevus surrounded by a halo of depigmentation (arrows).

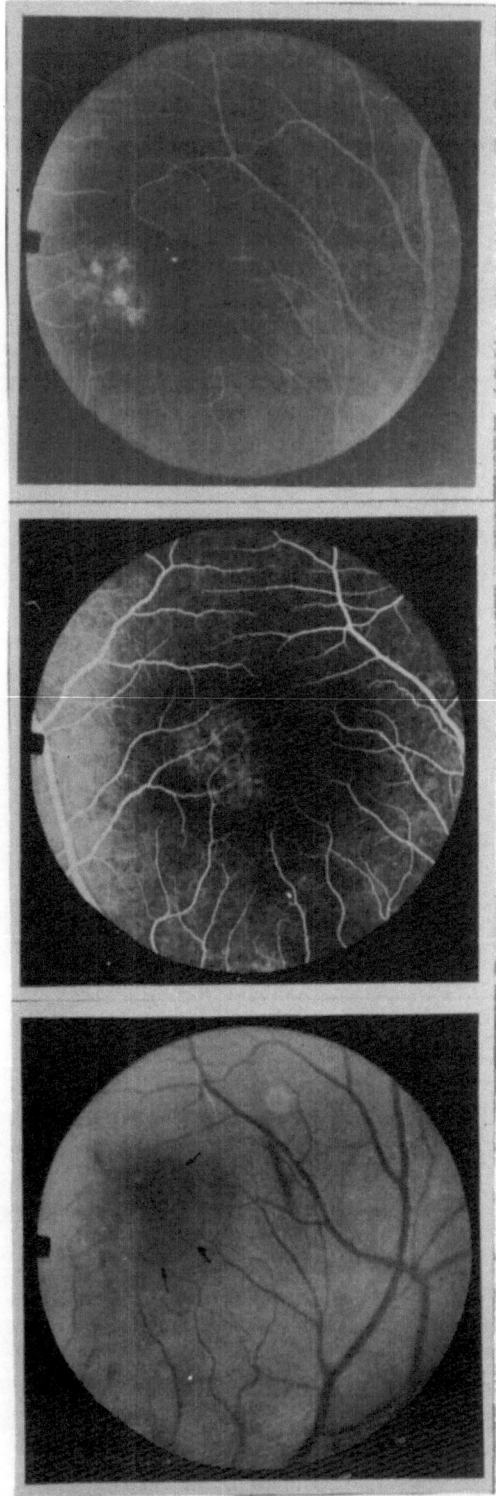

Fig. 3. Serous detachment associated with a suspected pigmented lesion (probably a naevus). Some staining at the late phase angiogram.

staining is seen at their level. Usually the limits of the lesion are better outlined by means of fluorescein angiography; the lesion appears larger than clinically suspected. More information, however, regarding the actual size of the lesion is obtained by taking fundus pictures with a red filter (Fig. 1). Fluorescein angiography and fundus pictures with red light are probably the most efficient methods for the regular follow-up of naevi.

Naevi are to be differentiated from hyperplasia of the pigment epithelium. The hyperplasias are sometimes congenital, sometimes secondary to inflammation. They are very sharply outlined and look darker than naevi. Some of them are homogeneously dark; others are unevenly pigmented and seem to have an irregular surface, surrounded by an area of depigmentation. Usually they are larger than the average naevi and their fluoroangiographic size correlates exactly with their ophthalmoscopic appearance (Fig. 4). Background fluorescence is completely blocked; retinal vessels pass undisturbed over the lesion, which has also no tendency to degenerate.

Melanocytomas are heavily pigmented tumours of the optic disc which are found usually in very pigmented individuals. However, they sometimes occur in Caucasians and we have had the opportunity to follow three cases. In one case the lesion was confined to the optic disc, whereas in the two others it extended into the nerve fiber layer (Fig. 5). One of them also had pigment epithelial changes surrounding the optic nerve. No progression was noticed during the observation period (one to three years). The diagnosis is mainly based on the typical location on the optic disc and the very heavy pigmentation. Melanocytomas are to be differentiated from malignant melanomas invading the optic disc.

II. MALIGNANT MELANOMAS OF THE CHOROID

Malignant melanomas of the choroid are most frequently found in the fifth decade but may occur at any age, even as young as 2 years (SCHEFFER et al., 1974). As is also the case for benign melanomas they are relatively more frequent in von Recklinghausen's disease (NORDMANN & BRINI, 1970).

The subjective complaints of the patients usually depend on the size and the location of the tumour. A localized reversible detachment of the macular neuroepithelium may be the first clinical sign of a small paramacular melanoma; as already mentioned, naevi as well as choroidal haemangiomas may cause the same complication.

Some authors have emphasized the diagnostic importance, especially in small flat malignant melanomas, of the accumulation of orange pigment (HAYREH, 1970, SMITH, & IRVINE, 1973). This material is probably lipofuscin contained in pigment epithelial cells or in macrophages overlying the tumour (WALLOW & TSO, 1972); it has, however, also been observed in other malignant tumours and even in naevi or localized detachments of the pigment epithelium (GASS, 1974). The presence of lipofuscin indicates a lesion of the pigment epithelium and is non-specific. Its colour varies with the colour of the lesion. Orange pigment is, however, more suggestive for a malignant melanoma (SHIELDS et al., 1974).

The fluorescein angiographic aspect of choroidal malignant melanomas depends on several different factors: 1. modifications of the pigment epithe-

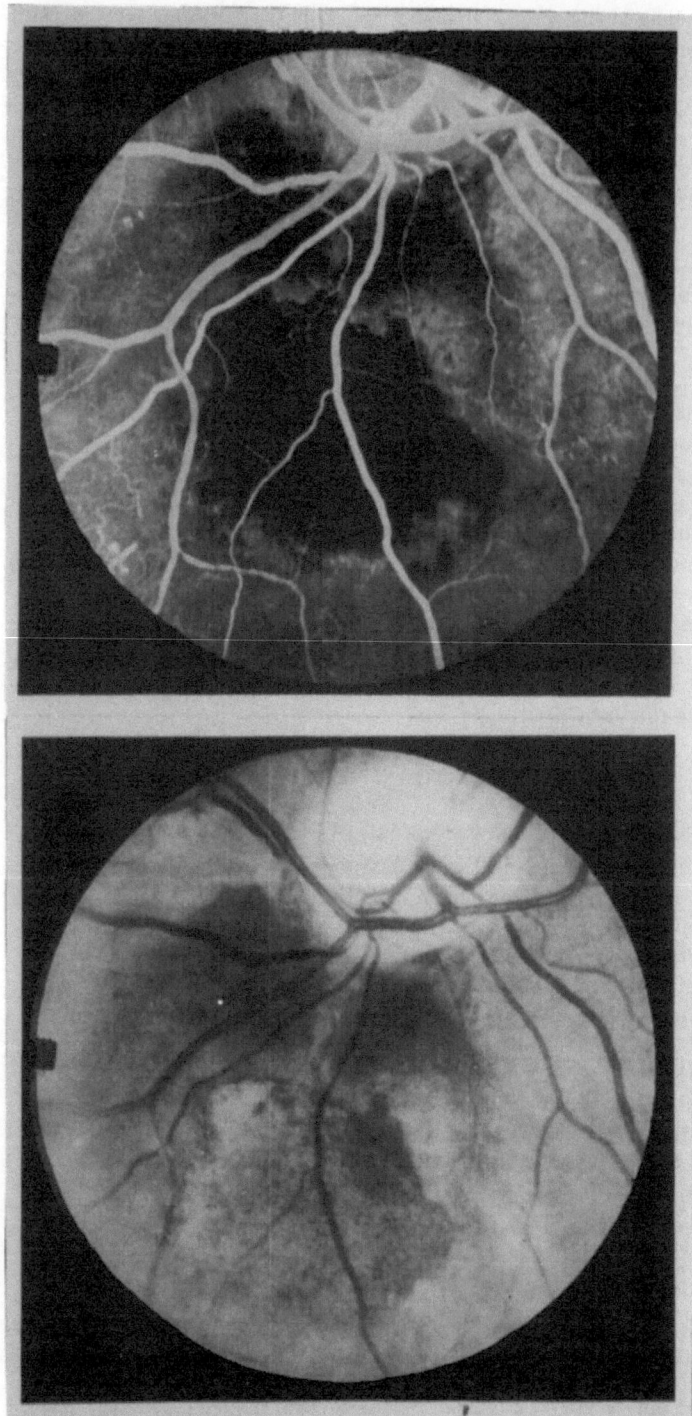

Fig. 4. Ophthalmoscopic and fluoroangiographic appearance of proliferation of the pigment epithelium.

226

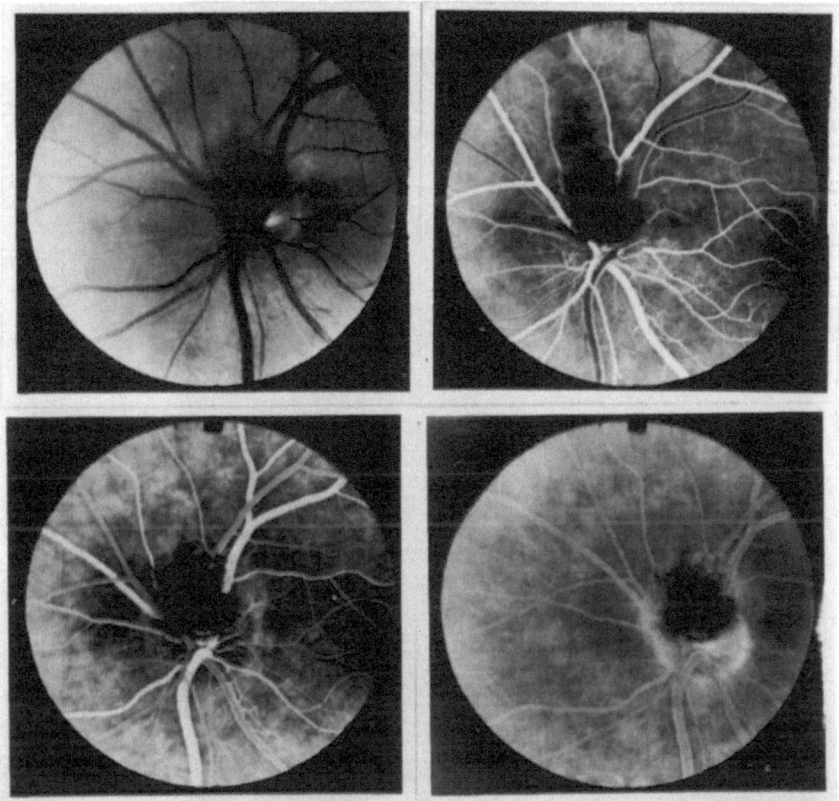

Fig. 5. Ophthalmoscopic and fluoroangiographic appearance of a melanocytoma.

lium. 2. vascularity of the tumour. 3. secondary detachment of pigment epithelium and retina. 4. ruptures in Bruch's membrane. 5. invasion of the retina and the vitreous. 6. haemorrhages.

Some melanomas fail to stain, because of massive hyperpigmentation (AMALRIC & BONNIN, 1969), because a large subsurface haemorrhage has prevented the appearance of fluorescein on the surface of the tumour (NADEL et al., 1970) or because the pigment epithelium over the tumour is still intact (SHIELDS et al., 1975).

Flat melanomas usually present an early fluorescence which does not necessarily increase in the later stages of the angiogram. Areas with orange pigment do not stain initially (Fig. 6); if they do, this is related to other secondary changes such as pigment epithelial detachments. In some cases small fluorescent dots appear in the venous time and become more obvious several minutes after injection. They are best seen at the limit of the lesion (Fig. 6). However, these dots are not characteristic for choroidal melanomas and they appear to be numerous also in metastases. We found them in about 30% of our malignant melanomas. Probably they represent small areas of elevation and destruction of the pigment epithelium (GASS, 1974;

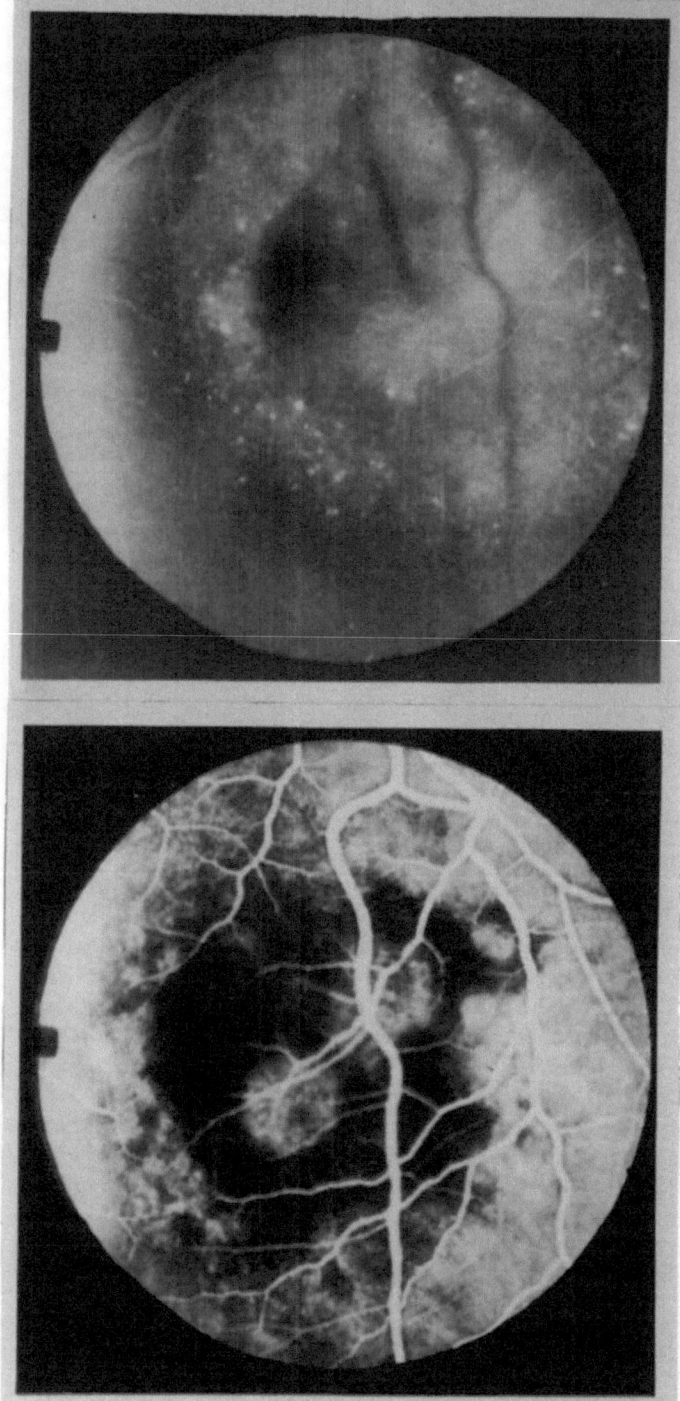

Fig. 6. Malignant melanoma. The areas of orange pigment do not stain in the early phases. 20 min after injection numerous fluorescent dots are seen especially at the limit of the lesion.

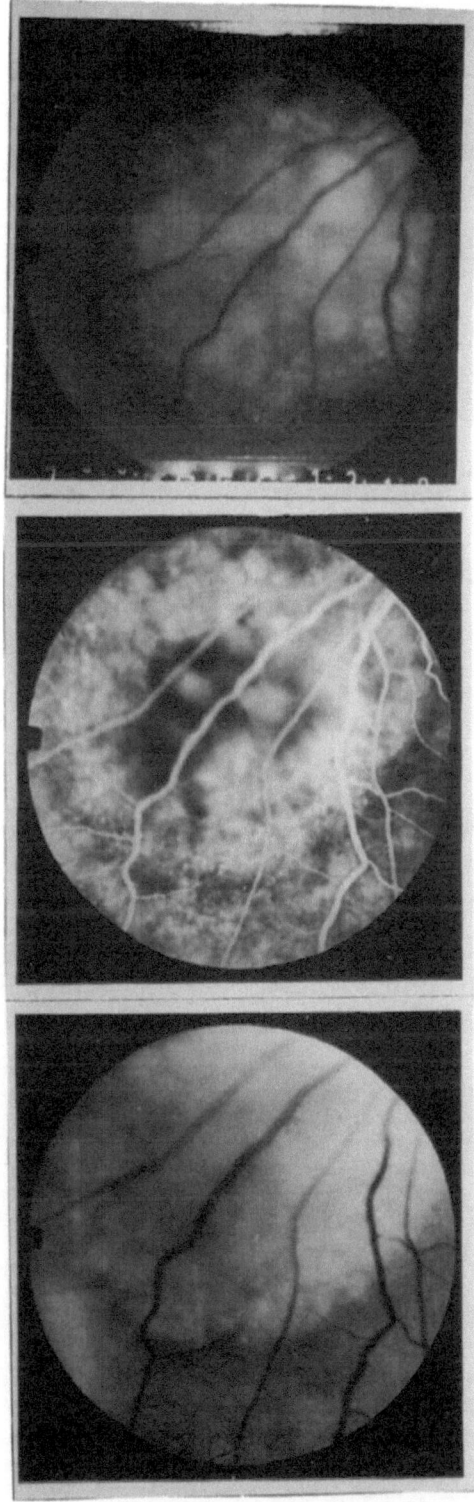

Fig. 7. Malignant melanoma. Progressive staining of the lesion.

229

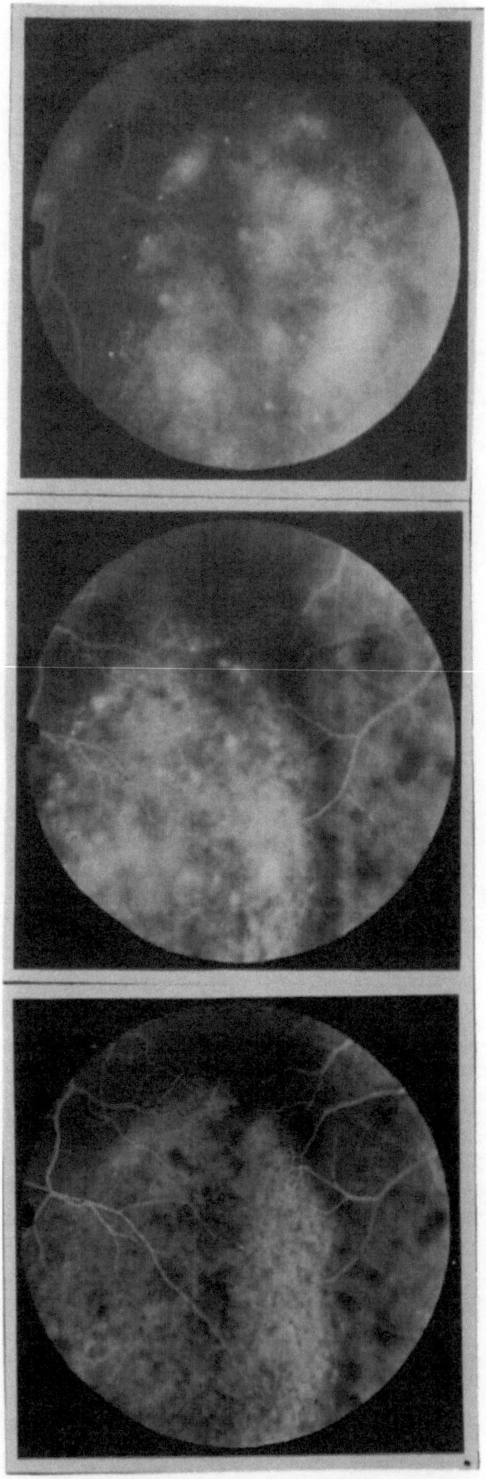

Fig. 8. Malignant melanoma with localized serous detachments.

HAYREH, 1974). Such dots are to be differentiated from drusen overlying choroidal naevi; however, they fluoresce later and much more intensely than drusen. Presence of these dots makes the diagnosis of naevus improbable.

Typically large melanomas display an early fluorescence with a mottled appearance, a progressive diffuse staining and long persistance of the fluorescence (Fig. 7). Localized pigment epithial detachments may be found. (Fig. 8) In elevated tumours the retinal capillaries appear dilated over the tumour. Signs of retinal perivasculitis may even been observed.

The tumour's own blood supply (so-called 'double circulation') can only be seen in large tumours when Bruch's membrane has been perforated (EDWARDS et al., 1969; HAYREH, 1974) (Fig. 9). Strangulation of the blood supply by the edge of the hole in Bruch's membrane may cause extensive congestion of the blood vessels in the tumour (WOLTER et al., 1973).

Late diffusion of the dye into the vitreous indicates perforation of the retina and invasion of the vitreous.

Circumpapillary extension of a malignant melanoma may cause papilledema.

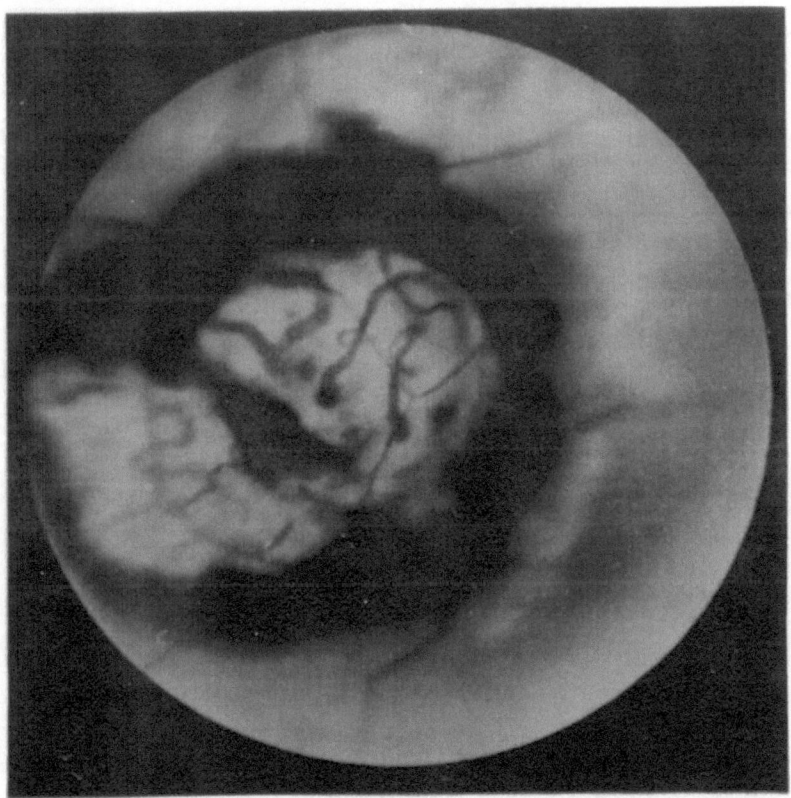

Fig. 9. So called 'double circulation' after rupture of Bruch's membrane. a. ophthalmoscopic appearance. b. fluoroangiography.

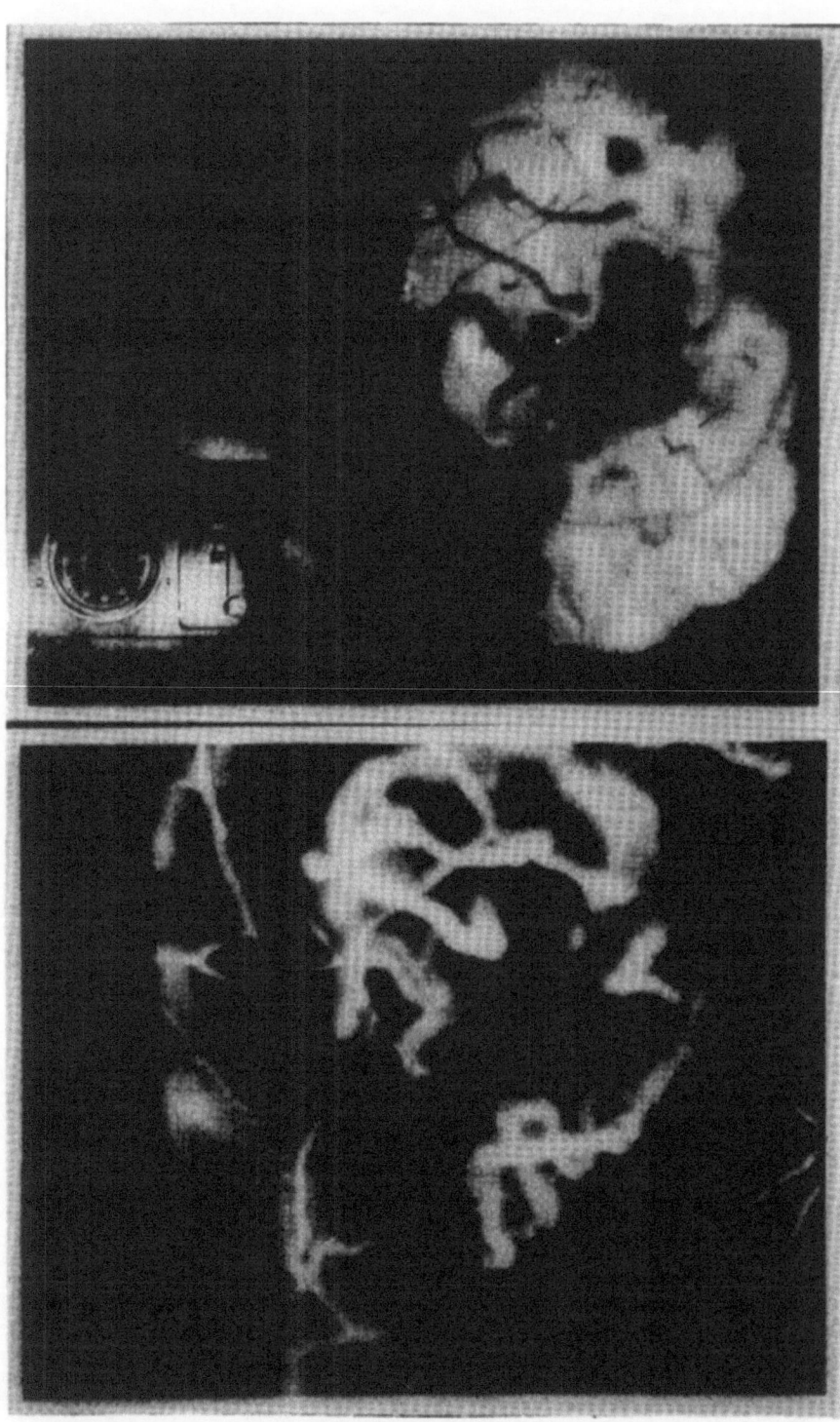

Fig. 9b.

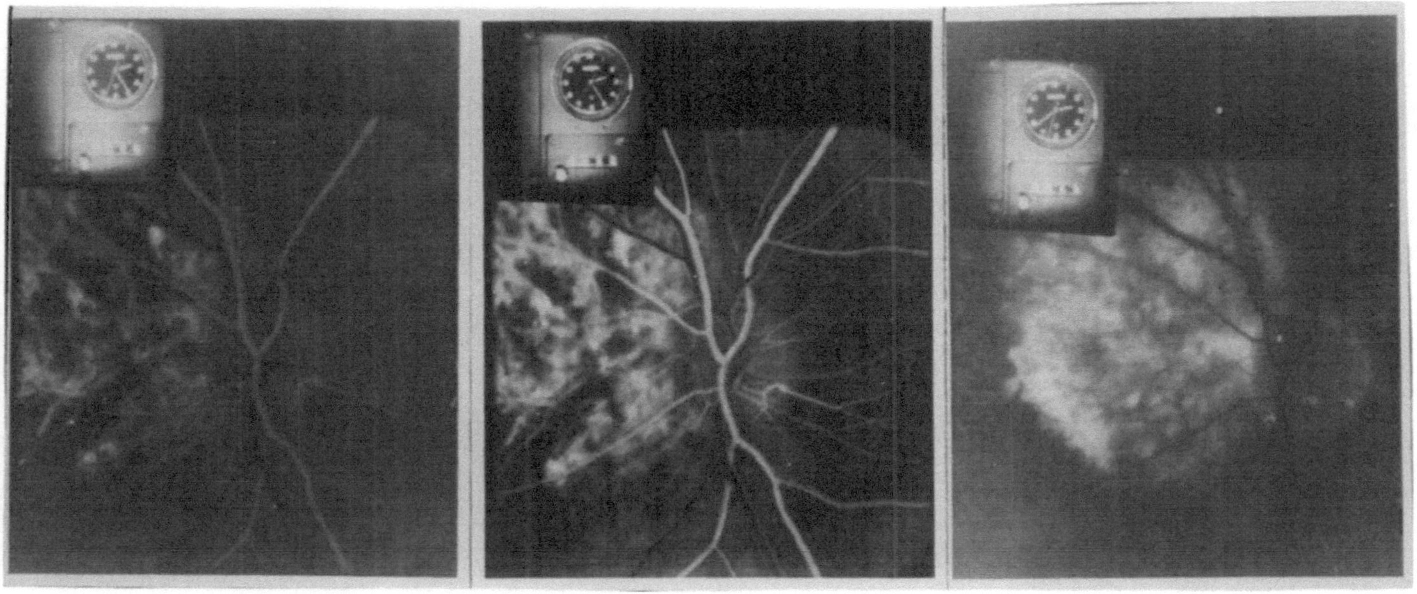

Fig. 10.   Haemangioma of the choroid.

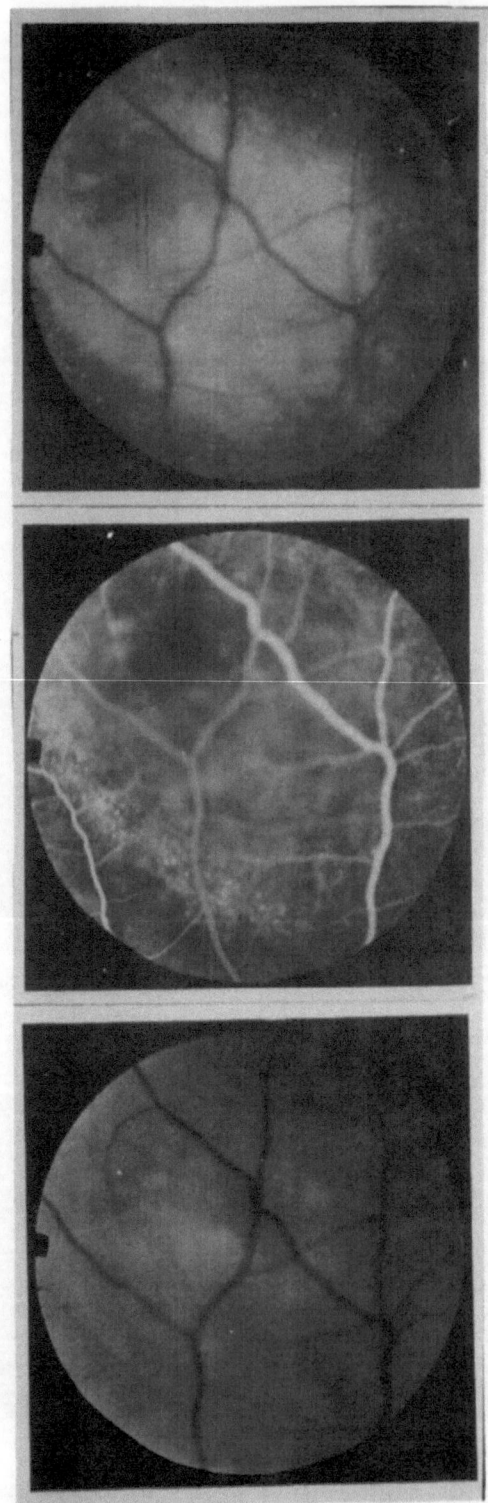

Fig. 11. Metastatic carcinoma of the choroid. Small fluorescent dots at the limit of the lesion. Aspect very similar to that of the malignant melanoma of Fig. 7.

Several lesions may be mistaken for malignant melanomas: most commonly this may be the case with choroidal naevi, metastatic tumours, choroidal haemangiomas, but sometimes also with subretinal haemorrhages, disciform macular degeneration or rhegmatogenous retinal detachment.

Although a typical early vascular pattern has been described in choroidal haemangiomas (WESSING, 1968; GASS, 1974), fluoangiographic differentiation with amelanotic melanomas is not always possible (Fig. 10). The diagnosis will depend on the clinical appearance, the negative P 32 test, the echography and the very slow progression.

Fluorescein angiography as well as the other diagnostic procedures is of questionable value in differentiating metastatic tumours from malignant melanomas. Small fluorescent dots at the limits of the lesion are perhaps more frequently found in choroidal metastases. (Fig. 11)

Fluorescein angiography, however, may be of great help in other suspected lesions. The peculiar fluorescein pattern of disciform macular degeneration or the absence of pathological staining in non-exsudative retinal detachment are important diagnostic signs. Differentiation between naevi and small melanomas may sometimes be difficult. The clinical appearance may be dubious; the value of perimetry is only very relative, as scotomas are no proof of malignancy. If the other diagnostic procedures, such as echography or P 32 uptake test also fail, (which is most likely to happen in cases of small tumours), the wisest thing to do is to closely watch the progression of the lesion, with the aid of fundus photography and fluorescein angiography. A malignant melanoma of the choroid is indeed not a surgical emergency (ZIMMERMAN, 1973). The small malignant melanomas measuring less than 5 disc diameters carry a favourable prognosis (FLOCKS et al., 1955), which thus allows some observation time. In fact, the size of the tumour seems more important regarding the prognosis than the cell type when only small melanomas are considered (DAVIDORF and LANG, 1974).

SUMMARY

Various clinical and fluoroangiographic aspects of naevi and melanomas of the choroid are discussed. Even though it is not always possible to differentiate with fluorescein angiography the different choroidal tumours, this method provides a number of informations regarding size and vascularity of the tumour and its influence on overlying structures. It is thus of primary importance in the follow-up of suspected lesions.

REFERENCES

AMALRIC, P. & BONNIN, P. L'angiographie fluorescéinique. *Bull. Soc. Ophthal. France.* Numéro spécial: *217-340* (1969).

BURTON, T.C. Iatrogenic breaks in Bruch's membrane in choroidal melanoma. *Trans. Amer. Acad. Ophthal. Otolaryng.*, in press.

DAVIDORF, F.H. & LANG, J.R. Small malignant melanomas of the choroid. *Amer. J. Ophthal.* 78: *788-793* (1974).

EDWARDS, W.C., LAYDEN, W.E. & MC DONALD, R. JR. Fluorescein angiography of malignant melanoma of the choroid. *Amer. J. Ophthal.* 68: *797-808* (1969).

235

FLINDALL, R.J. & DRANCE, S.M. Visual field studies of benign melanomata. *Arch. Ophthal. (Chicago)* 81: *41-44* (1969).
FLOCKS, M., GERENDE, J.H. & ZIMMERMAN, L.E. Size and shape of malignant melanomas of the choroid and ciliary body in relation to prognosis and histologic characteristics (a statistical study of 210 tumors). *Trans. Amer. Acad. Ophthal. Otolaryng.* 59: *740-758* (1955).
GASS, J.D. Differential diagnosis of intraocular tumors. A stereoscopic presentation. Ed. C.V. Mosby St. Louis, 1974.
HAYREH, S.S. Choroidal melanomata. Fluorescein angiographic and histopathological study. *Brit. J. Ophthal.* 54: *145-160* (1970).
HAYREH, S.S. Choroidal tumors: role of fluorescein angiography in diagnosis. In: Blodi F.C.: Current concepts in ophthalmology. Vol. IV. Ed. C.V. Mosby, St. Louis, 168-201, 1974.
MACLEAN, A.L. & MAUMENEE, A.E. Hemangioma of the choroid. *Amer. J. Ophthal.* 50: *3-11* (1960).
NADEL, A., O'CONNOR, P. & LINCOFF, H. Non fluorescent choroidal melanoma. *Amer. J. Ophthal.* 70: *748-752* (1970).
NAUMANN, G.O. Pigmentierte Naevi der Aderhaut und des Ziliarköpers. *Fortschr. Med.* 88: *334-336* (1970).
NAUMANN, G.O., HELLNER, K. & NAUMANN, L.R. Pigmented nevi of the choroid; clinical study of secondary changes in the overlying tissue. *Trans. Amer. Acad. Ophthal. Otolaryng.* 75: *110-123* (1971).
NAUMANN, G., ZIMMERMAN, L.E. & YANOFF, M. Visual field defect associated with choroidal nevus. *Amer. J. Ophthal.* 62: *914-917* (1966).
NORDMANN, J. & BRINI, A. Von Recklinghausen's disease and melanoma of the uvea. *Brit. J. Ophthal.* 54: *641-648* (1970).
OOSTERHUIS, J.A. & VAN WAVEREN, C.W. Fluorescein photography in malignant melanoma. *Ophthalmologica* 156: *101-116* (1968).
SCHEFFER, C.H., BINKHORST, P.G. & HAMBURG, A. Malignant melanoma of the choroid in a 2 year old infant. *Ophthalmologica* 169: *401-411* (1974).
SHIELDS, J.A., ANNESLEY, W.H. & TOTINO, J.A. Non fluorescent malignant of the choroid diagnosed with the radiactive phosphorus uptake test. *Amer. J. Ophthal.* 79: *634-640* (1975).
SHIELDS, J.A. & MAC DONALD, P.R. Improvement in the diagnosis of posterior uveal melanomas. *Arch. Ophthal. (Chicago)* 91: *259-264* (1974).
SHIELDS, J.A., RODRIGUES, M.M., SARIN, L.K., TASMAN, W.S. & ANNESLEY, W.H. JR Lipofuscin pigment over benign and malignant choroidal tumors. *Trans. Amer. Acad. Ophthal. Otolaryng.*, in press.
SMITH, L.T. & IRVINE, A.R. Diagnostic significance of orange pigment accumulation over choroidal tumors. *Amer. J. Ophthal.* 76: *212-216* (1973).
WALLOW, I.H.L. & TSO, M.O.M. Proliferation of the retinal pigment epithelium over malignant choroidal tumor. *Amer. J. Ophthal.* 73: *914-925* (1972).
WESSING, A. Fluoreszenzangiographie der Retina. Lehrbuch und Atlas. Ed. Georg Thieme, Stuttgart, 143-166, 1968.
WOLTER, J.R., SCHUT, A.L. & MARTONY, C.L. Hemangioma-like clinical appearance of a collar-button melanoma caused by the strangulation effect of Bruch's membrane. *Amer. J. Ophthal.* 76: *730-733* (1973).
ZIMMERMAN, L.E. Problems in the diagnosis of malignant melanomas of the choroid and ciliary body. *Amer. J. Ophthal.* 75: *917-929* (1973).

Key words: Fluorescein angiography, Choroidal naevus, Malignant melanoma of the choroid.

Author's address:
Department of Ophthalmology (Dir. Prof. Dr. J. François)
University of Ghent
de Pintelaan 135
Ghent, Belgium

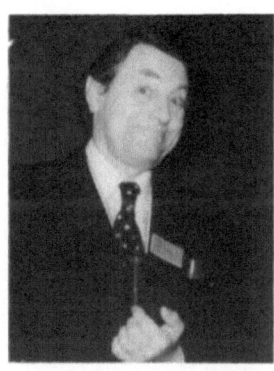

TECHNIQUES FOR THE LOCAL EXCISION
OF CHOROIDAL MELANOMAS

WALLACE S. FOULDS

(Glasgow, United Kingdom)

During the past seven years I have been exploring the feasibility and justifiability of excising locally primary tumours of the choroid and also large tumours of the ciliary body affecting the choroid secondarily by direct spread. Since SCHUBERT, in 1925, reported the removal of a leuco-sarcoma of the uvea with preservation of the eye, there have been sporadic reports mostly of single cases of choroidal tumours treated by local excision (STALLARD 1961, 1966, ALGAN et al, 1967, HAYE, 1968, FYODOROV, 1972; FOULDS, 1973). In recent years various techniques for full thickness eye wall resection have been investigated in experimental animals and in humans by PEYMAN and collaborators (PEYMAN & DODICH, 1972; PEYMAN et al, 1972, 1973, 1974).

In general techniques available for the exposure and excision of choroidal tumours have been developed from those used for partial cyclectomy with modifications necessitated by the more difficult access, the tendency of the incised choroid to bleed during or after the operation and the likelihood of collapse of the globe with gross vitreous loss associated with the extensive scleral opening required to clear the edges of the tumour.

LOCALISATION OF TUMOUR

Careful localisation and estimation of the size of the tumour is a necessary prerequisite to successful local excision. Localisation of the tumour preoperatively is made by binocular indirect ophthalmoscopy, threemirror slit lamp examination and B-scan ultrasonography. At the time of operation further localisation by trans-illumination is useful.

Access to tumours situated in the temporal choroid is easier than to those situated nasaly. Tumours in the inferior or superior choroid are more difficult of access than those affecting the temporal or nasal sectors. For tumours involving both ciliary body and choroid, raised intraocular pressure or visible involvement of more than 10 millimetres of the circumference of the angle of the anterior chamber are absolute contra-indications to local excision. Apart from involvement of the angle of the anterior chamber, the maximum size of tumours of the choroid, with or without ciliary body involvement which can be successfully resected is probably 12 millimetres in greatest diameter, although on occasion tumours of 13 or 14 millimetres diameter have been successfully tackled. Where local resection of such a large tumour is attempted the operation may have to be abandoned and enucleation of the eye performed because difficulty of access has made complete clearance of the tumour doubtful.

SURGICAL EXPOSURE

In early cases the author used a cruciate full thickness scleral incision centred over the choroidal mass allowing the development of four triangular flaps which could be enlarged until adequate exposure was obtained. Where the scleral incision indicated the likelihood of scleral involvement in the neoplasia, the flaps were excised and the defect made good by a full thickness hand cut scleral homo-transplant.

Later the initial technique was modified by substitution of lamellar dissection of the flaps with excision of the deep scleral lamella prior to dissection of the choroidal tumour if no adhesion was present between the sclera and the choroidal tumour or removal together with the tumour after dissection of the latter if scleral adherence was found. Currently a single large lamellar scleral flap, either limbus or fornix based, is used. With limbus based flaps the incisions are carried around the limbus on either side to improve the exposure. Where there is evidence of scleral penetration by the tumour a full thickness dissection is performed and the defect made good with a cadaver scleral homo-transplant.

The use of some support for the edges of the scleral opening has been variable but having rejected the use of a Flieringa ring after the first few cases (FOULDS, 1973) this device is now routinely used. It is carefully sutured to the sclera with multiple sutures so that its centre is concentric with the apex of the tumour. This may mean that the anterior edge of the ring passes across the cornea. In these cases it is sutured carefully at the limbus on either side. The use of a modified scleral support encompassing the limbus and extending posteriorly around the operation site may have much to commend it.

CHOROIDAL DISSECTION

When sufficient choroidal exposure has been obtained the choroidal tumour is usually easy to identify often having a distinctly lighter colour than the surrounding unaffected choroid. Indeed many melanomas of the choroid have a yellow or pinkish appearance when viewed from the scleral aspect.

Incision of unaffected choroid some 3-4 millimetres from the edge of the tumour is made with Vannas scissors and incision carried round the tumour under careful microscopic control. Bleeding from the incised choroid can be completely controlled by adequate hypotensive anaesthesia. Adequate anaesthesia with controlled hypotension is in the author's opinion a necessary prerequisite for this type of surgery.

Where possible the retina is left intact, the choroid containing the tumour stripping easily from the outer retinal aspect. Retinal involvement by choroidal melanomas of a size suitable for local resection seems to be very rare and when it occurs necessitates retinal resection also.

The usefulness of preoperative circumvallation with diathermy (STAL-

LARD, 1966) or photocoagulation or cryotherapy is debatable. None of these methods is required for haemostasis during surgery and all make it impossible to separate the choroid from the underlying retina. The usefulness of cryo-therapy applied at the time of surgery is currently being evaluated, particularly in those cases in which the retina is breached. In such cases a localised vitrectomy may help to avoid post-operative traction and retinal detachment, the latter complication occurring in a proportion of cases from organised haemorrhage occurring post-operatively or from inflammatory exudate.

RESULTS

To date local excision of choroidal tumours has been attempted in 14 cases. In two of the 14 the operations were abandoned at the time and enucleation performed. In one other case the affected eye was removed $1\frac{1}{2}$ years after local excision because of persisting low grade uveitis. In the other 11 cases the affected eye has been retained and in 4 the visual acuity is better than 6/12. In the remaining 7 cases visual acuity ranges from perception of light to 6/36. Of the 11 cases in which the tumour was successfully resected 6 developed cataract: in 3 of these good vision (6/12 or better) has been restored by subsequent cataract extraction. Of the remaining 3, 2 are awaiting cataract surgery and in the other, projection is poor probably from retinal detachment which has been confirmed by ultrasonography. In all, 3 patients developed retinal detachment and in one this was successfully treated by surgery, the patient retaining 6/12 vision with an aphakic correction.

The longest follow up is $7\frac{1}{2}$ years and the shortest 2 months. There have been no deaths from metastases nor any case with a local recurrence.

This paper is a preliminary report of the author's own experience of techniques used for the local excision of choroidal tumours. The difficult question of whether such surgery is justified and the selection of cases suited for what is an experimental form of therapy will be dealt with in another paper.

ACKNOWLEDGEMENTS

I wish to acknowledge my debt to the ophthalmologists in the West of Scotland who referred their cases to me.

REFERENCES

ALGAN, B., R. MIRGUET & F. MARTINELLE A propos d'un cas de choroidectomie partielle traitement conservateur d'un choriodoblastoma. *Bull. Soc. Ophthal. Fr.* 67: *944* (1967).
FOULDS, W.S. The local excision of choroidal melanomata. *Trans. Ophthal. Soc. U.K.* 93: *343* (1973).
FYODOROV, S.N. The ablation of a choroidal melanoma. *Ann. Ophthalmol.* 4: *510* (1972).

239

HAYE, C. Traitement chirurgical et radiothérapique des sarcomes de la choroide. *Arch. Ophthalmol.* 28: *873* (1968).

PEYMAN, G.A. & N.A. DODICH Full-thickness eye wall resection: An experimental approach for treatment of choroidal melanoma I. Dacron-graft. *Invest. Ophthal.* 11: *115* (1972).

PEYMAN, G.A. MAY, D.R., ERICSON, E.S. & M.F. GOLDBERG Full thickness eye wall resection: An experimental approach for treatment of choroidal melanoma. II. Homo- and hetero-graft. *Invest. Ophthal.* 11: *668* (1972).

PEYMAN, G.A., ERICSON, E.S. A.J. AXELROD & D.R. MAY Full thickness eye wall resection in primates. An experimental approach to treatment of choroidal melanoma. *Arch. Ophthalmol.* 89: *410* (1973).

PEYMAN, G.A., AXELROD, A.J. & GRAHAM, R.O. Full-thickness eye wall resection. An experimental approach for treatment of choroidal melanoma: Evaluation of cryotherapy, diathermy and photocoagulation. *Arch. Ophthalmol.* 91: *219* 1974).

STALLARD, H.B. Pigmented tumors of the eye. *Proc. R. Soc. Med.* 54: *463* (1961).

STALLARD, H.B. Partial choroidectomy. *Brit. J. Ophthal.* 50: *660* (1966).

Authors' address
Tennent Institute of Ophthalmology
University of Glasgow
Western Infirmary
Glasgow, United Kingdom

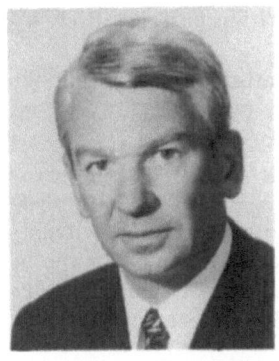

SURGICAL TREATMENT OF MALIGNANT TUMORS IN THE ANTERIOR SEGMENT OF THE EYE

T.N. WAUBKE

(Essen, Germany)

This paper reports on our indications for and operations of malignant tumors in the anterior segment of the eye.

Most of the tumors in this part of the eye are pigmented. In the past, the growth of pigmented tumors in the anterior segment seemed to be a sign of great malignancy as in cases of skin melanomas. Therefore, an extensive operation was held to be necessary: enucleation or even exenteration of the orbit.

This has changed completely during the last two decades. We try more and more -- even in cases of large tumors -- to conserve the bulbus. This has several reasons.

The main one is that the pathologists encouraged us to do so because their knowledge of malignant tumors has increased remarkably. This work is above all done by Lorenz ZIMMERMAN and his coworkers in Washington.

From our point of view the report of PAUL, PARNELL & FRAKER (1962) is especially important. They examined 2652 malignant melanomas of the choroid and ciliary body and found out the survival rates.

After 15 years 81.2% of the patients with melanomas of spindle cell type A were still alive and 73.6% of spindle cell type B; in cases of mixed and necrotic tumors the survival rate was 40.6%, in epithelioid cell type tumors 28.0%.

For our considerations it is important that in the anterior segment in most cases malignant tumors are of the spindle cell type A, not so often of spindle cell type B. The mixed and epithelioid types are observed rarely. In the posterior part of the eye it is exactly the other way around.

So from the point of the pathologist the operation of malignant tumors in the anterior segment of the eye seems to be justified.

Clinically, microsurgical progress allows very exact operations up to 40 times magnification. The technique of lamellar keratoplasty has improved and combined grafts of cornea and sclera are now a common technique.

In spite of these two essential points − histological findings and clinical possibilities − the indication for an operation has to be very strict.

Three points are important:

1. Growth of tumor must be proved either by reliable observations of the patient or continuous control by the doctor.

2. A total extirpation of the tumor must be possible.

3. It must be possible to control the area of operation postoperatively by biomicroscopy.

These essentials are important in order to get satisfying results with our treatment.

CONJUNCTIVA

In the conjunctiva we know two types of melanosis: diffuse and circumscribed. If no growth is observed there is no indication for an operation. In the conjunctiva we do not find the typical types of tumor cells such as in the iris and in the choroid. Therefore, it is very often difficult to distinguish between a benign and a malignant lesion.

If growth of the pigmentation has become obvious, the melanoma has to be extirpated and to be covered by conjunctiva. Normally this is easy in cases of circumscribed melanomas, but sometimes, if a melanoma grows diffusely, it may be very difficult, and a conjunctival graft from the second eye or with cadaver conjunctiva is necessary.

It is very important not to miss the right time of operation because local metastasis can be seen very often. Sometimes we observe massive tumor growth in the lids and in such cases an exenteration of the orbit is the only thing that can be done.

One should always think of the possibility of local or contact metastasis. This may cover a long time after removal of the primary tumor. We discovered metastasis in the lid as long as 7 years after operation of the primary tumor in the conjunctiva. The longest interval that has been described is even 28 years.

CONJUNCTIVA – CORNEA

If conjunctiva and cornea are affected by a tumor the operation will be much more complicated. Formerly the tumor part in the cornea was cauterised and then covered by conjunctiva. Today we extirpate the tumor completely and cover the corneal defect with a lamellar graft, and if necessary with a scleral part. Sometimes a tumor can be removed by normal trephining and the ensuing defect can be covered with a corresponding graft. The conjunctival excision has to be closed by a conjunctival graft.

However, in most cases the tumor growth is irregular. If we do not want to remove too much normal tissue, special techniques are necessary.

A scheme shows the various possibilities (Fig. 1). On the left the extent of a necessary extirpation can be seen. After having measured the line a, b and d we can cut out a metallic folia to find the right size of the graft. Such a folia is shown in the middle of the picture.

Because of the convexity of the cornea the preparation is sometimes very difficult. It is much easier to cut along a straight line. Therefore, we measure only the distance c and cut in the first step the whole segment of the donor's eye. In the second step we measure the distance a and d and cut along the line b. So it is possible to take the whole segment, to fix it in the operation field along the line a and then to cut off as much as necessary.

This technique proved to be succesful in several cases. It is particularly

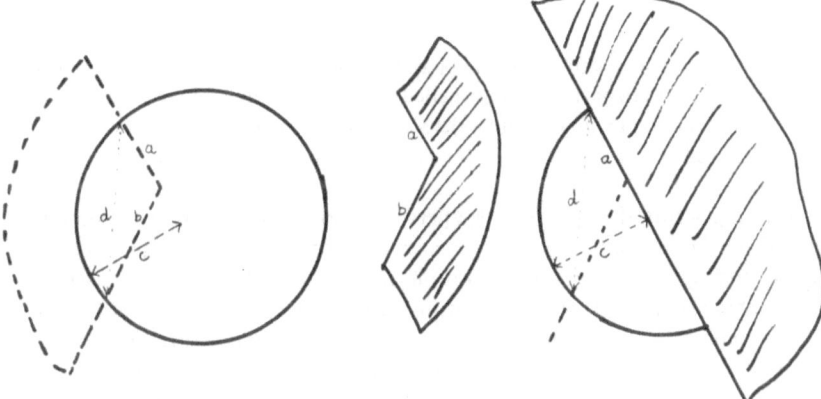

Fig. 1.

indicated in cases of recurrency that may often occur after many years. Sometimes very large grafts are necessary. In a case of a third recurrency of a melanoma of the conjunctiva and the cornea we used a graft of the half of the cornea with a wide scleral part. The visual results are mostly very satisfactory. In the above mentioned case the postoperative visual acuity was 0.9.

The prognosis of a growing diffuse melanosis of the conjunctiva is much worse. As an example I want to describe one particular case. A young patient of our clinic suffered from a malignant melanosis and she was operated 3 times, at last with a combined graft. In spite of this treatment large recurrency of a non pigmented tumor was seen. X-ray treatment was done in London by Dr. LEDERMAN. 4 months later a small tumor was extirpated again. 6 months later we saw no sign of recurrency in the conjunctiva of the eye, but contact metastasis in the upper lid. So an exenteration of the orbit became necessary.

The postoperative treatment is very important. We apply cortison locally as well as systemically. Sometimes growth of vessels occurs in lamellar grafts. In such cases x-ray treatment with Strontium 90 is very useful. It is important to realize, that only growing capillaries are sensitive to x-ray treatment, and not older vessels.

IRIS

In 125 iris tumors, ZIMMERMAN (1963) found 38 real malignant tumors, that means of the mixed and epithelioid type. He saw metastasis only in 3 cases. Since the iris tumors are mostly of spindle cell type A and B, local extirpation seems to be justified.

If a tumor does not reach the basis of the iris, only a total iridectomy is necessary. It is important to know, that dense pigmentation or deformity of the pupil is not a definite sign of malignancy. We often find benign lesions in such cases. If the iris tumor reaches the basis of the iris a scleral incision has to be performed in order to remove the tumor totally.

If an iris tumor has infiltrated the chamber angle or if a ciliary body tumor is found, total extirpation — a so called block excision — is also necessary. Tumor and chamber angle with sclera and cornea have to be removed and reconstructed by a corneal graft. Our technique is similar to that of FRIEDE & MÜLLER.

4 weeks before the operation we perform photocoagulation in the periphery of the fundus as prophylactic treatment in order to avoid retinal detachment after operation. Before operation the extent of the tumor is measured by diaphanoscopy. After having sutured a Flieringa ring, we cut with a 6 or 7 mm trephine. The trephined area is pushed down and a total graft is sutured in its place. Then we do the scleral resection with preplaced silk sutures. After lifting the scleral flap with the corneal graft the tumor and the trephined area are cut out. The scleral flap is sutured. After refilling the anterior chamber with air and saline, conjunctiva covers the operation wound.

In cases of iris and ciliary body tumor resections cataract develops very frequently even without preexisting lens opacity. We observed cataract development in about 50% of our cases, sometimes by lack of zonula fibers and also by a slight lens subluxation.

SUMMARY

Operations of pigmented tumors, even of a large extent in the anterior segment of the eye are justified, if we obey the following rules: a) strict indications; b) total extirpation of of the tumor from the clinical point of view and proved by histological examination, c) the operation field must be controlled for a long time after the operation as well as the whole eye and its adnexae.

REFERENCES

PAUL , PARNELL, & FRAKER, Int. Ophth. Clinics, Vol. 2, No 2, 1962. ZIMMERMAN, L. *Amer. Journ. Ophthalm.* 56: (1963).

Author's address:
Universitäts Augenklinik
Hufelandstrasse 55
Essen, Germany

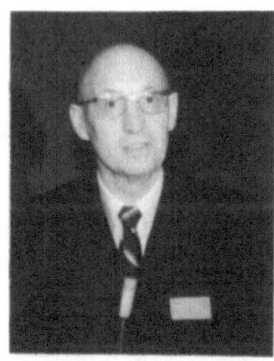

SCLERO–CORNEAL TREPHINING
(ELLIOT'S OPERATION)

F. HOLLWICH

(Münster, Germany)

Sclero-corneal trephining is already a very old technique. This procedure, published in 1914, was described by ELLIOT with the following sentence: 'The subject of this procedure is to tap the anterior chamber, to drain it permanently into the subconjunctival space, and, in doing so, to avoid, if possible, any interference with, or injury to the uveal tract'.

My personal approach to this operation started in 1935 when I entered the University Eye Clinic of Munich. I learned that this procedure is capable of lowering the increased intraocular tension of glaucoma patients in a high percentage of cases to permanently normal limits. This operation, skillfully performed by my first teacher WESSELY, was at that time a routine procedure in his clinic.

Also, it should be remembered that at that time, there were neither antibiotics nor corticosteroids available. WESSELY, therefore, limited the application of this procedure to those cases of glaucoma simplex in which the IOP was reducable by pilocarpine (maximum 2%) below 30 mm Hg. In

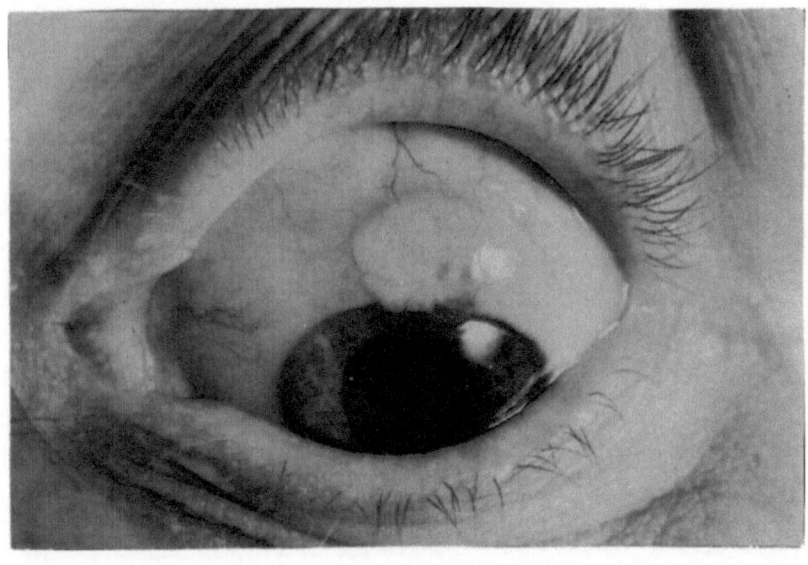

other words he used this procedure only in cases of a quiet and not yet decompensated eye. WESSELY used the trephine of 1,5 mm diameter.

My second teacher THIEL in Francfort 15 years later performed this procedure in every case of primary glaucoma. In congestive cases he first tried with local and systemic medication (corticosteroids, cocktail and diamox) to obtain a quiet eye with a round and narrow pupil before operation. THIEL used a trephine of 1.8 mm diameter.

DISADVANTAGES OF FILTERING OPERATIONS

As you see in the first picture, in a case of Elliot's trephining after five years of aqueous draining into the subconjunctival space: the conjunctiva, which represents the bleb over the seleral hole, became remarkably thin (Fig. 1). In about 2% of cases this thinning actually leads to potentially severe infection of the filtering bleb. It was, therefore, a great progress when the Greek ophthalmologist FRONIMOPOULOS and his coworkers introduced the so called 'protected Elliot' procedure. This procedure is very similar to the trabecutectomy (Cairns, Watson) and the so called 'double flap Scheie' procedure.

The next picture demonstrates the flat filtering bleb, which is characteristic in cases of 'protected Elliot' (Fig. 2). The aspect of the bleb being flat, is quite different from that we saw before in a case of original 'non-protected' ELLIOT.

Nevertheless, in performing the 'ELLIOT with scleral flap' there are two particular features which require attention:
1. splitting of the sclera is best performed with the microscope,
2. dissection of the limbus must be done in the same careful manner that ELLIOT pointed out in his first paper (slide): To avoid any interference with the ciliary body it is necessary that the limbus is completely free from conjunctiva and Tenon's capsule.

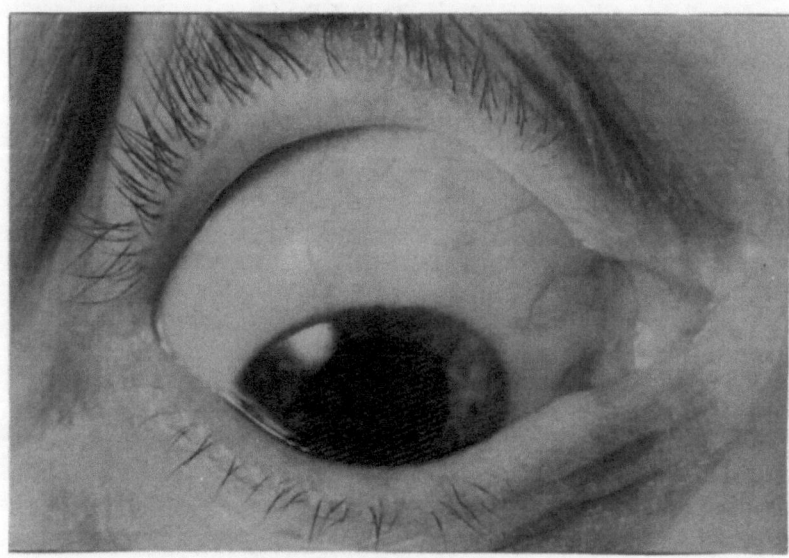

fig. 2

246

Sometimes, because two of the scleral emissary vessels penetrate parallel 5 or 6 millimeters posterior to the limbus (Fig. 3), it would be safer to place this flap in a transverse orientation instead of in the more conventional radial position (Fig. 4).

The trephine, then, can be placed halfway on the sclera, and halfway on corneal tissue (Fig. 5) as illustrated on this sketch. The drawing to the right is of ELLIOT's first publication (Fig. 6). The drawing to the left illustrates the technique of ELLIOT's trephining with scleral flap. The following film shows the procedure of 'ELLIOT's trephining with scleral flap' first in full, then with emphasis on certain specific details.

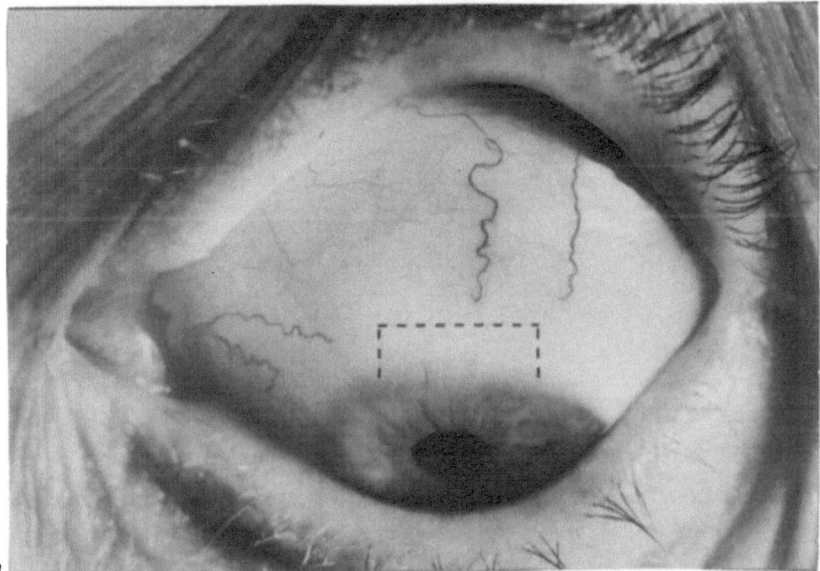

fig. 3

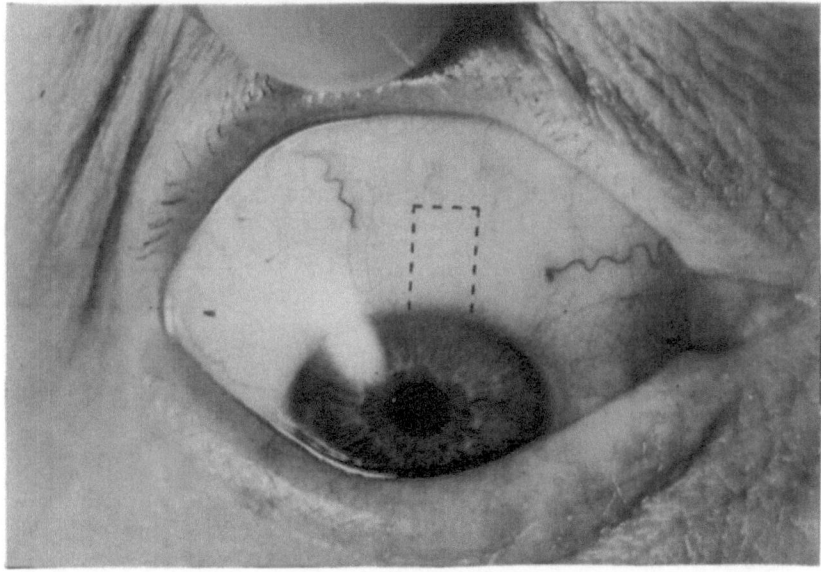

fig. 4

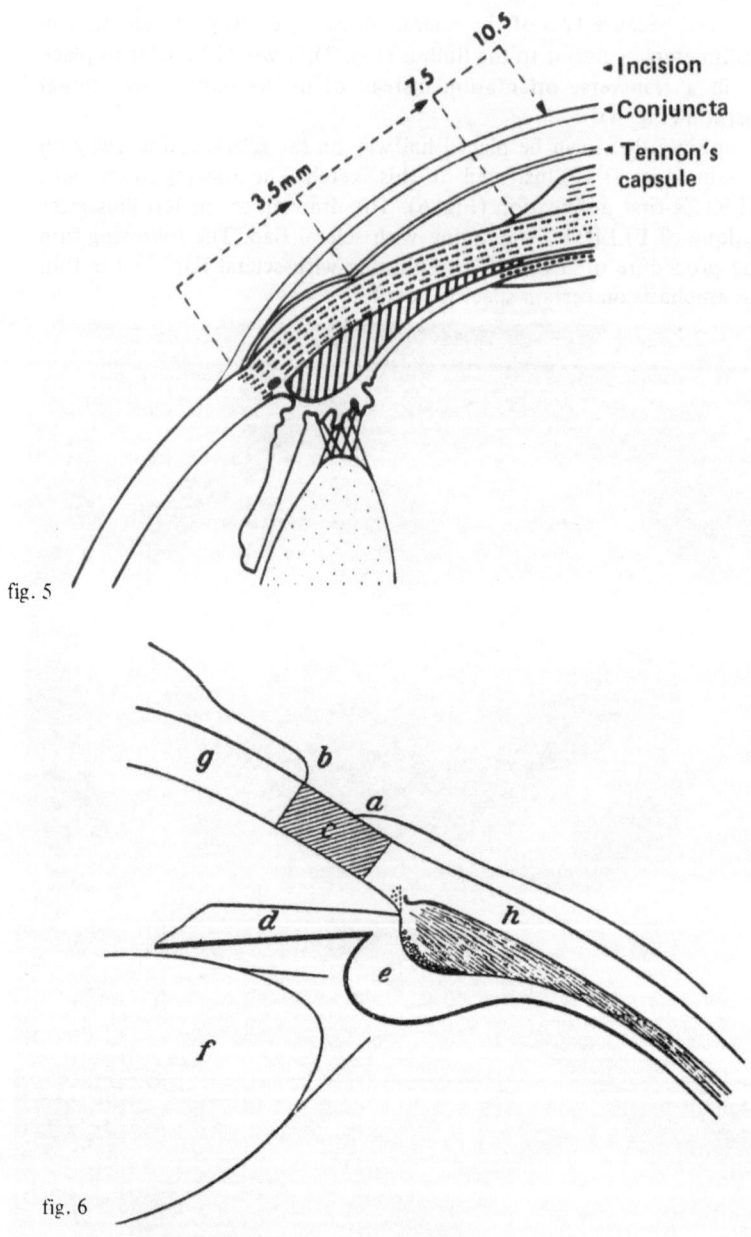

fig. 5

fig. 6

ELLIOT'S TREPHINING WITH SCLERAL FLAP

Part I

1. Bridle suture through the superior rectus muscle.
2. Limbus based conjunctival flap. Dissection of the limbus with the hockey knife after cauterisation of superficial episcleral vessels.

3. Trapdoor incision to perform a limbus based rectangular scleral flap of 2/3 thickness of the sclera avoiding to interfere with emissary vessels. The keratome and Paufique's knife is used.
4. The scleral flap is reflected towards the cornea.
5. Trephining at 12 o'clock using the 1.2 mm trephine. The scleral disc is removed with the Graefe knife.
6. The iris which buedges out is picked with toothed forceps and pushed back to permit slow outflow of aqueous. It is then slowly severed tangentially to avoid forceful outflow of aqueous. A small peripheral coloboma is seen. A remaining lamella of Descemet's membrane is visible; it is picked up with forceps and removed with scissors.
7. Resuturing of the scleral flap back into place with two Barraquer silk sutures at the corners distal to the limbus.
8. Closure of the conjunctival wound with running silk sutures beginning at 12 o'clock and running nasally and again from 12 o'clock running temporally. Only the conjunctiva is sutured and not Tenon's capsule.

The anterior chamber is free of haemorrhages. The pupil is over medium size due to almost continuous instillation of scopolamine $\frac{1}{2}$% and atropine 3% after viridectomy and during wound closure. Kanamytrex-drops, atropine, drops into the operated eye and pilocarpine into the other eye, binocular padding.

Part II

Immediately follows a second complete film
1. The scleral trapdoor incision is performed somewhat towards the nasal side to avoid interference with the emissary vessels.
2. Trephining at 12 o'clock. The buedging iris and the nearly totally severed button is seen which is severed entirely with Graefe knife.
3. Peripheral iridectomy, slowly done to avoid forceful outflow of aqueous. The iridectomy is not spontaneously visible, therefore a little massage is needed over the trephining hole.
4. Suturing of the scleral flap with two Barraquer silk sutures on its scleral side.
5. Suturing of the conjunctiva with two running sutures both beginning at 12 o'clock, the first runs nasally and the second temporally. Tenon's capsule is not sutured. The manner of conjunctival wound closure gives a certain physiological way of equal traction distribution, preventing external wound leak. The technique is performed by starting the suture at 12 o'clock and making a running suture first nasally and then starting again at 12 o'clock running temporally.

Part III

Specific details concerning button removal:
1. The button is hidden by the prolapsing iris. Therefore, the iridectomy is performed first. Then, the button still held in place by a few remaining unsectioned scleral fibres, is grasped and removed with scissors.

2. The button presents itself and is severed completely using a Graefe knife.

3. The button is removed and iridectomy is performed. A small portion of persisting lamella consisting of Descemet's membrane is grasped and it is severed and removed. Note that Elliot himself has already mentioned this phenomenon.

To finish this presentation, again a complete film is shown.

Part IV

1. Bridle suture through the conjunctiva. Dissection of the limbus using a hockey knife. Cauterisation of episcleral vessels.

2. Limbus based trap-door incision. To avoid interference with the scleral emissary vessels, the incision is performed in a transversal orientation instead of in the more conventional radiar direction.

3. The button presents itself at the side and is dissected and excised by means of a Graefe-knife. Under a continuous drip of scopolamine drops and of atropine the peripheral iridectomy is performed.

4. A small portion of persisting lamella consisting of Descemet's membrane is still visible and it is grasped and severed with scissors.

5. Closing of the scleral wound with two Barraquer silk sutures on the scleral side.

6. Closing of the conjunctiva without suturing Tenon's capsule.

Author's address:
Augenklinik der
Westfälischen Wilhelms-Universität
Westring 15
Münster, Germany

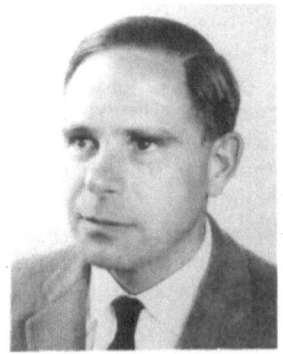

PSEUDOPHAKIA INTRACAPSULAR OR EXTRACAPSULAR TECHNIQUE? *

C.D. BINKHORST

(Terneuzen, the Netherlands)

Whereas extracapsular cataract extraction is the only technique practicable in young patients and in many patients with traumatic cataract, there is a choice between intracapsular and extracapsular extraction in patients with senile cataracts. During the past fifty years the intracapsular extraction has become the method of choice, although cautious surgeons always would advocate extracapsular extraction in case of retinal disease. With modern techniques for extracapsular nucleus and cortex removal time has come to re-evaluate our attitude in this matter. Lens implant surgery invites us even stronger to do so, because of the different features of the pseudophakic eye as compared with the aphakic eye.

We shall first examine the importance of stability of the lens implant and then compare the features of the aphakic eye after intracapsular and after extracapsular extraction.

Our own crystalline lens moves very little if at all around inside the eye and gives stability to the vitreous, the iris and the aqueous. Apparently the

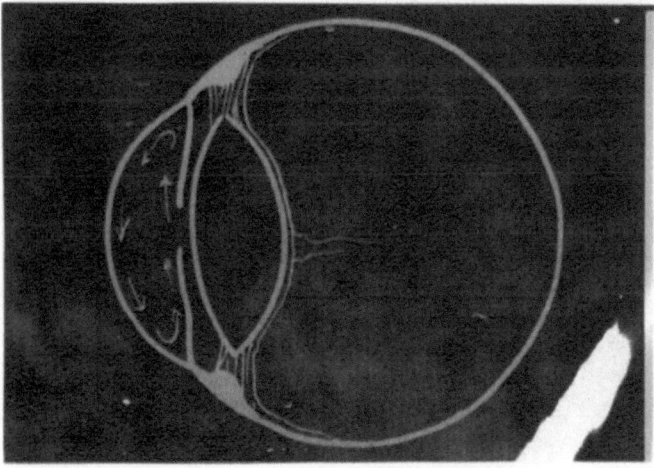

Fig. 1a. Section of phakic eye. There is a firm separation between the anterior and posterior segment. Quiet and regular current pattern in the anterior chamber.

251

eye is profiting from this stability and even the most vulnerable tissues such as the retina and the corneal endothelium, are well protected (Fig. 1a).

Intracapsular removal of the complete crystalline lens leaves the eye with a mobile aqueous and vitreous, and with a floating iris diaphragm (Fig. 1b). As the iris diaphragm in this eye is the last foothold for fixation of an intraocular lens, the latter will float with the iris. Pseudophako-donesis goes hand in hand with irido-donesis. Pseudophako-donesis even tends to reinforce irido-donesis. For some lens designs it can not be guaranteed that the corneal endothelium is never touched (Fig. 2). Moreover, the anterior cham-

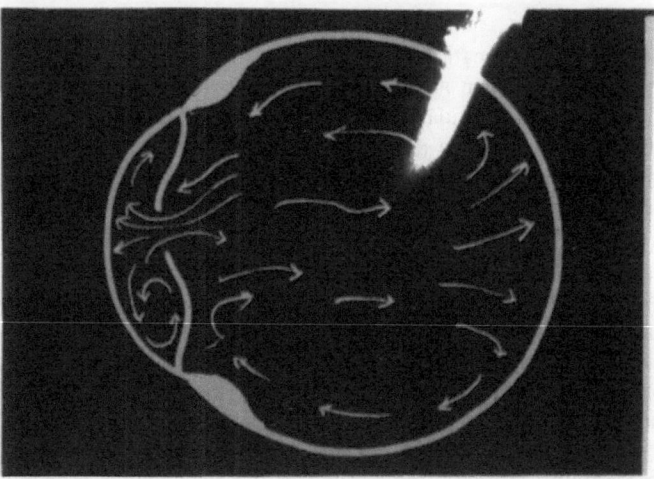

Fig. 1b. Section of intracapsular aphakic eye. No separation between anterior and posterior segment. Floating iris. Wild current patterns with heavy turbulences.

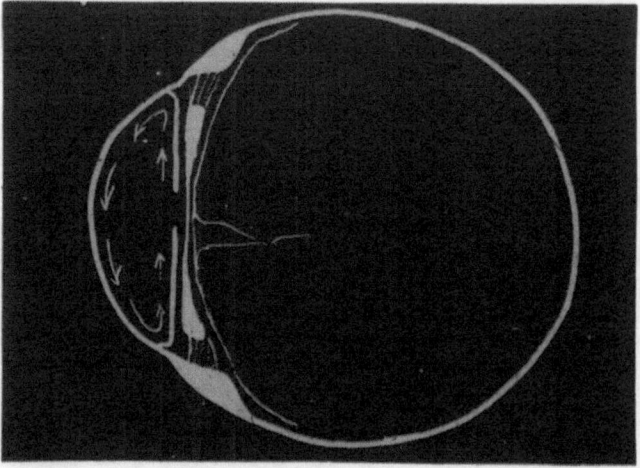

Fig. 1c Section of extracapsular aphakic eye. The vital characteristics of the phakic eye are preserved.

ber tends to shallowness, especially in the prone position, as has been demonstrated by Nordlohne (Fig. 3). This also favours corneal endothelium contact. The floating iris has a pupillary opening of unpredictable width, and this can give rise to decentering of the lens.

As far as a lens is merely held by the sphincter muscle, it can decenter in any direction when the pupil is of inadequate width (Fig. 4). Excessive decentering in all these cases, moreover, can lead to dislocation of the lens with even more disastrous consequences (Fig. 5). Lenses sutured to the iris generally ride in the direction of the suture when the pupil dilates (Fig. 6). Lenses hooked in a peripheral coloboma do not necessarily ride high in a dilated pupil (Fig. 7), but can decenter sidewards (Fig. 8). Decentered lenses are a potential danger for the corneal endothelium. Although the iris has turned out to be more resistent to touch, to manipulation, and to the burden of an intraocular lens than we ever thought in the past, the limit to this all is set by its atrophy. This can occur at the pupillary border by the pressure of haptics, the more so after prolonged use of miotics (Fig. 9). Iris atrophy has also occurred with iris sutures chaving through (Fig. 10). The round-the-clock-movements of the iris promote its atrophy everywhere where pressure is enough (Fig. 11). Iris atrophy favours decentration and dislocation of a lens with its possible consequences. The conclusion therefore is that any lens merely supported by the iris after intracapsular surgery, without or with dislocation and without or with iris atrophy, can endanger the cornea.

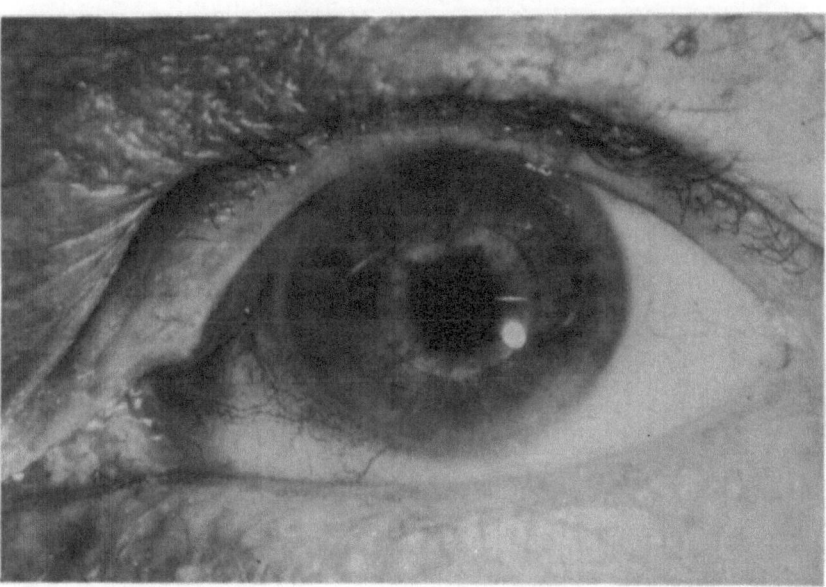

Fig. 2. Horizontally placed four-loop lens after intracapsular surgery. Loop contact dystrophy of the cornea nasally.

Extracapsular surgery fits the eye out with a capsular membrane that steadies vitreous and aqueous, and to some extent also the iris (Fig. 1c). The iris in this case becomes a slightly more acceptable support for a lens (Fig. 12), but the ideal support for a lens is the capsular membrane itself (Fig. 13, 14). Pseudophako-donesis is absent, the anterior chamber is slightly deeper, fixation is independent of the pupil size, iris atrophy can not

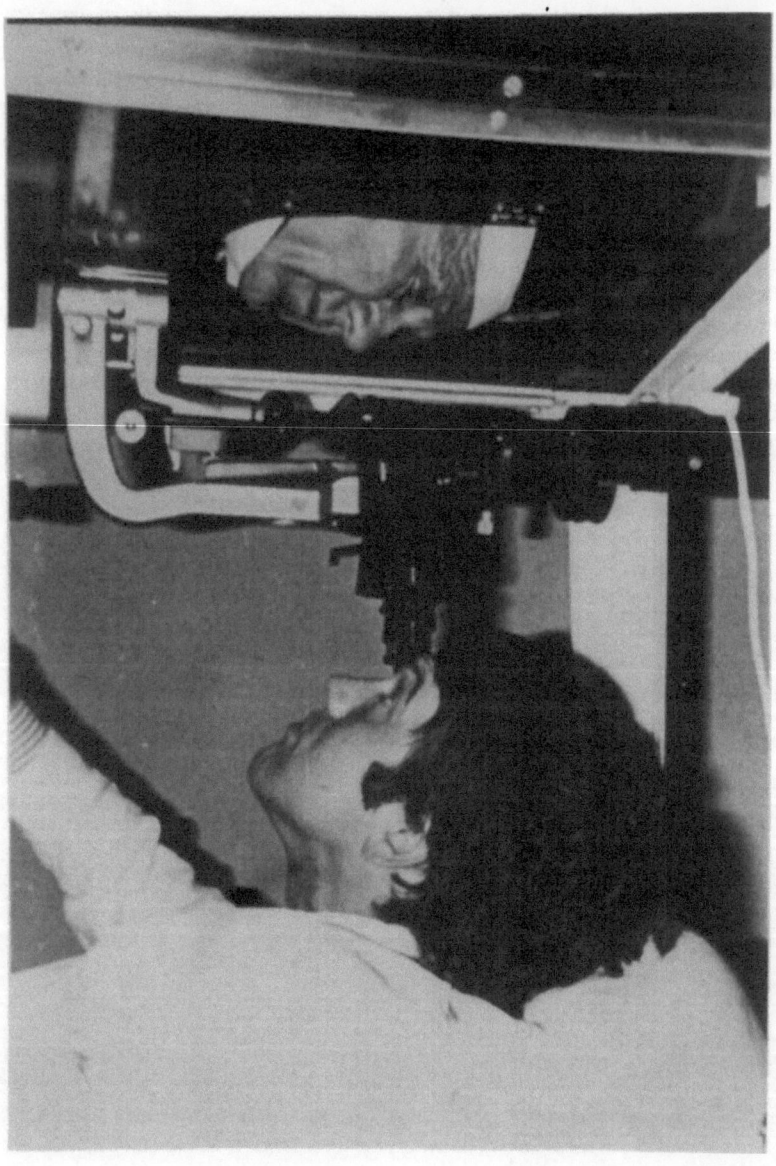

Fig. 3. Anterior chamber depth measurement in the prone position (courtesy Dr. M.E. NORDLOHNE).

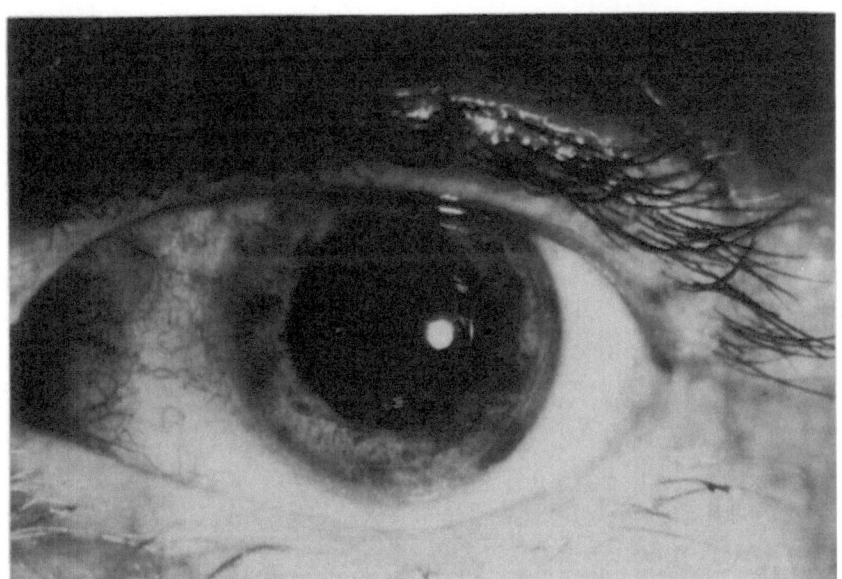

Fig. 4.   Dislocated four-loop lens in dilated pupil after intracapsular surgery.

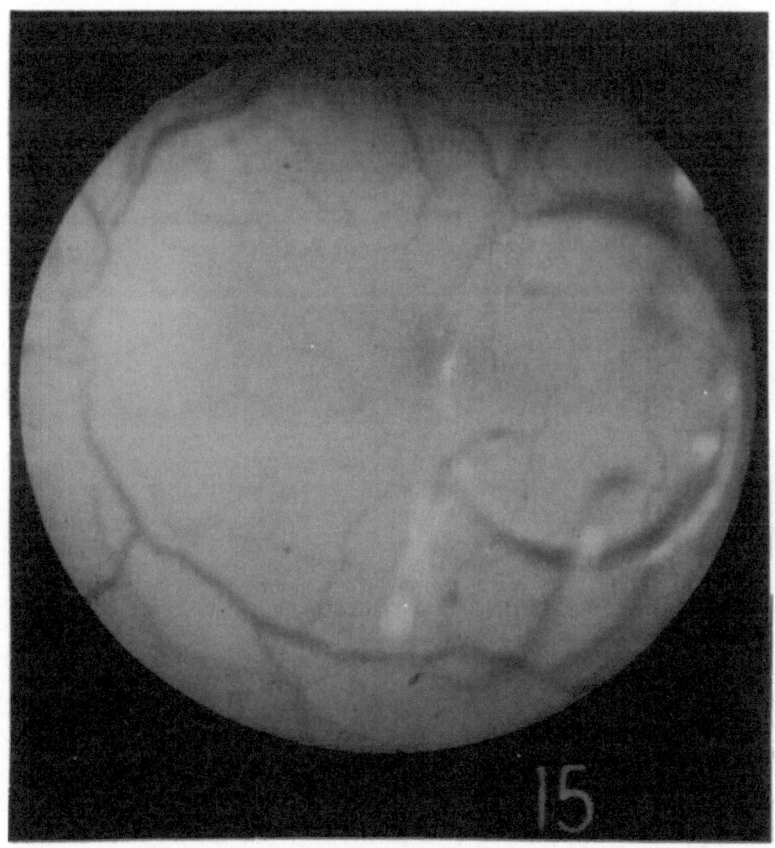

Fig. 5.   Posterior dislocation of four-loop lens.

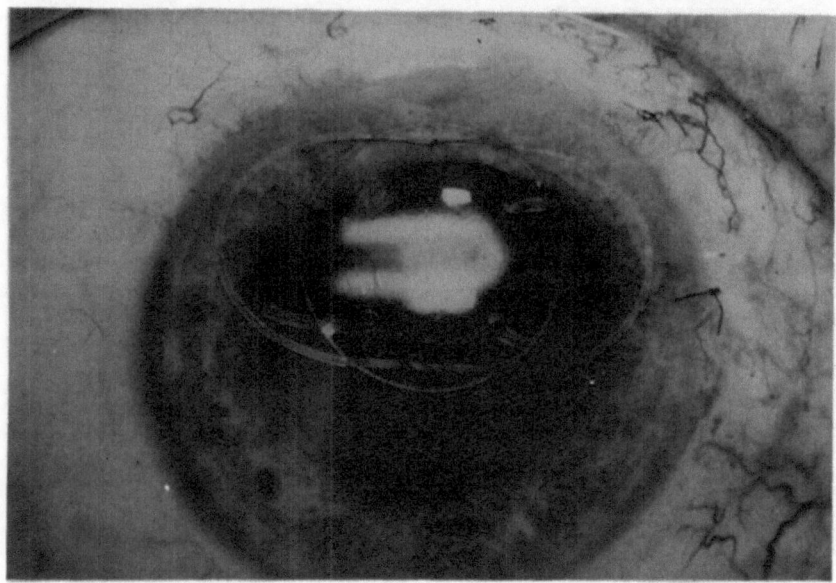

Fig. 6. Four-loop lens after intracapsular surgery, sutured to the iris. The lens rides high after pupil dilatation.

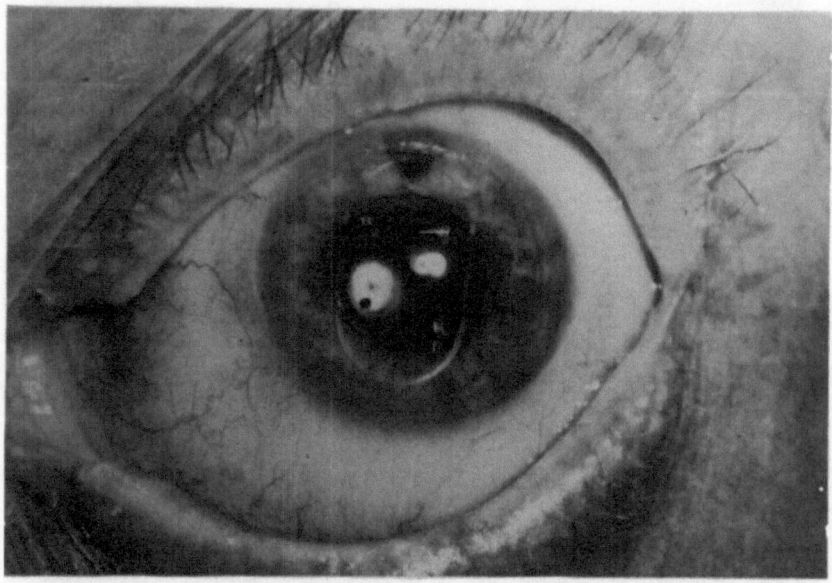

Fig. 7. Vertically placed four-loop lens after intracapsular surgery. The lens remains centered in dilated pupil (loop suture).

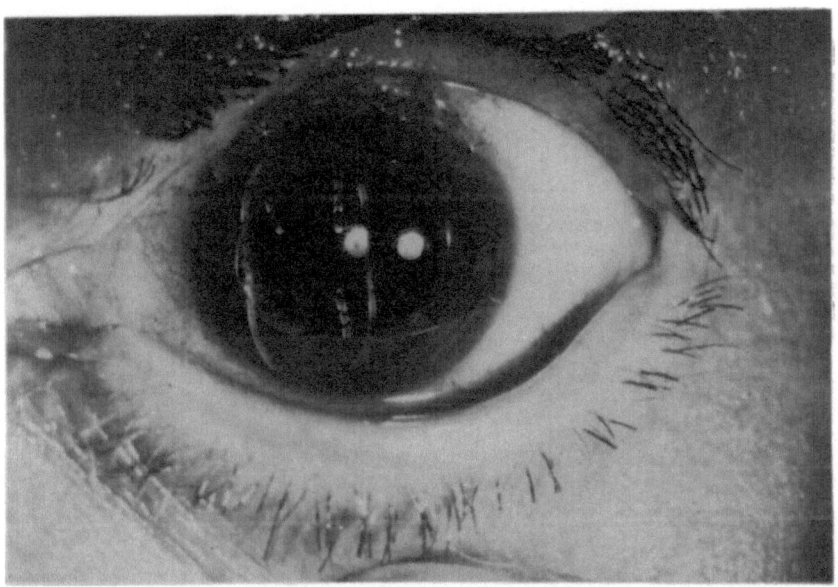

Fig. 8. Vertically placed four-loop lens after intracapsular surgery. The lens falls sidewards when the pupil is dilated (loop suture).

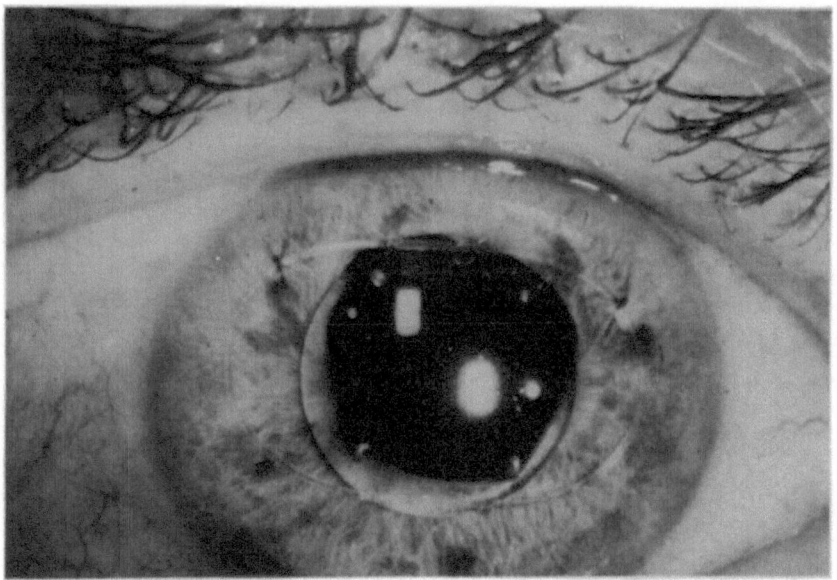

Fig. 9. Marked pupillary border iris atrophy with incompetent sphincter muscle action after prolonged use of miotics. After dislocation the lens had to be sutured to the iris.

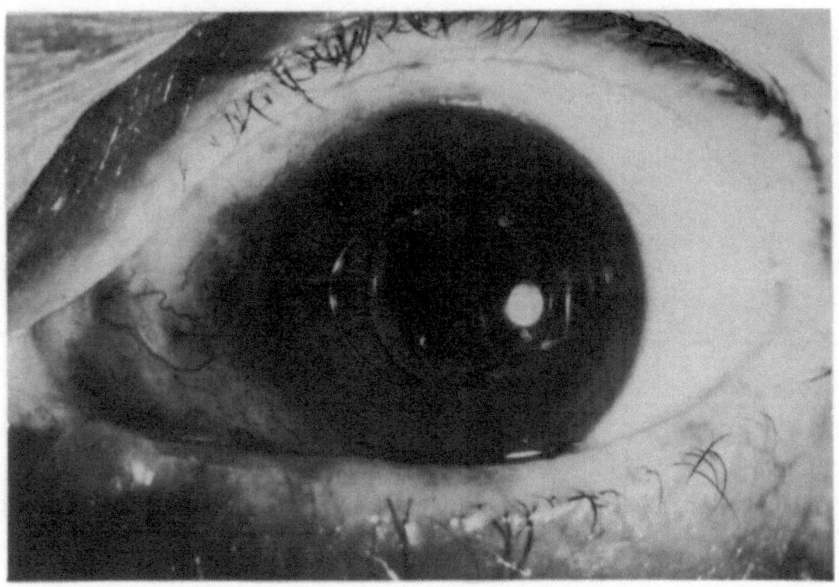

Fig. 10. Four-loop lens after intracapsular surgery. The nasal anterior loop is sutured to the iris and is chaving through. The temporal posterior loop is dislocated.

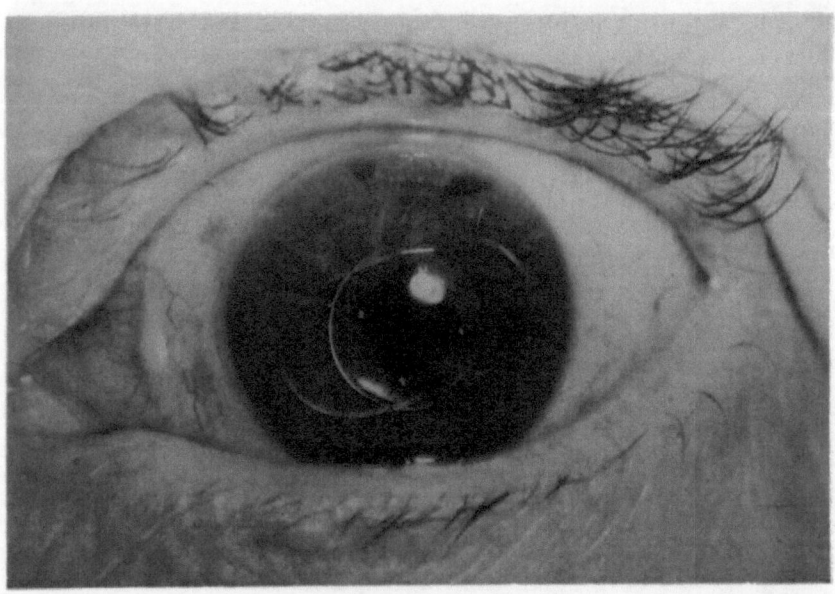

Fig. 11. Horizontally placed four-loop lens after intracapsular surgery. The nasal anterior loop tip has caused some iris atrophy.

occur. The capsular membrane is an avascular membrane, extremely suitable to hold implant material. Corneal pathology in my personal series of over 600 implantations after extracapsular extraction has almost completely been ruled out.

Let us turn again to the crystalline lens (Fig. 1a). Apart from providing stability inside the eye, the crystalline represents a separation of the contents of the anterior and posterior segment of the eye.

Intracapsular extraction and depriving the eye of this separation means that these contents can mix up to some degree. Vitreous can enter the anterior chamber, aqueous can penetrate into the posterior segment, some forward displacement of the iris root is likely to happen. It is easy to accept that all this can have consequences. We know of vitreous keratopathy, we know of vitreous degeneration, we know of aphakic pressure rise, we know of persistent flares in the anterior chamber, and Worst has attractive ideas about a deleterious effect of aqueous on the retina. Whereas the crystalline lens accounts for a fixed pattern of slow currents inside the eye, current patterns after intracapsular surgery, due to the floating iris and vitreous, become wild and develop into turbulences, which may promote pressure differences that never existed before (Fig. 1b). Intracapsular extraction really brings the eye in a deplorable state. It has been said that in this situation a lens in the pupil or in front of the pupil restores more or less normal conditions, but this is only true in as far as mushrooming of the vitreous through the pupil is prevented On the contrary, combined irido- and pseudophako-donesis probably accentuate these pathological hydrodynamics. The finer structures of the eye as the macular area and as the corneal endothelium could suffer in the long run. This 'concussion theory' could explain cases of late corneal decompensation in intracapsular aphakia and could also explain instances of aphakic macular oedema, which, according to some people, occurs even more frequently in intracapsular pseudophakic eyes than in intracapsular aphakic eyes.

Extracapsular surgery leaves the separation of the anterior and posterior segment of the eye intact (Fig. 1c). It guarantees the same quiet current pattern in the eye and prevents mixing up of the contents of the eye. Many of the deleterious effects of intracapsular surgery are absent in extracapsular surgery. The beneficial effect of extracapsular surgery manifests itself already during the early postoperative days. Some characteristics of the recovering eye tend to be more favourable after extracapsular surgery than after intracapsular surgery. Surgical uveitis, pressure decompensation, and corneal endothelial decompensation (striate keratitis) are usually less pronounced after extracapsular surgery. The eye quiets down faster, cornea's generally are more clear. Also the longterm fate of the eye is more favourable after extracapsular surgery than after intracapsular surgery. Late corneal breakdown has not yet been encountered in my personal series. Clinical evidence of a much lower rate of retinal complications after extracapsular than after intracapsular surgery has been present for many years in these series. We could clearly confirm this in a selective study that has been presented elsewhere. (Retinal accidents in Pseudophakia. Intracapsular

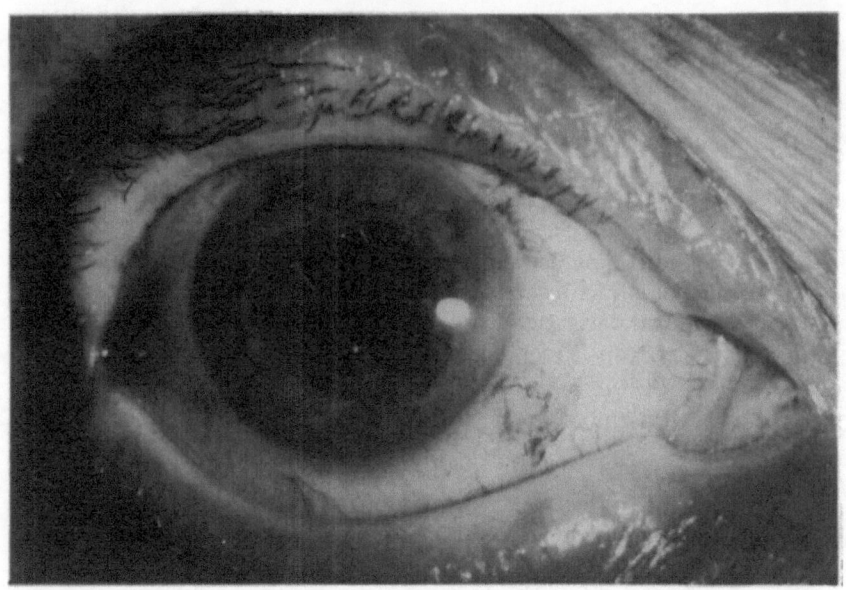

Fig. 12. Two-loop lens after extracapsular extraction, merely adhering to the iris. Pupil dilatation.

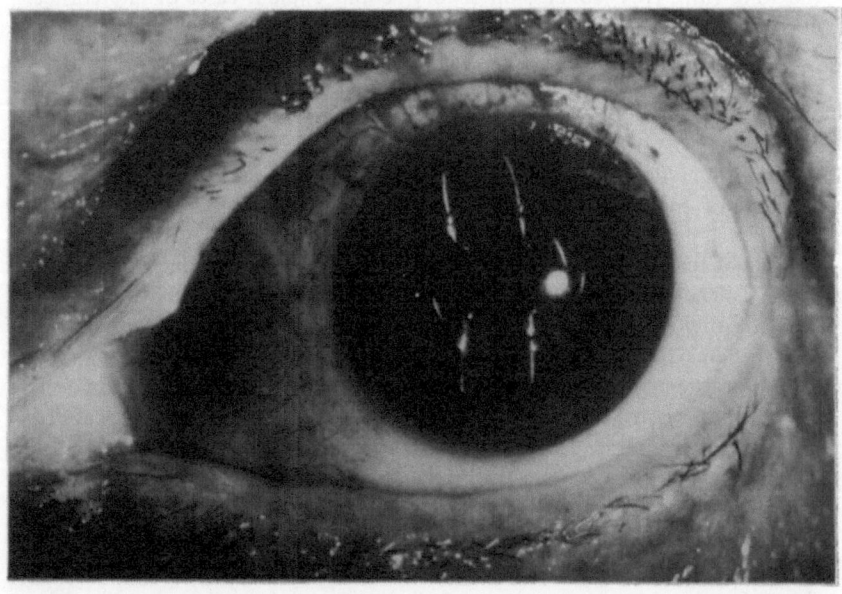

Fig. 13. Two-loop lens after extracapsular extraction, with loops adhering in the capsular bag. Pupil dilatation.

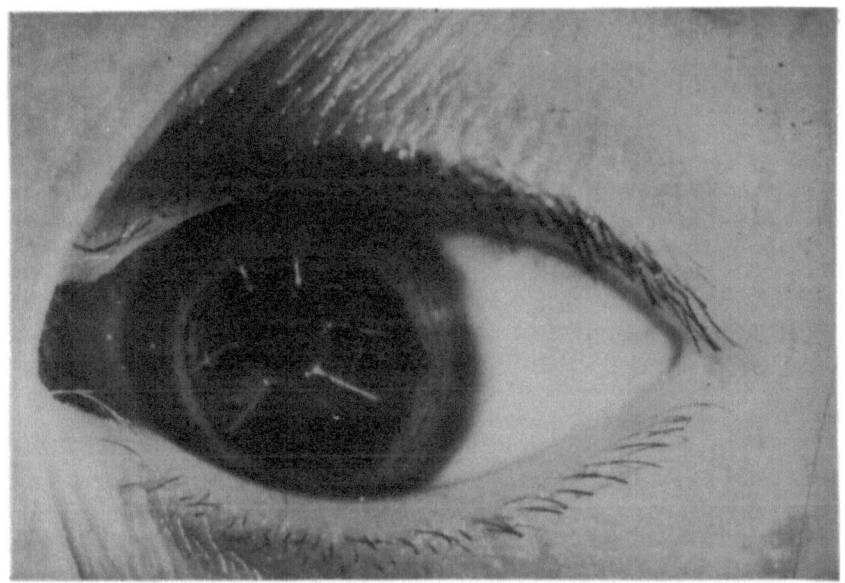

Fig. 14. Three-loop lens after extracapsular extraction with loops adhering in the capsular bag. Pupil dilatation.

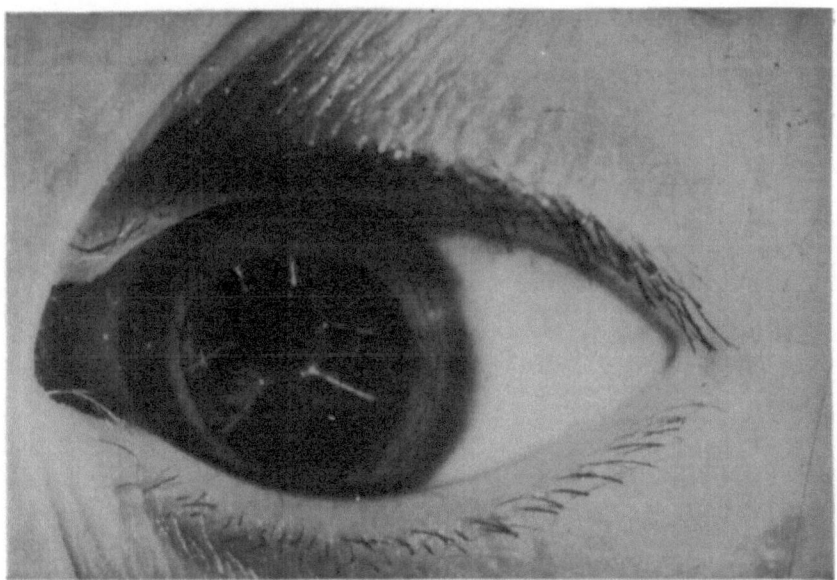

Fig. 15. Abundance of cortical material. Fourth day postoperatively. Pupil dilatation. Aspiration indicated.

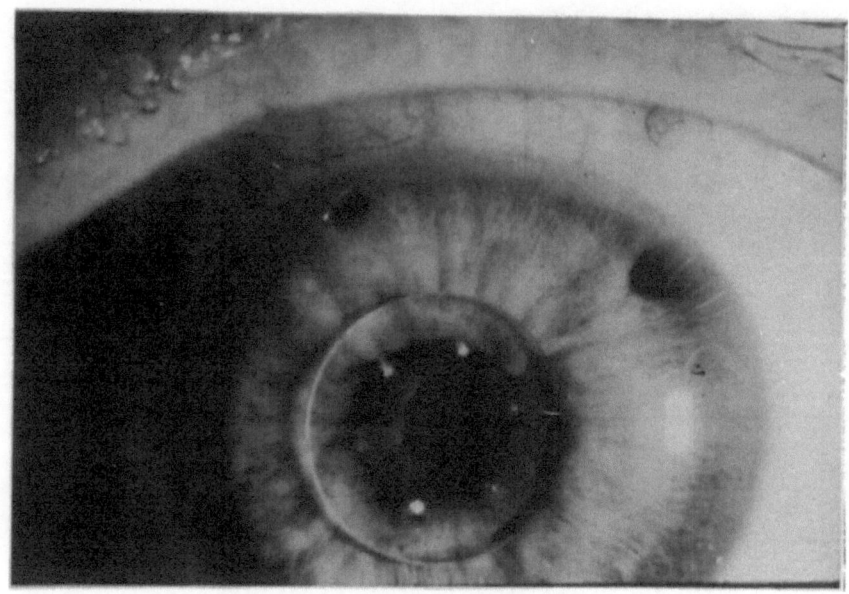

Fig. 16. Capsular membrane after needling.

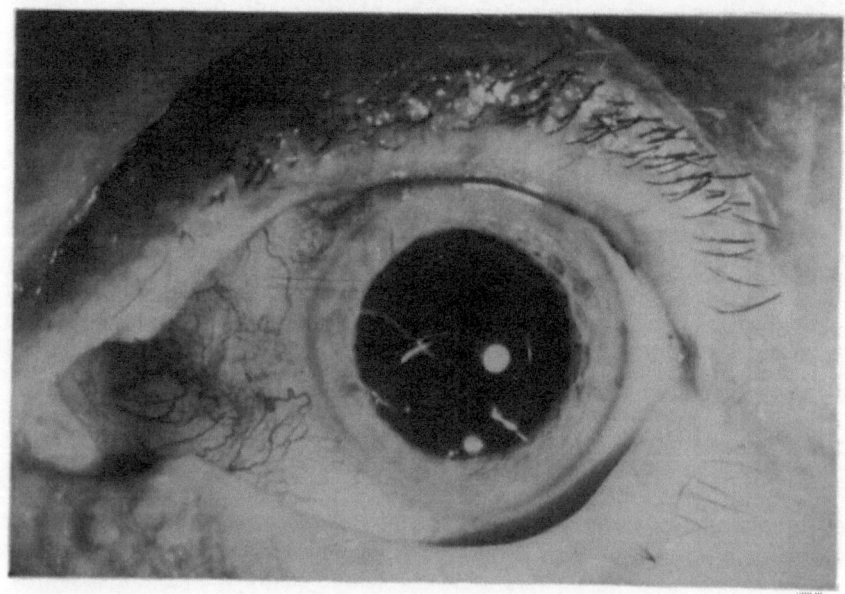

Fig. 17. Two-loop lens after extracapsular surgery. Fourth day postoperatively. Capsular adhesions have not (yet) been formed.

versus extracapsular surgery. Presented before the Amer. Acad. Ophthal. Otolaryngol., Dallas 21-25 Sept. 1975). Whereas the mechanism of aphakic macular oedema is still under discussion, whether its cause is vitreous strands, inflammation, toxicity of the aqueous (Worst) or concussion of the retina, its cure-all seems to be the extracapsular cataract extraction.

Extracapsular cataract extraction means low-risk surgery. Due to shorter incision and vitreous protection surgical and postsurgical accidents are less likely to happen, even in less favourable circumstances of anaesthesia and nursing. Vitreous prolaps and its complications can almost completely be ruled out. Also for this reason should extracapsular surgery be the technique of choice for lens implantation. However, as it is now, extracapsular extraction may seem more difficult than the intracapsular extraction, and its technical perfection is not yet up to the level of the latter. Secondary cataract remains some problem (Fig. 15, 16), as well as the few lenses that do not adhere to the capsular membrane (Fig. 17). Aspiration of cortical material or needling of the capsular membrane in case of secondary cataract, and suturing of the lens to the iris in case of non-adhering of the lens, are the answers for the moment being. The interest of competent surgeons and advanced technical aids are necessary for further improvement and acceptance of the extracapsular technique. And this, I feel, is very much worth while.

SUMMARY

The advantages of extracapsular over intracapsular cataract extraction in pseudophakia are discussed. As well the fixation of the implant as the long-term fate of the eye are favourably influenced by extracapsular surgery.

Author's address:
Axelsestraat 54
Terneuzen, The Netherlands.

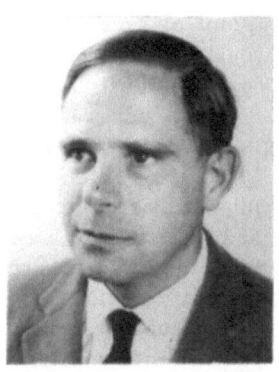

RETINAL ACCIDENTS IN PSEUDOPHAKIA
INTRACAPSULAR VERSUS
EXTRACAPSULAR SURGERY*

C.D. BINKHORST, A. KATS, T.T. TJAN
& L.H. LOONES

(Terneuzen, the Netherlands)

The technical perfection of intracapsular cataract extraction to-day is such that complications have been reduced to a minimum. Retinal complications such as retinal detachment and cystoid macular oedema seem to be accepted as inevitable. However, these complications continue to discredit the long-term fate of many intracapsular aphakic eyes.

Since its definition by IRVINE (1953) and GASS (1966) postsurgical macular oedema turned out to be of increasing importance and its incidence is reported with increasing percentages, depending on the criteria and the methods of detection used.

In the past most extracapsular extractions were failures of intracapsular extraction and as such their results can not be compared with the results of intracapsular extraction. New approaches to extracapsular hard nucleus and cortex removal led to a revival and thorough improvement of Daviel's original extraction technique (BINKHORST et al., 1972). Time has come to re-evaluate the extracapsular technique against the intracapsular technique.

Because we were impressed by the superior fixation possibilities for intraocular lenses after extracapsular extraction as compared to intracapsular extraction we have built up since 1963 to date a series of over 600 intentional extracapsular extractions combined with iris clip or irido-capsular lens implantation. This has enabled us to compare the long-term results of extracapsular surgery to those of intracapsular surgery. In earlier publications we already mentioned that after extracapsular extraction of senile cataract retinal detachment had not occurred and that cystoid macular oedema was unknown (BINKHORST 1972, 1973). NORDLOHNE (1974), in a thorough study of our complete series up to January 1st, 1972, comprising 864 eyes, found an incidence of retinal detachment of 2.07 per cent after intracapsular extraction of senile cataracts, and an incidence of zero per cent after extracapsular extraction of senile cataracts. He found an incidence of cystoid macular oedema of 3.96 per cent after intracapsular extraction of senile cataract, and only one case after extracapsular extraction of senile cataract. It had been necessary to needle a capsular membrane in the latter case. In 16 uncomplicated cases out of his own first 72 iris clip lens implantations after intracapsular extraction visual acuity was found increasing between 4 and 18 months postoperatively, and he speculated that this could be due to

* Read before the Amer. Acad. Ophthal. Otolaryngol., Dallas 21-25 sept. 1975.

subsiding macular oedema. We felt that further proof of a deleterious influence of intracapsular surgery on the retina would be useful (BINK-HORST, 1973). Not only gross retinal accidents such as retinal detachment and cystoid macular oedema were searched for, but our study was also meant to register the influence of minor, possibly recurrent macular accidents, unnoticed by the patient and the surgeon.

For our purpose only cases of uncomplicated senile cataract undergoing primary implantation with uncomplicated surgery and recovery have been chosen such that a comparison between intracapsular and extracapsular surgery could be made with optimal reliability. It was very important that the observation period for both types of surgery was as equal as possible. This was the case nearly ideally in 3 groups of patients with unilateral surgery, and satisfactorily in 3 groups of patients with bilateral surgery. The situation of comparison in the same patient who underwent different surgical procedure in both eyes, is most favorable.

One hundred and twenty eyes of eighty-five patients with an average age of 68 years at the time of examination were involved. The study was concluded on April 1, 1975. In one group of patients (group IV) it was undertaken to describe macular appearance. In all groups macular function was tested with visual acuity, with Amsler's test for the central visual field, and with Haidinger's brushes phenomenon. The perception of Haidinger's brushes has been registered in a different way for bilateral and for unilateral cases. In bilateral cases it was tried to compare both eyes by listing the best eye with ++++ and rewarding the fellow-eye with + + + + (equally well), + + + (slightly less), + + (definitely less), + (hardly seen), and in case of a completely negative answer with −. Purposely, the intracapsular eye or the extracapsular eye with capsulotomy was given the best chance by always testing the other eye first. In unilateral cases comparison with the other eye was not undertaken and the answers were simply registered as positive or negative.

RESULTS IN UNILATERAL SURGERY (GROUP I TO III)

About equal numbers of patients with about equal observation period, that underwent different surgical procedures were found amongst those operated upon between April 1, 1971 and April 1, 1972. In that year as many times intracapsular surgery as extracapsular surgery had been performed. The observation period, consequently, was 3 to 4 years, with very slight differences. All patients were called in and about 70 percent could be re-examined, totalling 50 patients.

Group I. Eighteen patients with unilateral intracapsular surgery

The average observation period was 44 months.

Retinal detachment occurred in two eyes. Visual acuity with spectacle correction ranged from light perception to 1.0 and over (average 0.73). With Amsler's test there was no performance in 2 cases with poor vision and metamorphopsia in a third case.

Haidinger's brushes (Table I, group I): When presented to the operated

TABLE I

HAIDINGER'S BRUSHES. UNILATERAL PSEUDOPHAKICS.

GROUP I (intracaps.)		GROUP II (extracaps.) (c.caps.)		GROUP III (extracaps.)	
C537	positive	IC169	positive	C519	positive
C538	positive	IC158	positive	C526	positive
C536	positive	IC143	positive	C512	positive
C560	positive	IC162	positive	IC1032	positive
C579	positive	IC1030	positive	IC1031	positive
C568	positive	IC156	positive	IC170	positive
C558	negative	IC157	positive	IC153	positive
C545	positive	IC121	positive	IC141	positive
C523	positive	IC166	negative	IC139	positive
C565	positive	IC104	positive	IC1028	positive
C562	positive	IC106	negative	IC173	positive
C551	negative	IC129	negative	C491	positive
C550	negative	IC137	positive	IC226	positive
C566	negative	IC103	negative	IC195	positive
C535	positive	IC111	positive	C563	positive
C530	positive	IC117	positive	IC176	positive
C544	positive				
C523	positive				

eye 4 patients gave a negative answer, whereas they performed well with the fellow-eye.

Group II   Sixteen patients with unilateral extracapsular surgery with capsulotomy

The average observation period was 42 months. Capsulotomy had been performed with an average of 35 months prior to the re-examination, in 3 eyes twice.

Retinal detachment occurred in one eye. Visual acuity with spectacle correction ranged from 0.25 to 1.0 and over (average 0.81). The Amsler test revealed metamorphopsia in one case.

Haidinger's brushes (Table I, group II) were not perceived by 4 patients with the operated eye, but only with the fellow-eye.

Group III. Sixteen patients with unilateral extracapsular surgery without capsulotomy

The average observation period was 40 months.

Retinal detachment did not occur in this group. Visual acuity with spectacle correction ranged from 0.5 to 1.0 and over (average 0.91). The Amsler test revealed no irregularities.

Haidinger's brushes (Table I, group III) were perceived by all patients, as well with the operated eye as with the fellow eye.

A number of 35 patients could be traced that had been operated on both eyes between 1963 and 1974.

Group IV. Twenty-three patients with intracapsular surgery in one eye and extracapsular surgery without capsulotomy in the other eye

The observation period at the time of re-examination ranged from 8 to 118 months (average 51 months) for the intracapsular eyes, and from 7 to 88 months (average 35 months) for the extracapsular eyes.

Retinal detachment had occurred in one eye 3 months after intracapsular surgery. Visual acuity with spectacle correction ranged from 0.02 to 1.0 and over (average 0.68) for the intracapsular eyes, and from 0.10 to 1.0 and over (average 0.67) for the extracapsular eyes. It has to be taken into account that 4 extracapsular eyes had poor visual acuity due to secondary membrane formation and that the remaining extracapsular eyes had visual acuity ranging from 0.33 to 1.0 and over (average 0.78). Amsler's test revealed definite metamorphopsia in 5 intracapsular eyes, whereas in 2 extracapsular eyes the test pattern was said to be 'irregular'. This could have been caused by secondary membranes.

Haidinger's brushes (Table II, group IV): Four out of 23 patients did not perceive Haidinger's brushes with neither eye and this was certainly not due to severe maculopathy. Consequently, comparison between both eyes was

TABLE II

HAIDINGER'S BRUSHES. BILATERAL PSEUDOPHAKICS.

GROUP IV				GROUP V			
Intracaps.		Extracaps.		Intracaps.		Extracaps. (c caps.)	
C588	–	C564	+ + + +	C17	+ +	C388	+ + + +
C534	+ + +	IC267	+ + + +	C1098	–	IC137	+ + + +
C603	+ + +	IC1038	+ + + +	C315	+ +	C296	+ + + +
C482	+ + + +	IC150	+ + + +	C1090	+ + + +	IC146	+ + + +
C639	+ + +	IC1066	+ + + +	C521	+ + + +	IC161	+ + + +
C569	+ +	IC204	+ + + +	C1053	+ + +	IC337	+ + + +
C640	+ + +	IC382	+ + + +	C593	+ + + +	IC221	+ + + +
C376	+ + + +	C457	+ + + +				
C177	-	IC39	+ + + +	GROUP VI			
C471	+ +	C450	+ + + +	Extracaps. (c caps.)		Extracaps.	
C352	+ +	C297	+ + + +				
C1076	+ + +	C1049	+ + + +	IC1081	+ + +	IC1084	+ + + +
C391	+ + + +	IC112	+ + + +	IC138	+ + +	IC340	+ + + +
–	+ + + +	IC399	+ + + +	IC192	+ + +	IC155	+ + + +
C286	+ +	C477	+ + + +	C419	+ + +	IC219	+ + + +
C587	+ + + +	IC224	+ + + +	IC107	+ +	IC123	+ + + +
C509	+ + + +	IC182	+ + + +				
–	+	C641	+ + + +				
C452	+	IC212	+ + + +				

only possible in the remaining 19 patients. Of these 19 patients 6 patients performed equally well with both eye, whereas 13 patients performed best with the extracapsular eye. Two intracapsular eyes did not perceive the phenomenon at all whereas the extracapsular fellow-eyes did. We estimated that the average perception of Haidinger's brushes with the intracapsular eyes was only 66 percent of the perception with the extra-capsular eyes.

Fundoscopic appearance. In this group we assessed the fundoscopic appearance of the macula and found that only in 10 out of 23 intracapsular eyes the macular appearance was normal or almost normal, whereas this was the case in 16 out of 19 extracapsular eyes (4 extracapsular eyes could not be assessed due to secondary membranes). The typical appearance of cystoid macular oedema was not encountered, in a few cases however the appearance was suggestive of previous macular oedema, consisting of a dry macula with a small central 'pepper and salt' area.

Group V   Seven patients with intracapsular surgery in one eye and extracapsular surgery with capsulotomy in the other eye

The observation period at the time of re-examination ranged from 33 to 190 months (average 76 months) for the intracapsular eyes and from 13 to 88 months (average 45 months) for the extracapsular eyes. Posterior capsulotomy had been performed from one to 85 months (average 35 months) prior to re-examination, in 7 cases once and in 2 cases twice.

Retinal detachment did not occur in this group. Visual acuity with spectacle correction ranged for the intracapsular eyes from 0.25 to 1.0 and over (average 0.76) and for the extracapsular eyes from 0.5 to 1.0 and over (average 0.93).

Amsler's test revealed metamorphopsia in two intracapsular eyes.

Haidinger's brushes (Table II, group V): Comparison was possible in all 7 eyes. Three patients had equal perception in both eyes. The remaining 4 patients had good perception with the extracapsular eyes. One intracapsular eye did not perceive Haidinger's brushes at all, another intracapsular eye could hardly perceive it, and 2 intracapsular eyes perceived it definitely less than the extracapsular fellow-eyes. We estimated the perception with the intracapsular eyes at only 68 percent of the perception with extracapsular eyes.

Group VI   Five patients with bilateral extracapsular surgery and with capsulotomy in one eye

The observation period for the eyes without capsulotomy ranged from 9 to 44 months (average 27 months) and for the eyes with capsulotomy from 10 to 66 months (average 39 months). Posterior capsulotomy had been performed from 9 to 44 months (average 20 months) prior to re-examination, in each eye only once.

Retinal detachment did not occur in this group. Visual acuity with spectacle correction for the eyes without capsulotomy ranged from 0.5 to 1.0 and over (average 0.68), and for the eyes with capsulotomy from 0.33 to 1.0 and over (average 0.80).

Amsler's test revealed no abnormality.

Haidinger's brushes (Table II group VI): Comparison was possible in all 5 patients. The brushes were readily seen with both eyes in each patient, but each patient stated slightly worse perception with the eye that did undergo capsulotomy, which could be estimated at 70 percent as compared with the eyes without capsulotomy.

DISCUSSION

A follow-up of 48 pseudophakic eyes after intracapsular surgery, and 72 eyes after extracapsular surgery (28 eyes with capsulotomy and 44 eyes without capsulotomy) for senile cataract revealed that retinal detachment had occurred in 3 eyes after intracapsular surgery and in one eye after extracapsular surgery. In that eye posterior capsulotomy had been performed. In no instance had retinal detachment complicated extracapsular surgery without capsulotomy. The incidence of retinal detachment is clearly in favour of extracapsular surgery. Further methods of examination in the same series aimed at the diagnosis of maculopathy. In group IV in which the fundoscopic appearance of the macula could be compared in an optimal way we found that maculopathy occurred in 13 out of 23 intracapsular eyes whereas only in 3 out of 19 extracapsular eyes. The average visual acuity after extracapsular surgery was always superior to that of intracapsular surgery, also if posterior calsulotomy had been performed (Table III). This difference was most convincing in bilateral cases with different procedures in both eyes.

Also the Amsler test results were in favour of extracapsular surgery (Table IV).

TABLE III

Average visual acuity

–	intracaps. (48 eyes)	0.70
–	extracaps. c caps. (28 eyes)	0.84
–	extracaps. (44 eyes)	0.82

TABLE IV

Amsler test. Metamorphopsia. Review of the complete material.

–	intracaps. (48 eyes)	10
–	extracaps. c caps. (28 eyes)	1
–	extracaps. (44 eyes)	–

TABLE V

Haidinger's brushes not perceived. Review of the complete material.

–	intracaps. (48 eyes)	7
–	extracaps. c caps. (28 eyes)	4
–	extracaps. (44 eyes)	–

The use of Haidinger's brushes in this study asks for further comment. The perception of a brush-like phenomenon, when polarized light is falling upon the macula, was first described by HAIDINGER as far back as 1844. Outstanding physiologists, amongst others VON HELMHOLTZ (1909, 1911), have since been fascinated by its origin. BÖHM (1940) pointed to the radial arrangement of the structural elements of the macula, such as Henle's fiber layer and Müller's supporting fibers in the outer plexiform layer of the normal retina. He assumed an analyzer normally being present in the macula. Von Tschermak-Seysenegg linked the phenomenon to the yellow pigment present in the above mentioned structures and explained the phenomenon with its double-refracting properties. The view that the brushes phenomenon was dependent on the presence and on the regular and radial arrangement of the double-refracting yellow macula pigment molecules, acting as an analyzer for light of short wavelength (470 nm) was held in later publications (GOLDSCHMIDT, 1950): FORSTER, 1954; STANWORTH & NAYLOR, 1955; SHERMAN & PRIESTLEY, 1962). STANWORTH & NAYLOR clearly specified that the phenomenon suffered, amongst others, in conditions interfering with the analyzing function of the macula as well as in conditions interfering with the receptor function that should be good for better than 20/200 visual acuity. Although FORTIN (1926) had mentioned the value of polarized light for the detection of disorganization of Henle's fiber layer as far back as 1907, it was GOLDSCHMIDT (1950), who from 1950 onwards stimulated the clinical use of the brushes phenomenon through the construction of his so-called 'Macula Deficiency Tester'. Interesting clinical investigations have been published in subsequent years (GOLDSCHMIDT, 1950; FORSTER, 1954; STANWORTH & NAYLOR, 1955; PRIESTLEY & FOREE, 1055-1956; SHERMAN & PRIESTLEY, 1962). Apart from macular defects considerable attention has been paid to the value of the test in various oedematous conditions of the macula. GOLDSCHMIDT (1950) was the first to stress this point. FORSTER (1954) described its extinction already in the early stage of oedema, when visual acuity was not affected and the fundoscopic appearance of the macula was normal. The importance of the test for macula oedema, being simple and rapid, is stressed by STANWORTH & NAYLOR (1955), as well as by PRIESTLEY & FOREE (1955, 1956).

In relation to cataract surgery the test has been used by SHERMAN & PRIESTLEY (1962) to help evaluate macular function preoperatively. Reports about the postoperative use of the test are so far lacking in literature. We have used the test to detect macular pathology, including oedema and underline the statement of STANWORTH & NAYLOR (1955) that the brushes can remain extincted even when the oedema has disappeared and visual acuity has been restored.

In our study we used the instrument known as 'Cüppers Cheiroscop Koordinator' (Fa. Oculus, 6331 Dutenhofen, Wetzlar (Germany)). The polarization plane can rotate at variable speed and in variable direction, which gives good control of the patient. Four patients out of a total of 85 patients examined gave negative answers with both eyes and were excluded from this study. The aim of our study was to compare the recognition of Haidinger's brushes after intracapsular and after extracapsular surgery, the latter with and without posterior capsulotomy.

The conclusion about 50 patients with unilateral surgery (Table I) was as follows. Of 18 patients after intracapsular surgery 4 patients did not perceive Haidinger's brushes. Of 16 patients after extracapsular surgery with capsulotomy also 4 patients did not, whereas all 16 patients after extracapsular surgery without capsulotomy did perceive the phenomenon. All 31 patients with bilateral surgery (Table II) perceived Haidinger's brushes with the extracapsular eye, whereas with the intracapsular eye 3 patients did not at all and 2 patients did hardly perceive it. In group IV and V all patients perceived equally well or better with the extracapsular eye than with the intracapsular eye, in group VI perception was always better with the extracapsular eye without capsulotomy than with the eye with capsulotomy. Table V reviews the complete material.

There was a total number of 15 patients that either indicated metamorphopsia with the Amsler test (4 patients) or did not perceive Haidinger's brushes (4 patients), only 7 patients did both. Apparently the site of the lesion is decisive in this respect. Exclusive involvement of the receptor layer may cause metamorphopsia whereas Haidinger's brushes test remains positiv. Exclusive involvement of Henle's fiber layer causes a negativ Haidinger's brusher test without metamorphopsia. More extensive involvement of the retina affects both tests. Thus Haidinger's test seems to complement Amsler's test. The above mentioned hypothesis is supported by the average visual acuity of our patients with metamorphopsia (0.24) in comparison with that of our patients with negative Haidinger's test (0.55).

Fundoscopic findings and all functional tests (visual acuity, Amsler test, Haidinger's brushes) point to better protection of the retina and including the macular area, by extracapsular surgery than by intracapsular surgery. Posterior capsulotomy seems partly to compromise this protection.

It has to be remembered that experienced and careful surgeons have always chosen for extracapsular cataract surgery in case of a delicate (high myopia, history of detachment) or diseased (diabetic retinopathy) retina.

Though a comparison could not be made between cataract extraction without and with lens implantation, it is firm belief that the conclusion from our study holds true in case intracapsular aphakics are compared with extracapsular aphakics without lens implantation.

SUMMARY

A follow-up of 120 pseudophakic eyes of 85 patients that underwent surgery for senile cataract showed a definite superiority of extracapsular surgery over intracapsular surgery as far as the long-term fate of the retina concerns. Comparable series have been chosen.

Retinal detachment did not occur in extracapsular eyes that never had posterior capsulotomy, and occurred most often after intracapsular surgery. Signs of previous or existing maculopathy were searched for with the usual tests (fundoscopy, visual acuity, Amsler test) and moreover with Haidinger's brushes test. The macula turned out to have least suffered after extracapsular surgery without capsulotomy and most after intracapsular surgery.

Haidinger's brushes test is a valuable tool for the detaction of postoperative macular oedema.

REFERENCES

BINKHORST, C.D., KATS, A. & LEONARD, P.A.M. Extracapsular pseudophakia: Results in 100 two-loop iridocapsular lens implantations. *Am. J. Ophthal.* 73: *625-636* (1972).

BÖHM, G. Über makulare (Haidingersche) Polarisationsbüschel und über einen polarisations-optischen Fehler des Auges. *Acta Ophthalm.* 18: *109-142* (1940).

FORSTER, H.W. The clinical use of the Haidinger's brushes phenomenon. *Am. J. Ophthal.* 38: *661-665* (1954).

FORTIN, E. Entoptische Vorrichtungen für die entoptische inspektion. *Rev. Espec.* 1: *238-275* (1926).

GASS J.D.M. & NORTON, E.W.D. Cystoid macular edema and papilledema following cataract extracting. A fluorescein fundoscopic and angiographic study. *Arch. Ophthal.* 76: *646-661* (1966).

GOLDSCHMIDT, M. A new test for function of the macula lutea. *Am. Arch. Ophthal.* 44: *129* (1950).

HAIDINGER, W. Über das direkte Erkennen des polarisierten Lichtes. *Ann. Phys. Chem.* 53: *29-39* (1844).

HELMHOLTZ, H. VON. Handb. physiol. Optik. Bd 1, 2, 3. Voss, Hamburg und Leipzig. 1909, 1911.

IRVINE, S.R. A newly defined vitreous syndrome following cataract surgery. *Am. J. Ophthal.* 36: *599-619* (1953).

NORDLOHNE, M.E. The intraocular implant lens. *Documenta Ophthalmologica* 38: issue I (1974).

PRIESTLEY, B.S. & FOREE, K. Clinical significance of some entoptic phenomena. *Am. Arch. Ophthal.* 53: *390-397* (1955).

PRIESTLEY, B.S. & FOREE, K. A new entoscope. *Am. Arch. Ophthal.* 55: *415-416* (1956).

SHERMAN, M.E. & PRIESTLEY, B.S, The Haidinger brush phenomenon. A new clinical use. *Am. J. Ophthal.* 54: *807-812* (1962).

STANWORTH, A. NAYLOR, E.J. The measurement and clinical significance of the Haidinger effect. *Trans. Ophthal. Soc. United Kingdom* 65: *67-79* (1955).

TSCHERMAK–SEYSENEGG, A. VON. Über anomale Sehrichtungsgemeinschaft der Netzhäute bei einem Schielenden. *v. Graefes Arch. Ophthal.* 47: *508-540* (1899).

TSCHERMAK-SEYSENEGG, A. VON. Physiologisch-optische Studien II über das Sehen im polarisierten Licht. *Doc. Ophth.* 2: *26-40* (1948).

Key words:
Retinal detachment
Maculopathy
Cataract extraction
Pseudophakia
Intracapsular surgery
Extracapsular surgery
Haidinger's brushes

Author's address:
Axelsestraat 54
Terneuzen, The Netherlands

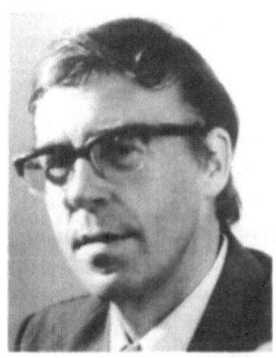

THE BURSA INTRAVITREALIS PREMACULARIS

JAN G.F. WORST

(Haren (Gr.), the Netherlands)

This is a report on a highly characteristic anatomical structure, situated in the vitreous in front of the macula. Its presence has been demonstrated in anatomical specimens by means of selective white Indian ink injections. This anatomical structure, for which the name *Bursa Intravitrealis Premacularis* is proposed (abbreviated as bursa premacularis), is a sacklike, slightly oval, horizontally oriented space filled with a clear fluid. The bursa premacularis communicates with the area of Martegiani by way of a short 'canal'. A second, wider, 'canal' enters the premacular bursa from Cloquet's canal. The bursa premacularis is a normal component of any adult eye. It is absent in neonatal and infantile eyes and is subject to important changes in the course of senile involution of the vitreous.

ANATOMICAL PROCEDURES FOR DEMONSTRATING THE BURSA PREMACULARIS

Both fresh anatomical specimens and formaline fixed eyes may be used. Several natural and artificial causes may lead to damage of the premacular bursa, changing it beyond recognition. This is one of the reasons why this elusive structure has been discovered so late. Its presence is also difficult to demonstrate with histological techniques, as the twodimensional histological slide makes it difficult to demonstrate threedimensional membrane relations.

The fact that histologically prepared eyes have been conserved at zero pressure inevitably means a total collapse of the bursa, which makes it unidentifiable.

Four variations in anatomical technique have been used:

1. Filling of Cloquet's canal with white Indian ink through the anterior route.
2. Translental injection into Berger's space.
3. Retrograde filling through the optic nerve and Martegiani's area.
4. Cannulation of the premacular bursa and filling of it under direct transvitreal observation.

The drawings of Fig. 1 and Fig. 2 are semischematic representations of the premacular bursa, and are not to scale.

The top of the bursa is formed by a narrow canal which seems to branch off from Cloquet's canal, but may also be interpreted as a direct continuation of it. The bifurcation is situated slightly below the equatorial plane (Fig. 2, 10). The top of the sac is supported by its connection with Cloquet's canal (Fig. 2, 9), around which it may 'twine' with an incomplete spiral. Distant support to the double canal system is provided by the insertion of the walls of Cloquet's canal on the posterior surface of the lens

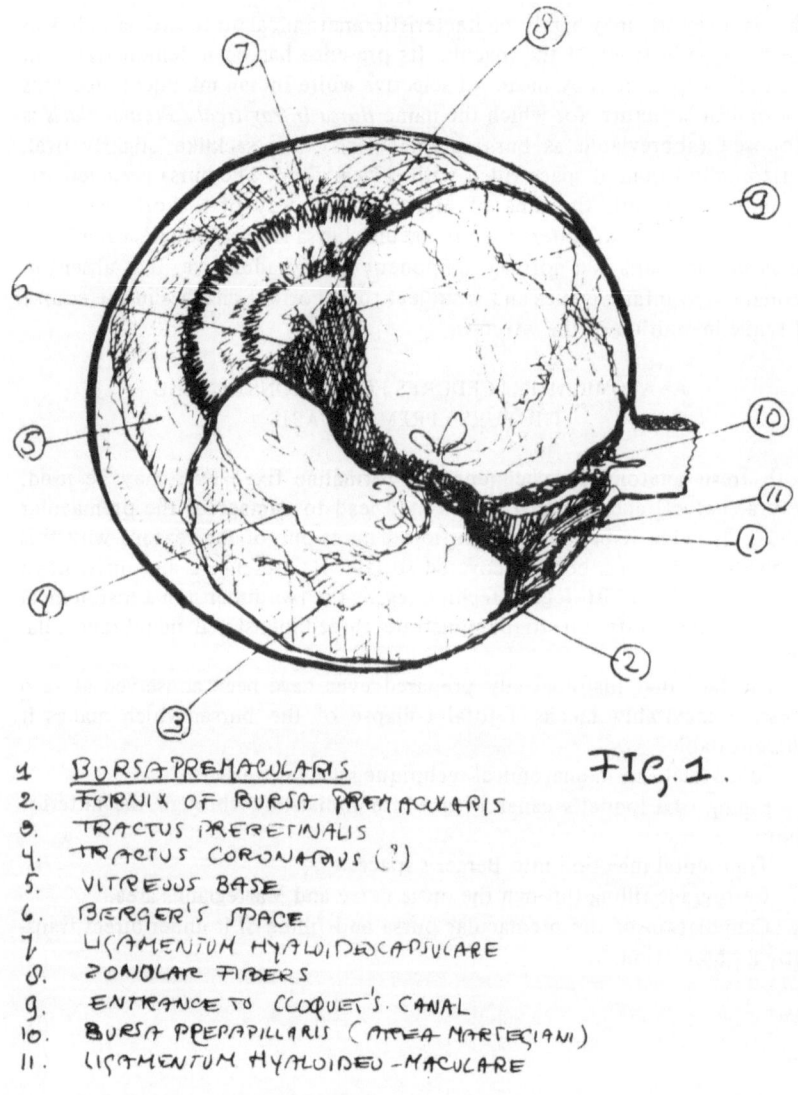

FIG. 1.

1. BURSA PREMACULARIS
2. FORNIX OF BURSA PREMACULARIS
3. TRACTUS PRERETINALIS
4. TRACTUS CORONARIUS (?)
5. VITREOUS BASE
6. BERGER'S SPACE
7. LIGAMENTUM HYALOIDEOCAPSULARE
8. ZONULAR FIBERS
9. ENTRANCE TO CLOQUET'S CANAL
10. BURSA PREPAPILLARIS (AREA MARTEGIANI)
11. LIGAMENTUM HYALOIDEO-MACULARE

(ligamentum hyaloideo-capsulare of Wieger (Fig. 1, 7)). An intravitreal membrane (Fig. 1, 4) of which the origin at the vitreous base is difficult to trace (tractus coronarius?) joins the entrance to the bursa, forming highly characteristic 'petals' (Fig. 2, 11) around it. In case of total collapse of the bursa, the midvitreal ring may become more conspicuous (Fig. 3). the entrance to the bursa is physiologically situated below the central visual axis, and partakes in the typical S-shaped configuration of Cloquet's canal. The bursa widens funnellike towards the macula.

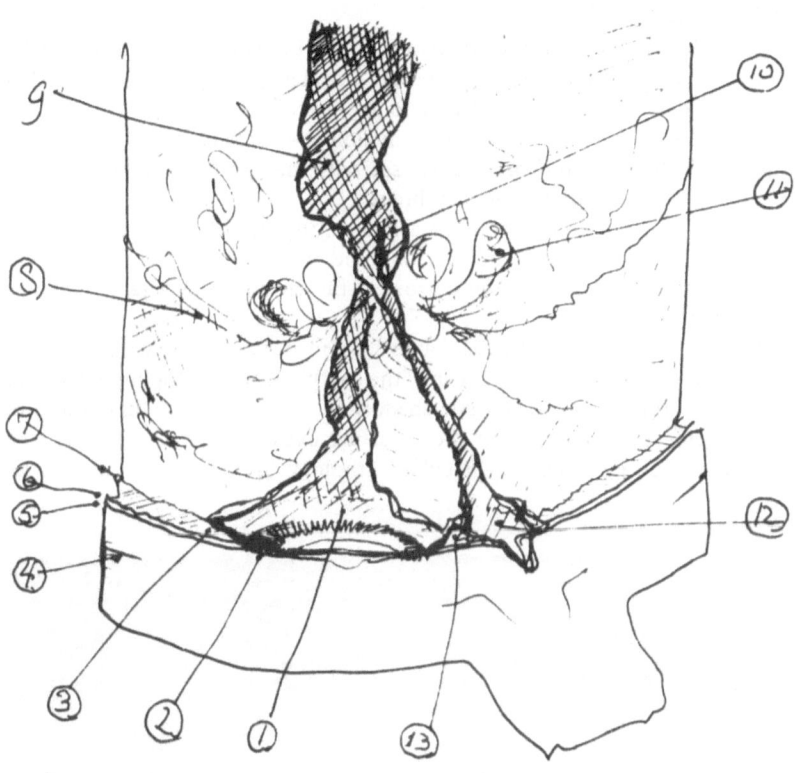

1. BURSA PREMACULARIS
2. LIGAMENTUM HYALOIDEO-MACULARE
3. FORNIX OF PREMACULAR BURSA
4. RETINA
5. MEMBRANA LIMITANS INTERNA
6. MEMBRANA HYALOIDEA POSTERIOR
7. TRACTUS PRERETINALIS
8. TRACTUS CORONARIUS (?)
9. CANALIS CLOQUETI.
10. BIFURCATION
11. "PETALS'
12. BURSA PRERAPILLARIS (AREA MARTEGIANI)
13. COMMUNICATING CHANNEL

Fig. 2.

Its conical shape is evident in preparations, but under more physiological pressure relations the bursa assumes a balloonlike shape. The wide part of the bursa, the fornix (Fig. 2, 3) is situated a few tenths of a millimeter in front of the retina. This part of the bursa is clearly suspended and extended by a vitreous 'membrane' (Fig. 2, 7). This membrane is probably an extension of the tractus preretinalis (Fig. 1, 3). The fornix has an oval shape with a vertical diameter of 4 mm, and a horizontal diameter of 6 mm. Below the peripheral ring formed by the fornix the bursa narrows sharply. Its sharply inwards sloping wall inserts on the rim of the macula with a fairly wide bending bend (Fig. 2, 2).

In analogy to the anterior insertion of the insertion of the wall of Cloquet's canal on the hyaloideocapsular ligament, its posterior insertion should be called the ligamentum hyaloideo-maculare.

The adherence of the ligamentum hyaloideo-maculare is quite strong. It joins the bottom of the premacular sac with the posterior vitreous membrane and the internal limiting membrane.

In case of posterior vitreous detachment, rupture of the bottom of the premacular bursa usually occurs along the outer rim of the ligamentum hyaloideo-maculare, leaving the bottom of the sac partly or totally adherent to the macula.

This creates the typical large round hole in the posterior vitreous membrane. If the bursa is filled with ink, the sharply inwards sloping bottom of the sac will throw a characteristic shadow on the retina. The dimensions of the oval ring of the fornix of the bursa are extremely constant. It can be retraced in several types of macular pathology as the outer limit of the

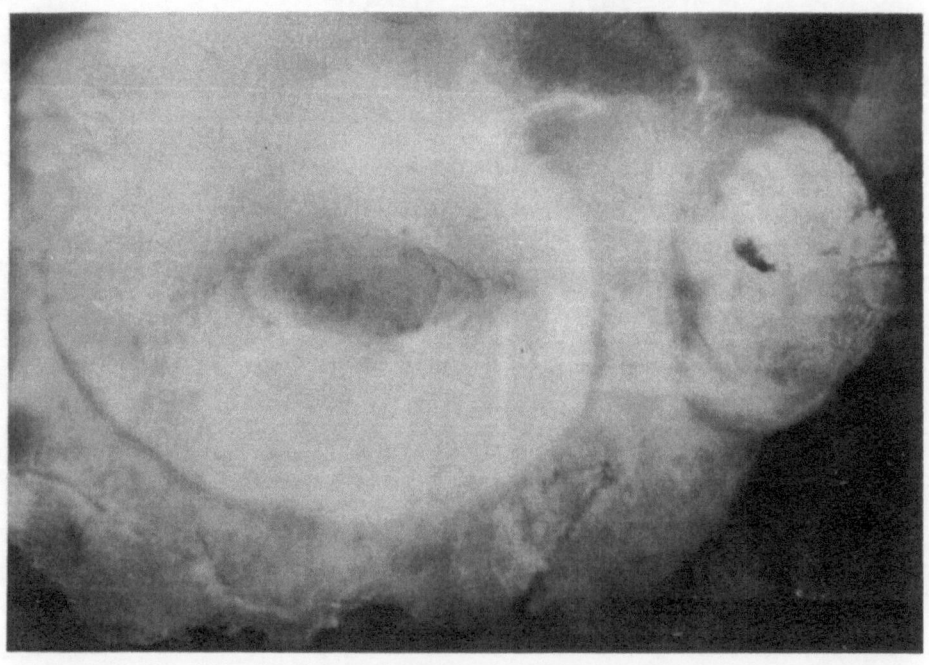

visible pathological lesions. Shrinkage of the remaining central elements of the premacular bursa in vitreous detachment causes macular pucker.

Fig. 3 shows the typical aspect of a collapsed premacular bursa. Martegiani's area is clearly outlined. The connecting canal is vaguely visible. The central oval ring is accentuated by the overlying collapsed funnel. Folds in the membrane indicate its slackness. There is a beginning posterior vitreous detachment around the bursa, which is made visible by the ink which has run into it. Posterior vitreous detachments often start at a local defect in the bottom of the premacular burs (not shown here).

SUMMARY

A new anatomical structure in front of the macula has been demonstrated by means of stereomicroscope dissection of the vitreous body. This new structure is a fluid saclike space for which the name bursa intravitrealis premacularis is proposed (bursa premacularis).

Special white Indian ink injections have been used.

REFERENCES

EISNER, G. Biomicroscopy of the Peripheral Fundus. Springer-Verlag, Berlin, Heidelberg, New York. 1973.

Author's address:
Department of Ophthalmology
Refaja Clinic
Stadskanaal, the Netherlands

Reprint requests to J.G.F. Worst, M.D., Julianalaan 11, Haren (Gr.), the Netherlands.

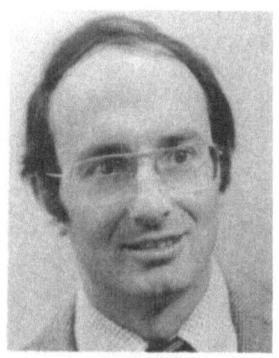

UNEXPECTED FINDINGS IN HEREDITARY MACULAR DYSTROPHY

AUGUST F. DEUTMAN

(Nijmegen, The Netherlands)

Although I have been studying hereditary determined macular dystrophies with great interest for many years already, unexpected findings and unusual types of macular dystrophy do still appear.

1. VITELLIFORM DYSTROPHY

Vitelliform dystrophy or *Best's disease*, is a well known autosomal dominant type of macular dystrophy characterized in almost all cases by a markedly subnormal electro-oculogram (EOG) (DEUTMAN, 1971). Although I speculated originally that leaking vessels were very uncommon in this and other types of macular dystrophy, we found over the last few years a few interesting cases that did show evidence of fluorescein leakage.

The three classic macular fluorescein leakage patterns of central serous choroidopathy, serous detachment of the retinal pigment epithelium and haemorrhagic detachment of the retinal pigment epithelium could be found in several patients suffering from Best's disease.

a. Best's disease with central serous choroidopathy.

In one patient we found a point-like leak at the site of the eggyolk lesion, increasing in size throughout the angiography procedure (Fig. 1).

b. Best's disease with serous detachment of the retinal pigment epithelium.

In another patient with Best's disease, whom I followed a long time already, visual acuity decreased rather suddenly after many years of observation. His vitelliform lesion appeared to be enlarged and around his old lesion there was the typical appearance of serous detachment of the retinal pigment epithelium (Fig. 2).

c. Best's disease with haemorrhagic detachment of the retinal pigment epithelium

Haemorrhages have been seen rather frequently in vitelliform lesions and they appeared to have their origin in the choriocapillaris (DEUTMAN, 1971).

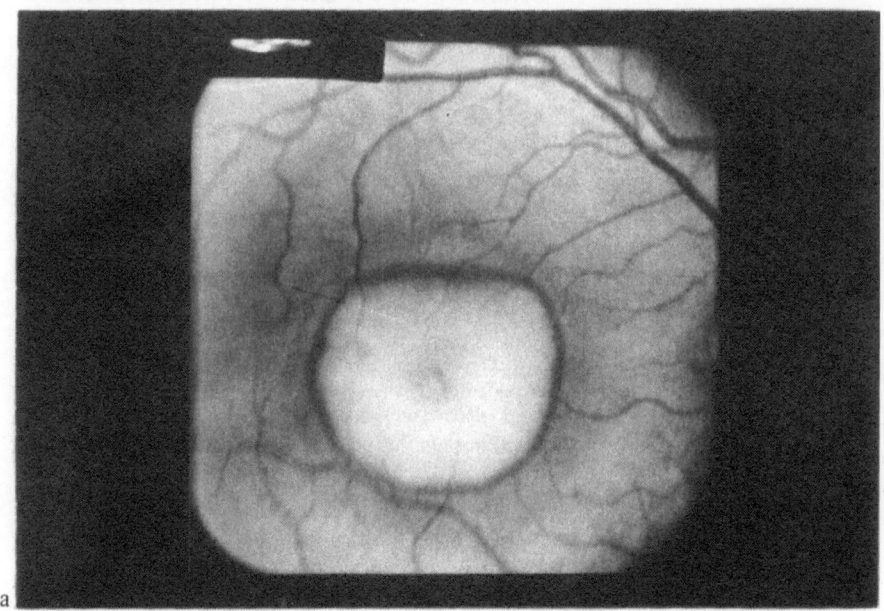

a

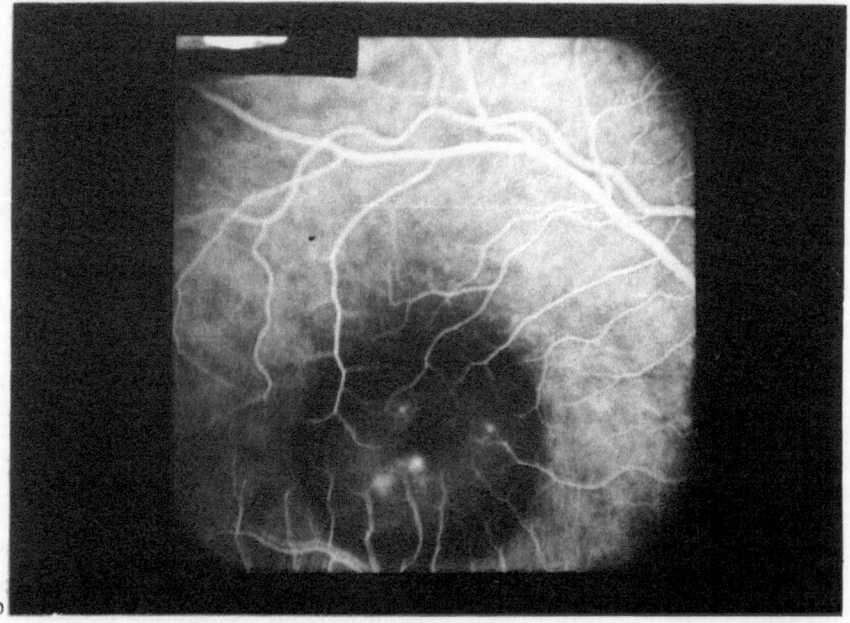

b

Fig. 1. Central serous choroidopathy-like leakage in vitelliform dystrophy (Fig. 1abc). Note the hypofluorescence at the site of the vitelliform lesion in the fellow eye with an additional extrafoveal vitelliform structure (Fig. 1de). Only in the later stages of angiography there is some hyperfluorescence (Fig. 1f).

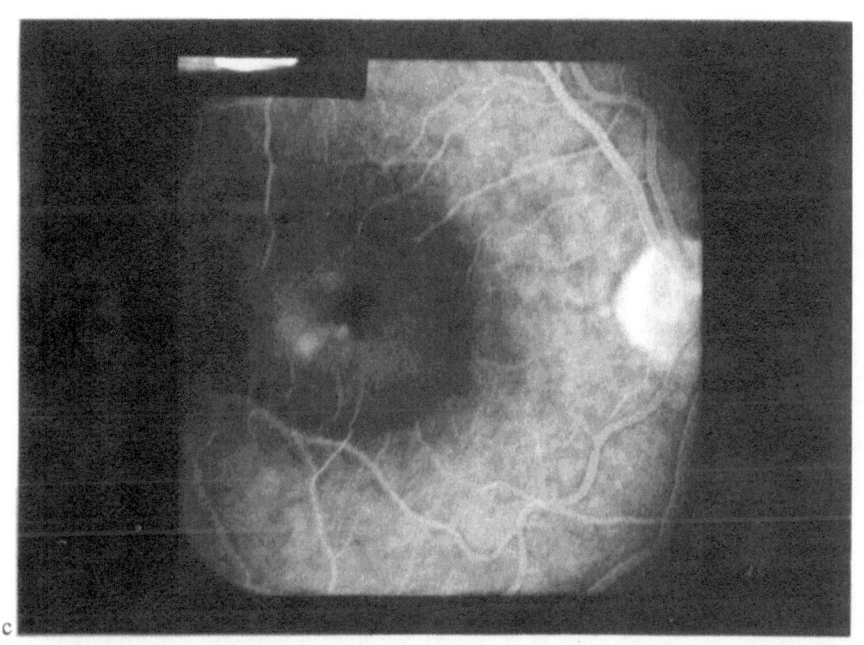

c

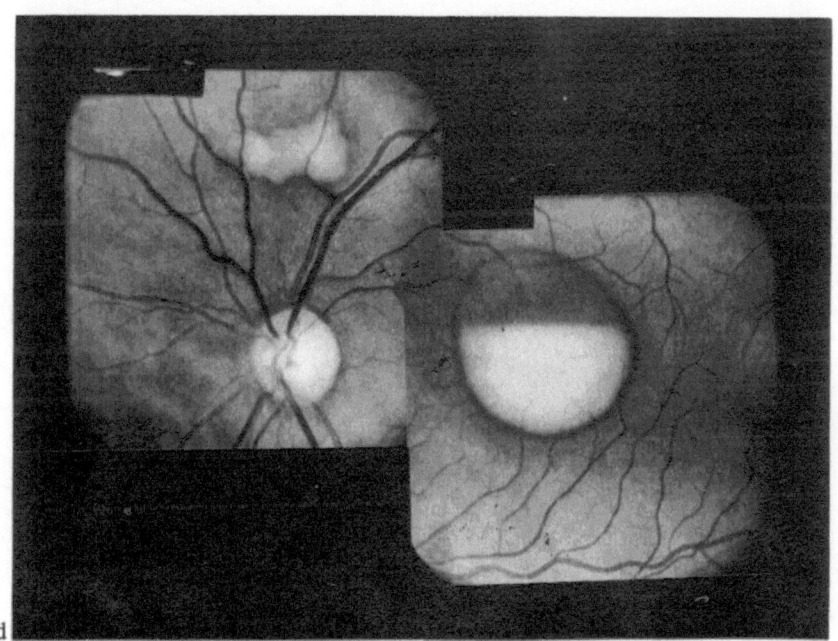

d

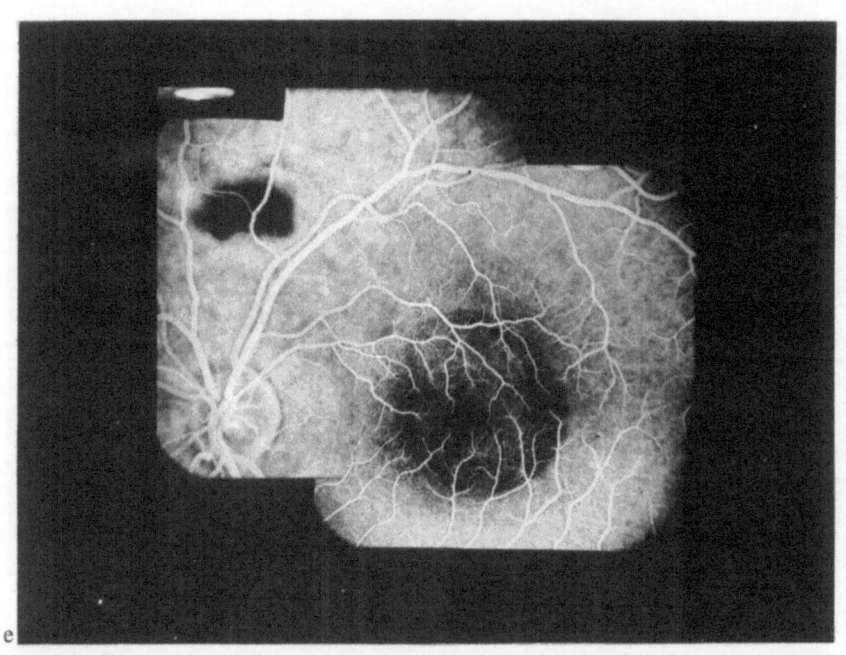

e

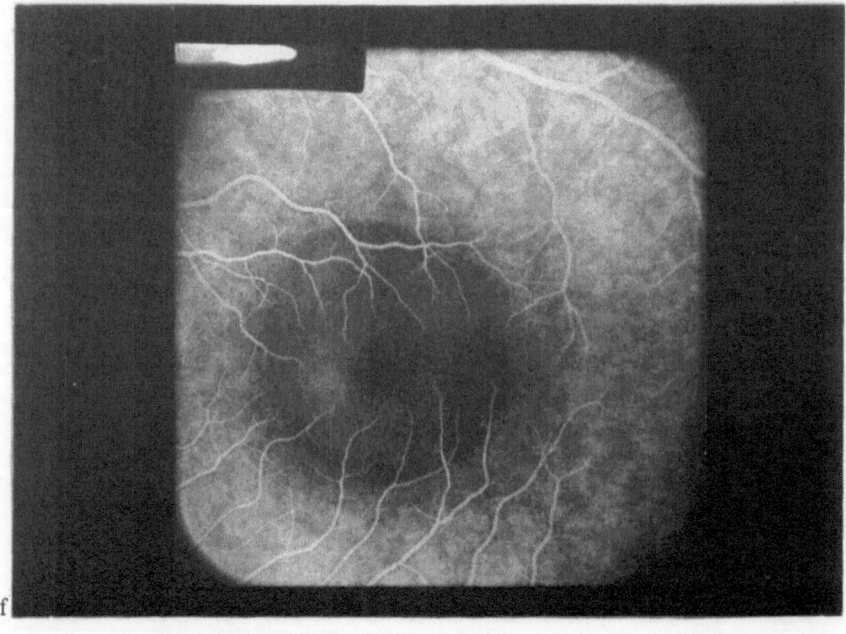

f

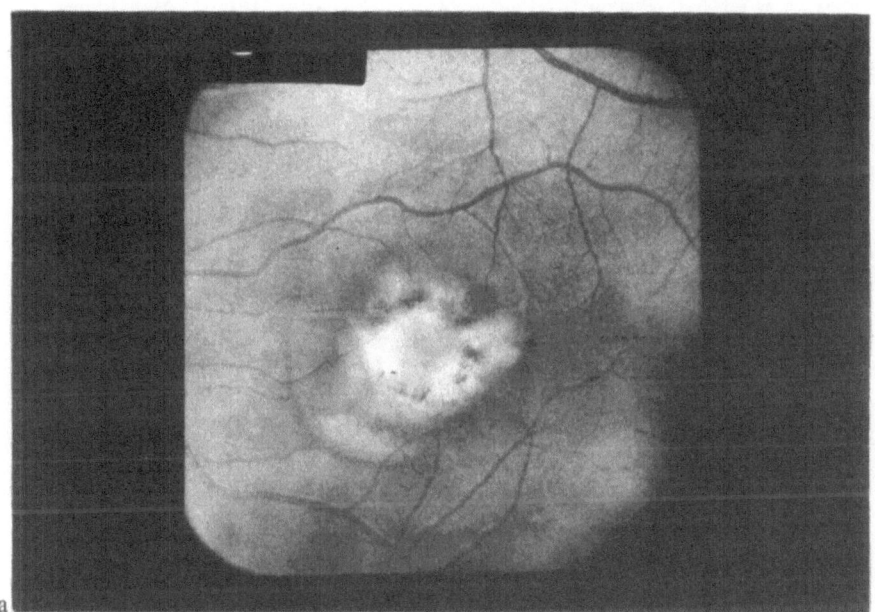

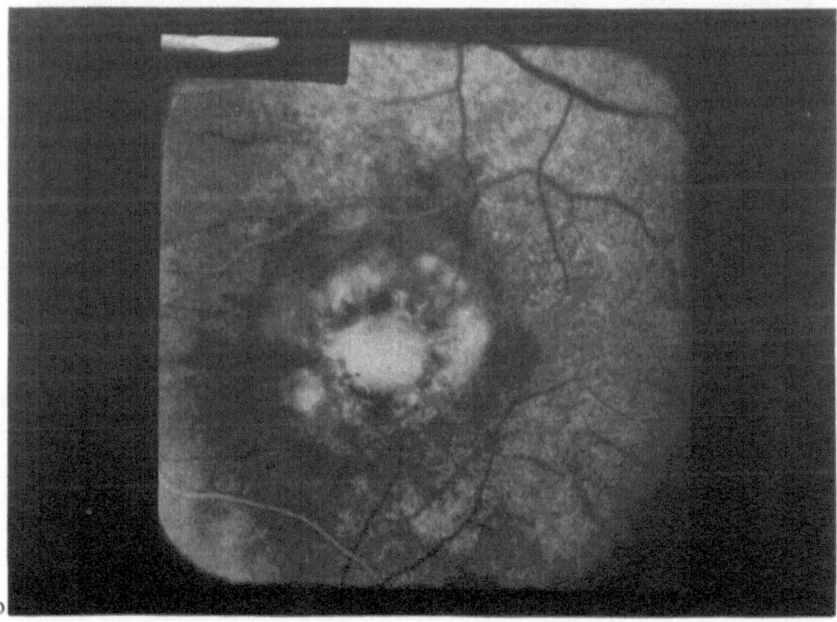

Fig. 2. Serous detachment of the retinal pigment epithelium in vitelliform dystrophy. A zone of rpe-detachment developed rather suddenly around a central vitelliform lesion, that had been there for a long time (Fig. 2abc). Argon laser coagulation flattened the pigment epithelial detachment (Fig. 2def).

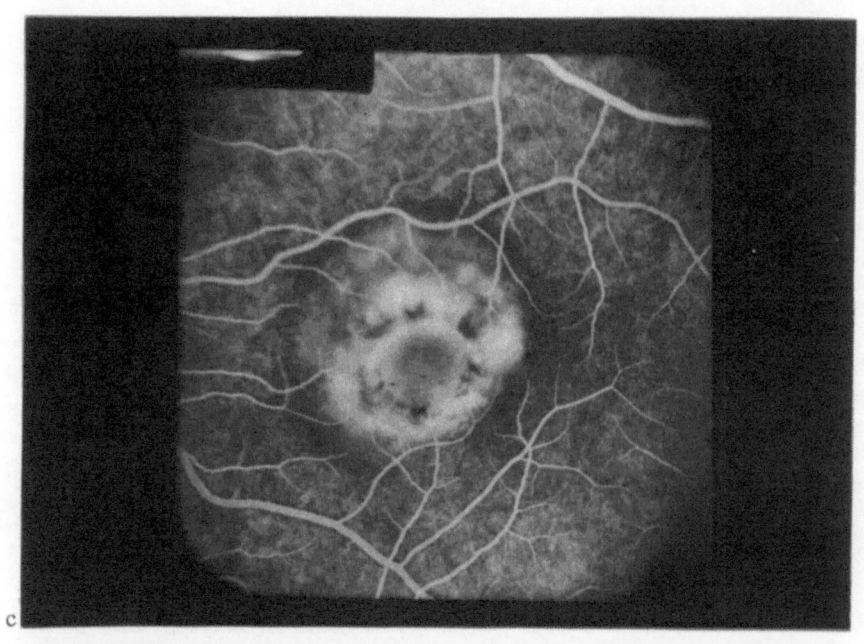

c

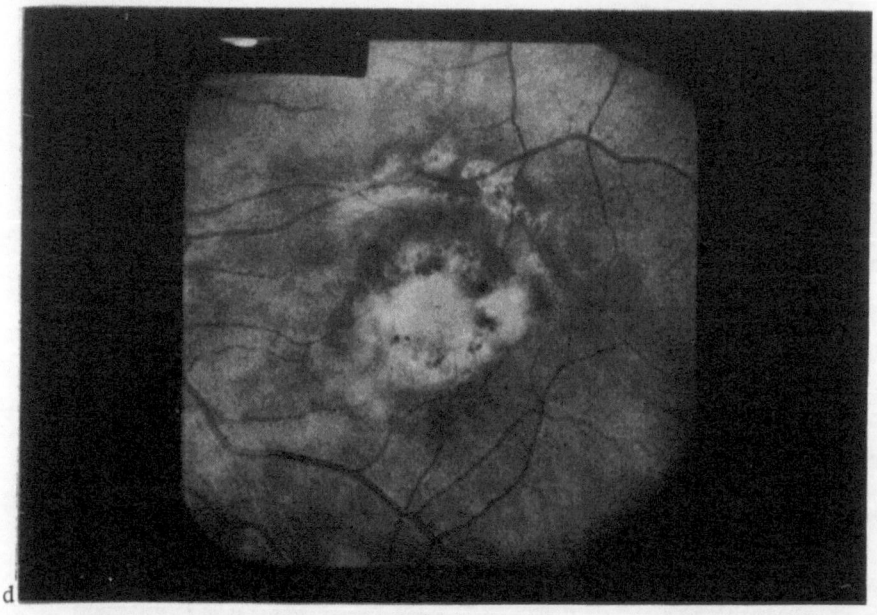

d

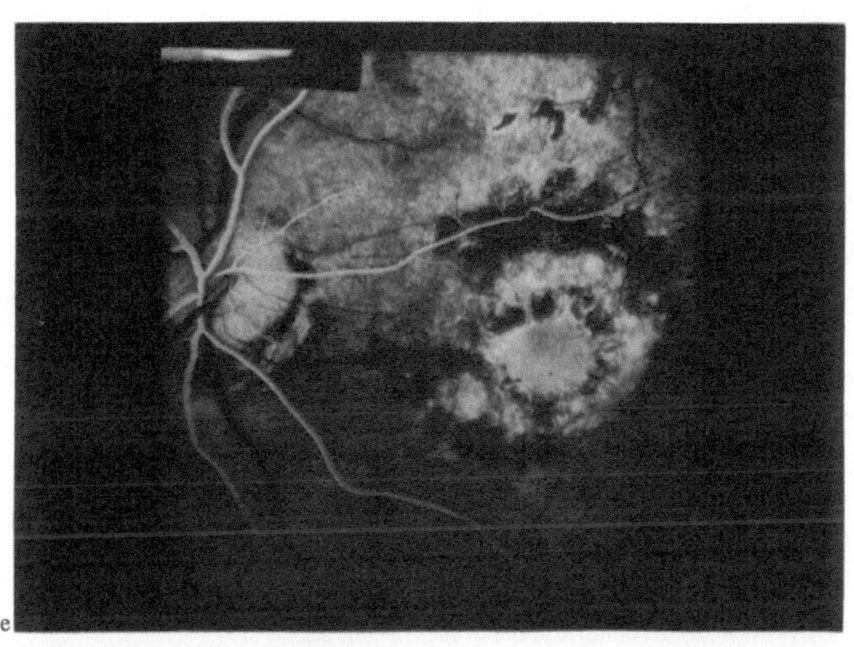

e

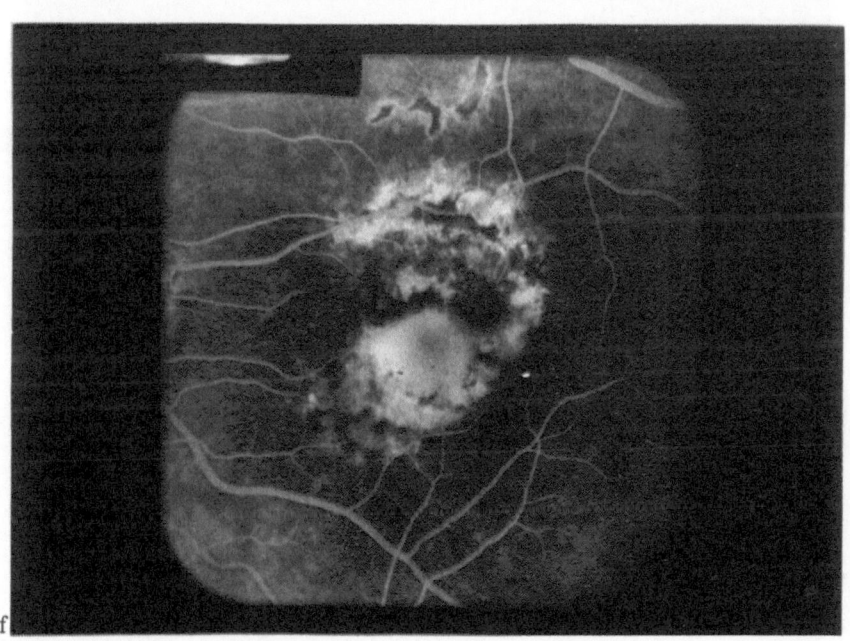

f

287

Not long ago cases with subretinal neovascularisation were presented in Best's disease (BENSON et al, 1975) and we have also seen such cases. The appearance of the lesion, may be almost exactly like the one in presumed histoplasmin choroiditis (Fig. 3). Decompensation, of the Bruch membrane-retinal pigment epithelium complex obviously leads to these three types of fluorescein leakage from the choriocapillaris through the choriodoretinal diffusion barrier.

It is questionable if photocoagulation may be of some help in these cases.

BRALEY (1966) treated some of his patients with xenon arc photo-coagulation with questionable results. We only treated the patient with the serous detachment of the retinal pigment epithelium with the Argon laser when his serous detachment did not subside and the complaints remained. We could flatten the macula in this patient (Fig. 2 def.)

2. DOMINANT CYSTOID MACULAR OEDEMA (DYSTROPHY)

Over the last few years we have observed in our institute five different pedigrees, in which an apparently autosomal dominant macular dystrophy occurred with the predominant abnormality of leaking perimacular capillaries. Personally I examined three of these pedigrees.

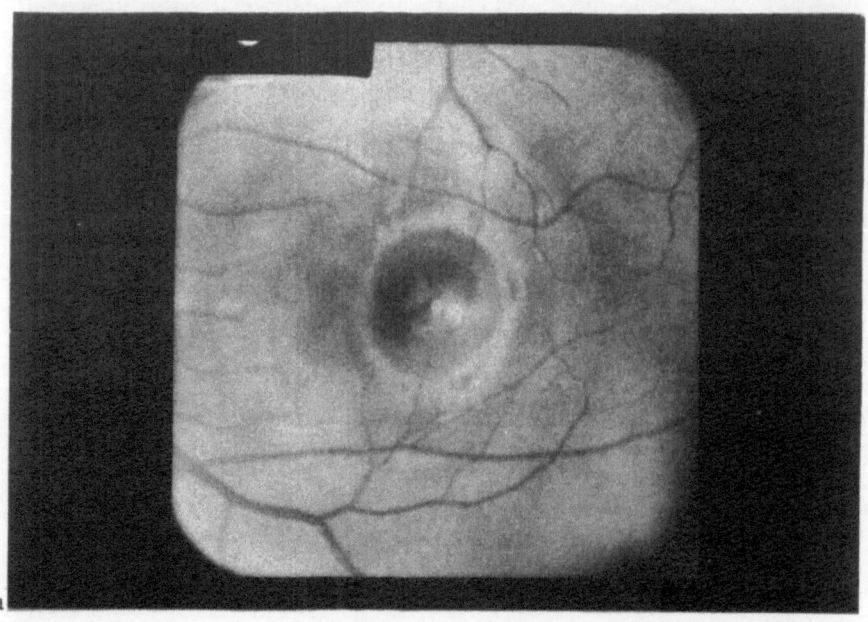

a

Fig. 3. Haemorrhagic detachment of the retinal pigment epithelium, indistinguishable from presumed histoplasmin choroiditis in a young patient with vitelliform dystrophy. There is typical subretinal neovascularisation. Note the atrophic vitelliform lesion in the other eye (Fig. 3e).

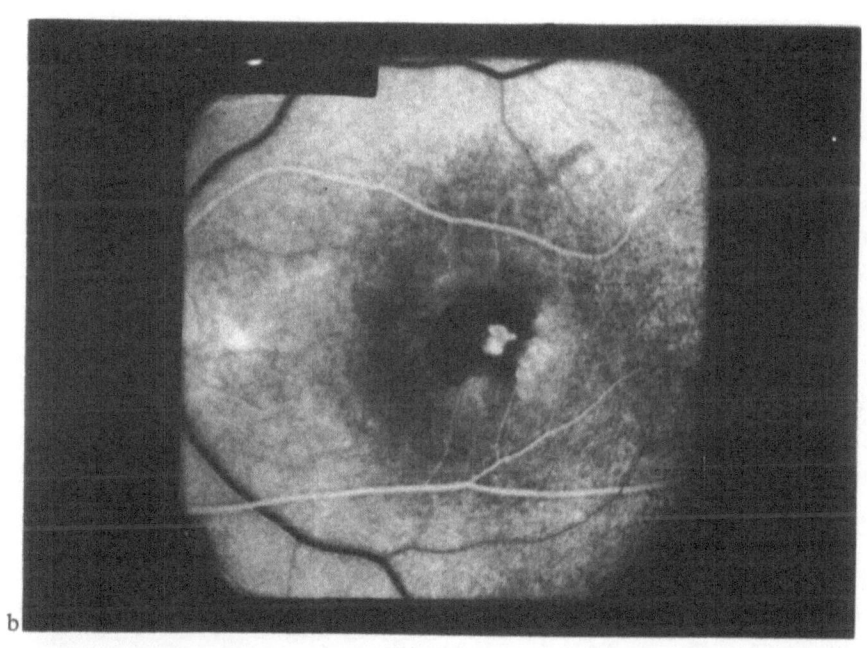

b

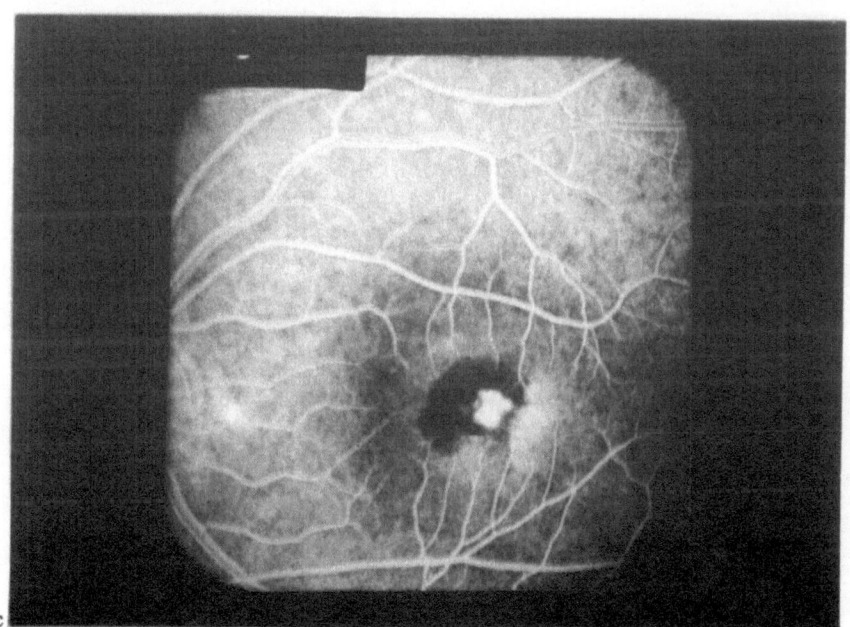

c

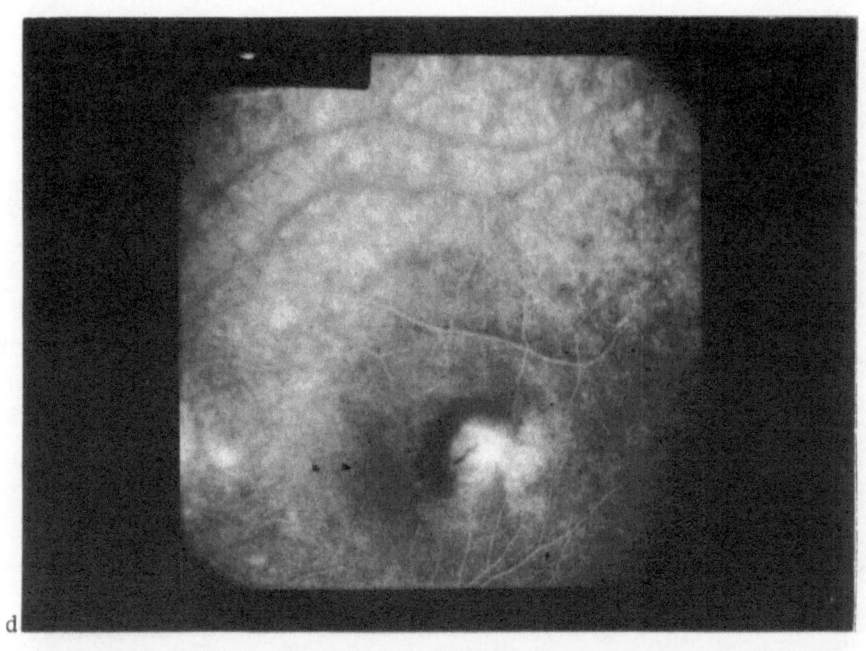

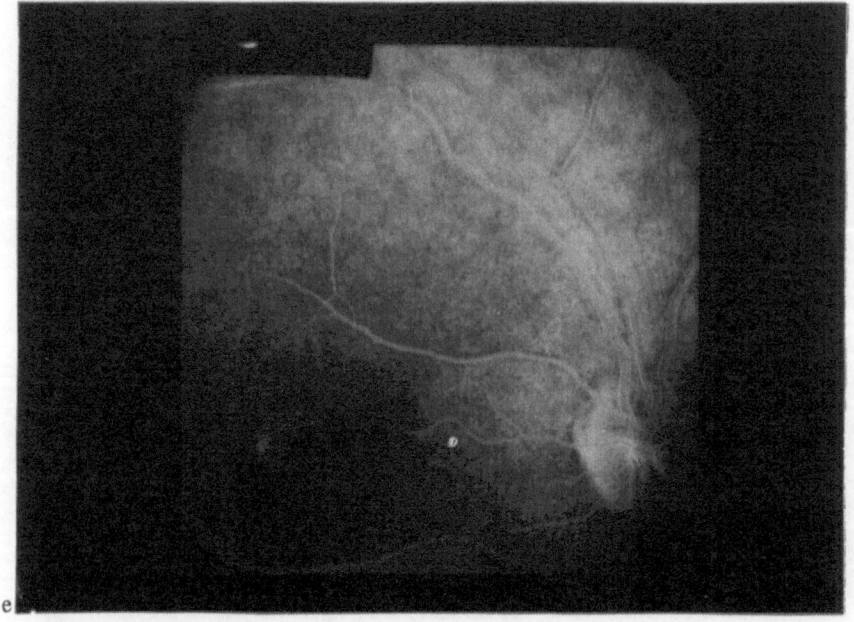

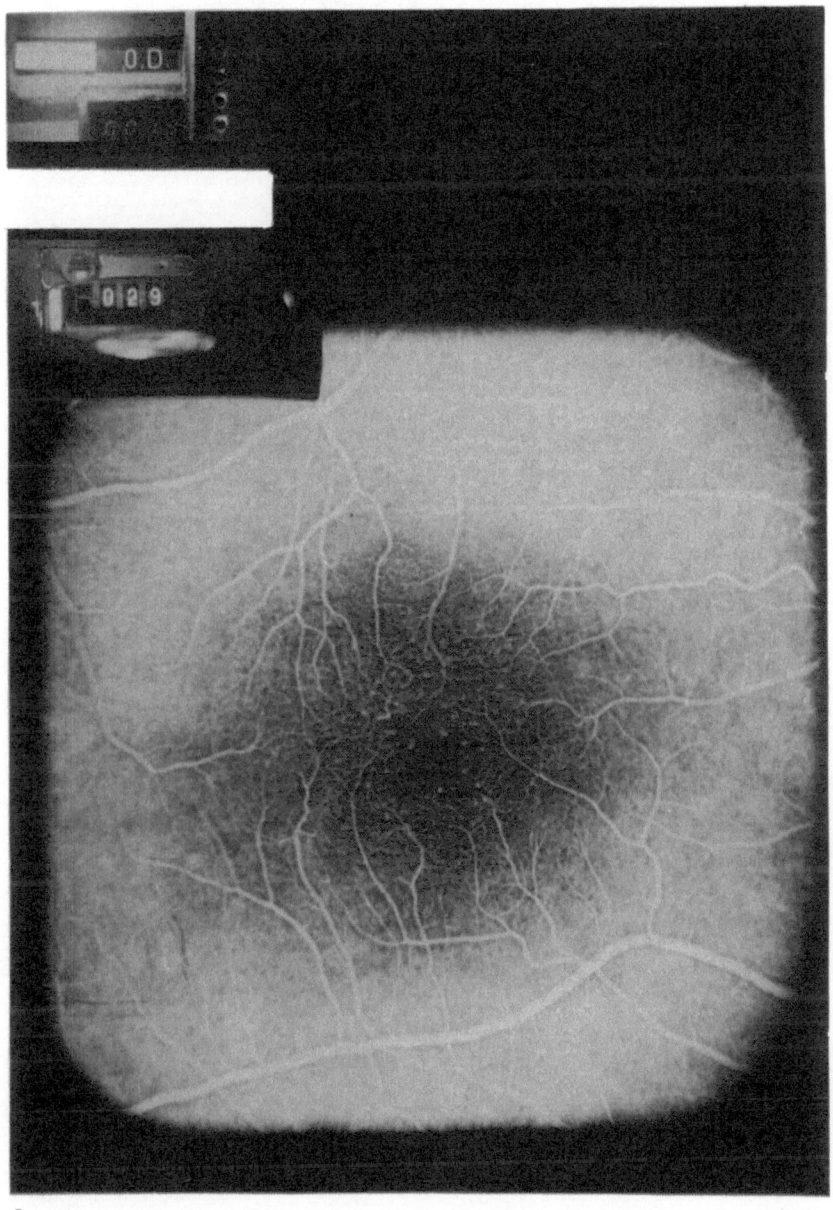

a

Fig. 4. Cystoid macular edema in a 10-year-old girl with hereditary macular dystrophy showing the well-known pattern of dilated and leaking perimacular capillaries (abcd).

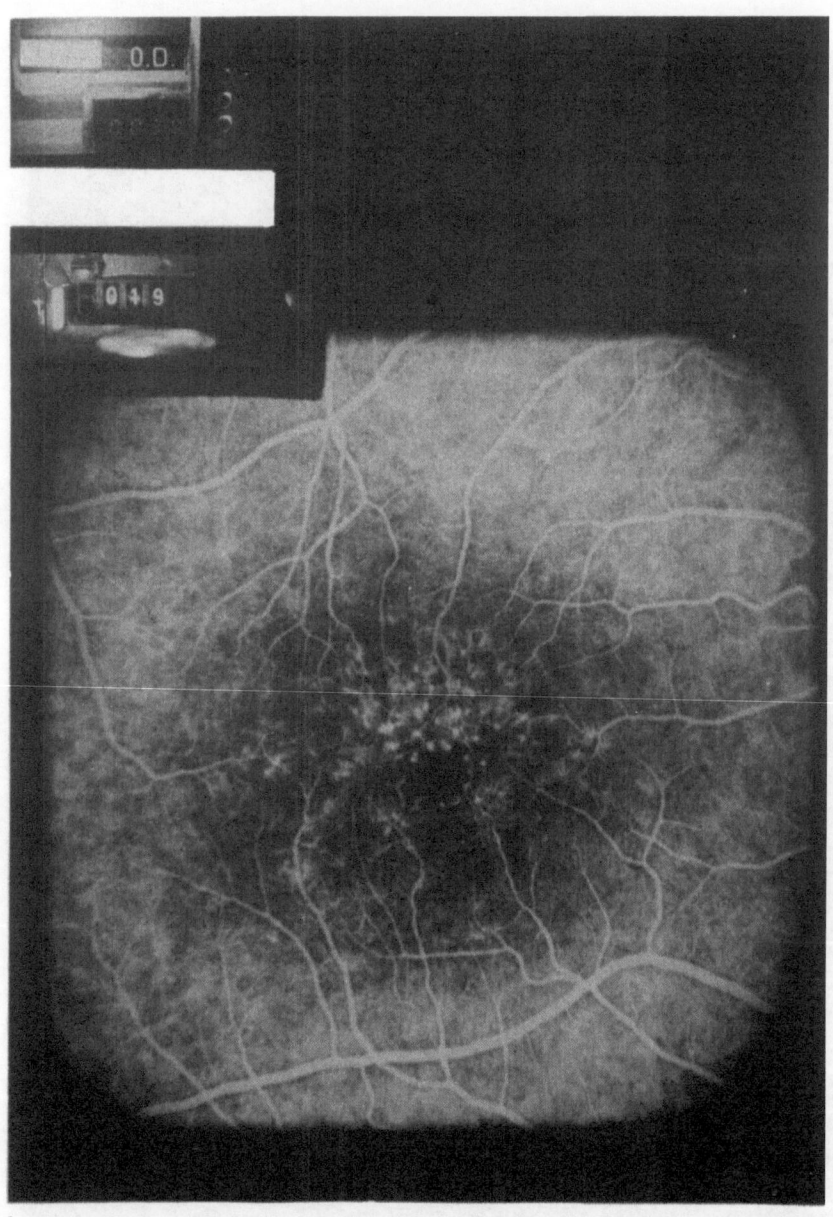

b

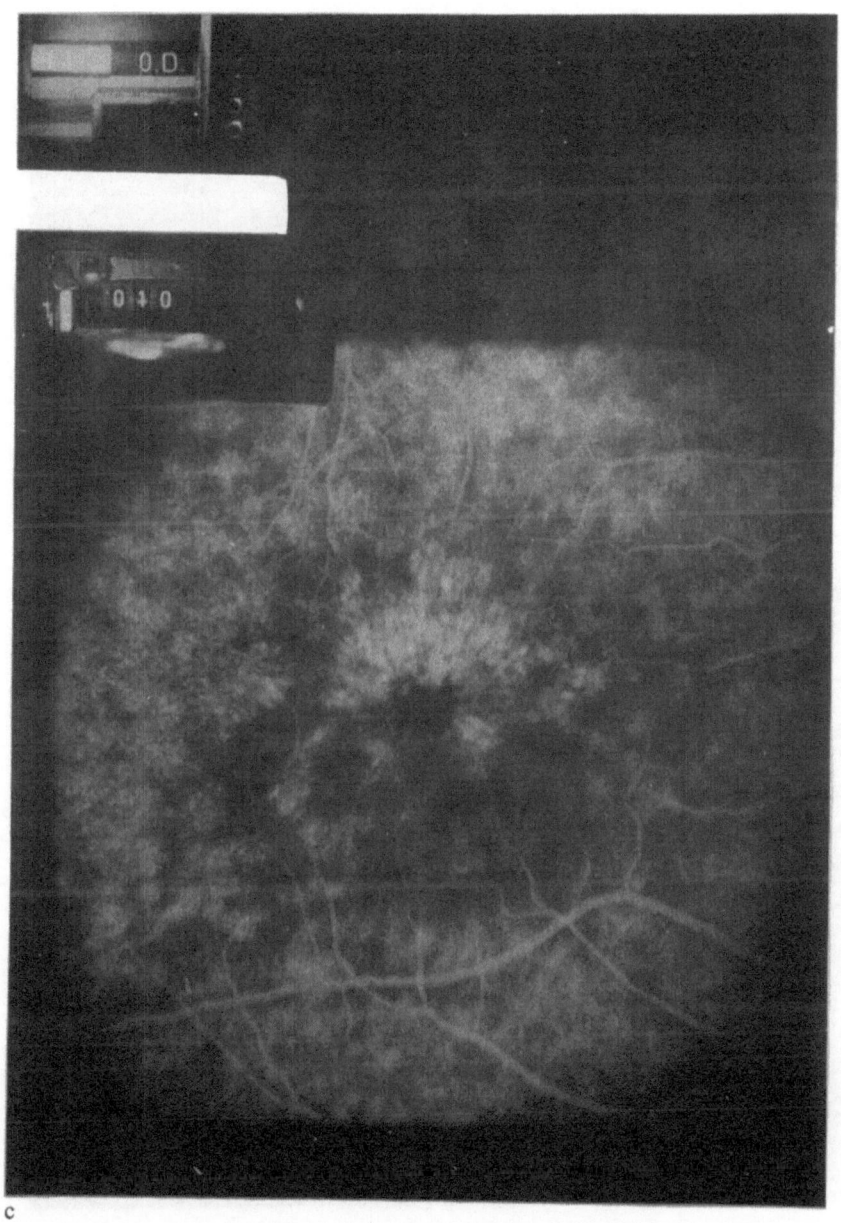

c

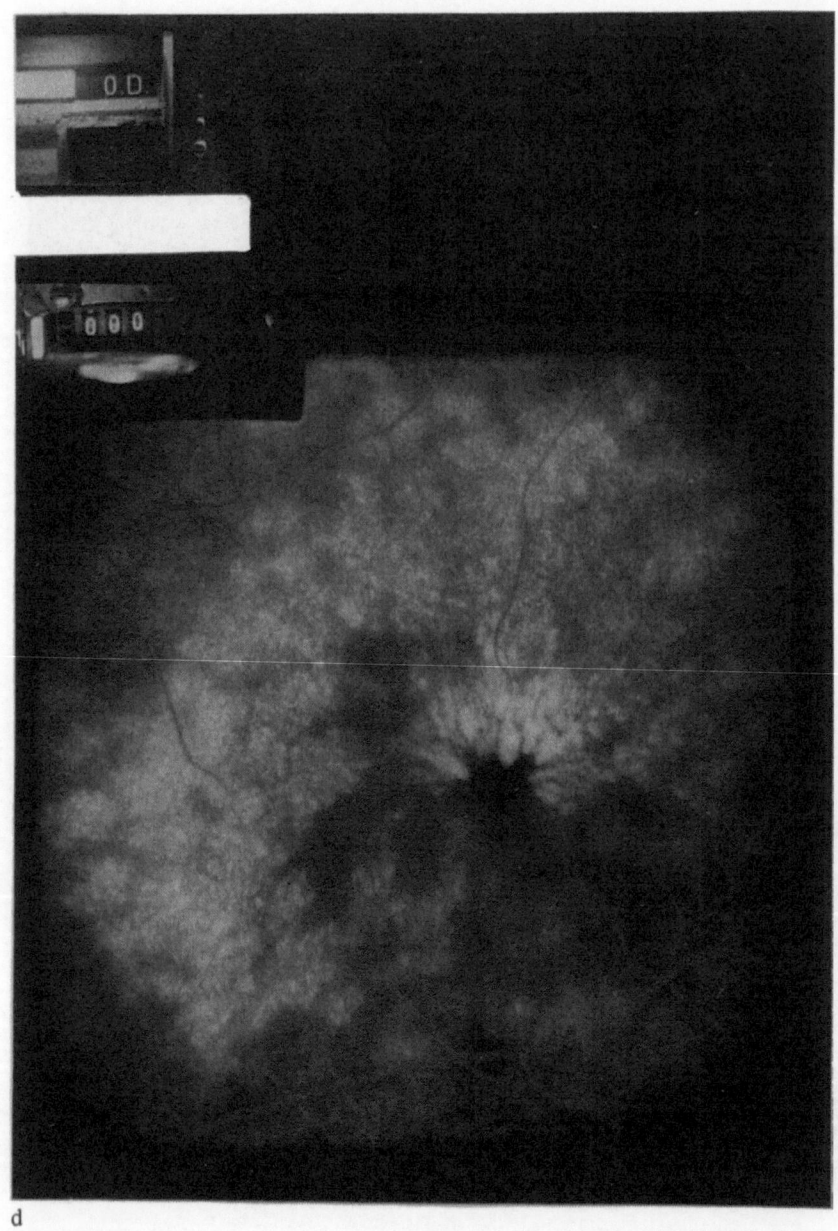

d

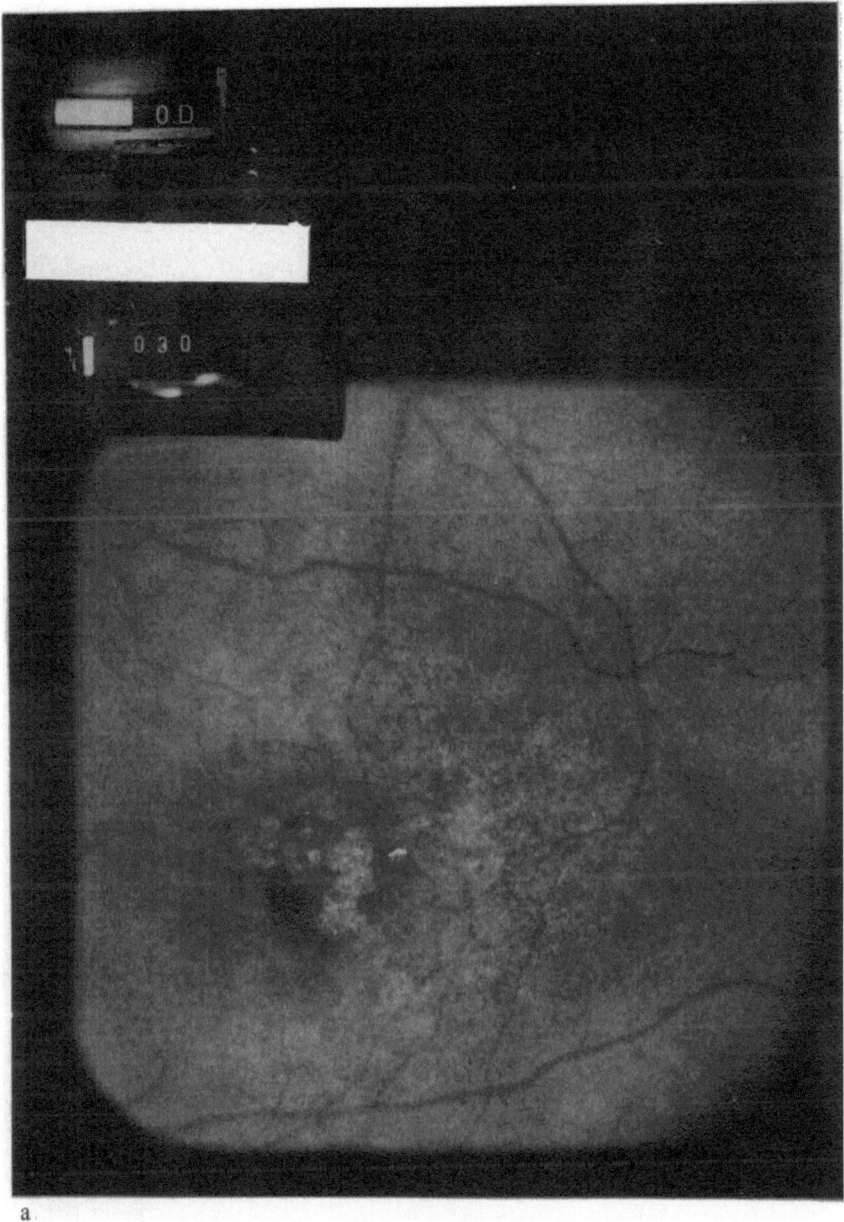

a

Fig. 5. Atrophic macular degeneration in the mother of the girl, whose fundus pictures are depicted in Fig. 4. There are some dilated and leaking retinal capillaries around the central zone of pigmentepithelial atrophy (abc: left eye, d: right eye).

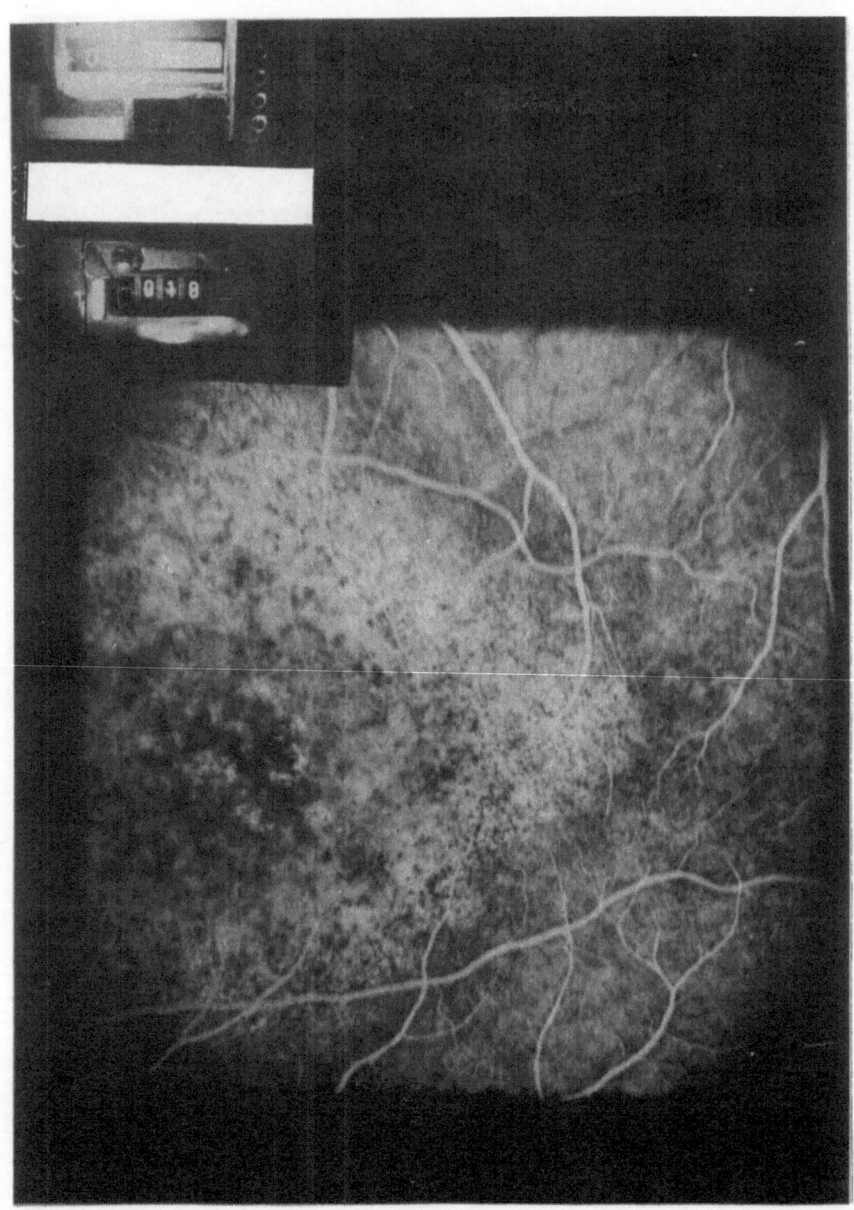

b

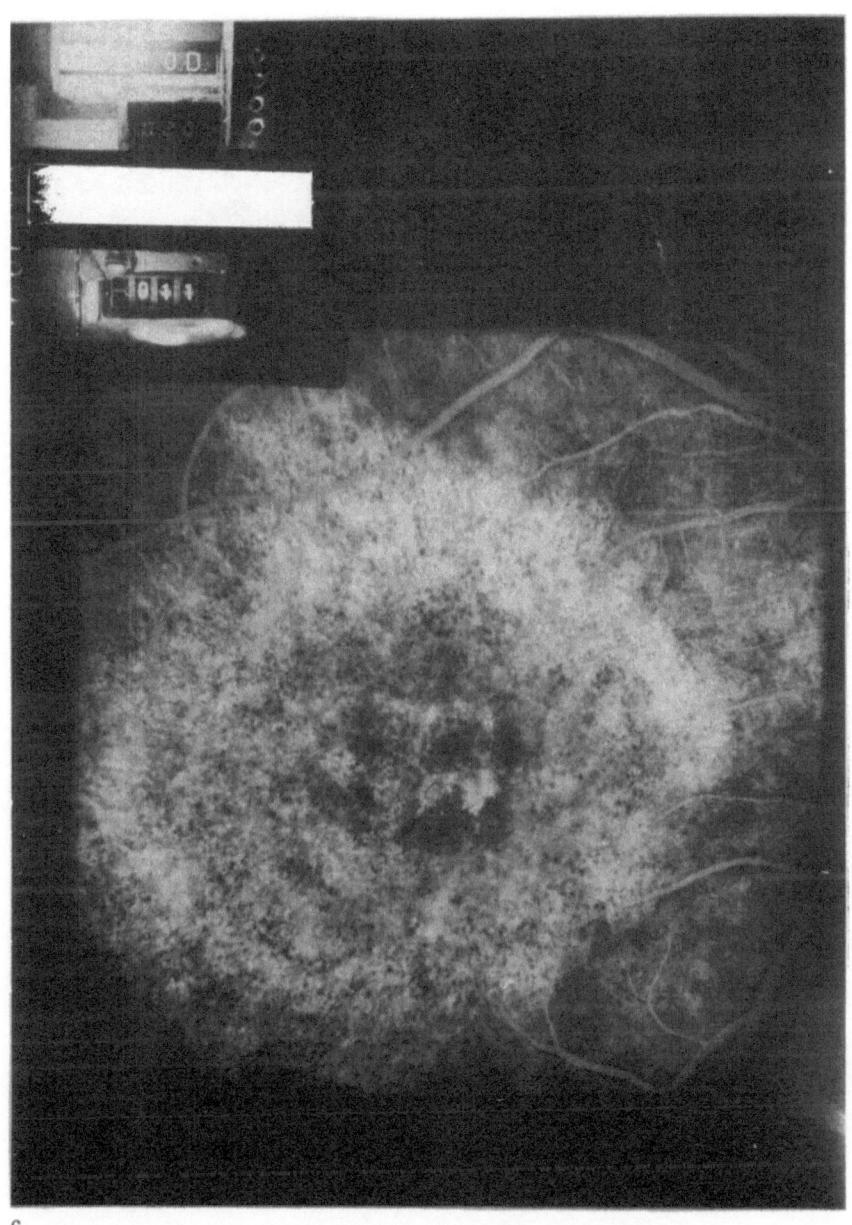

c

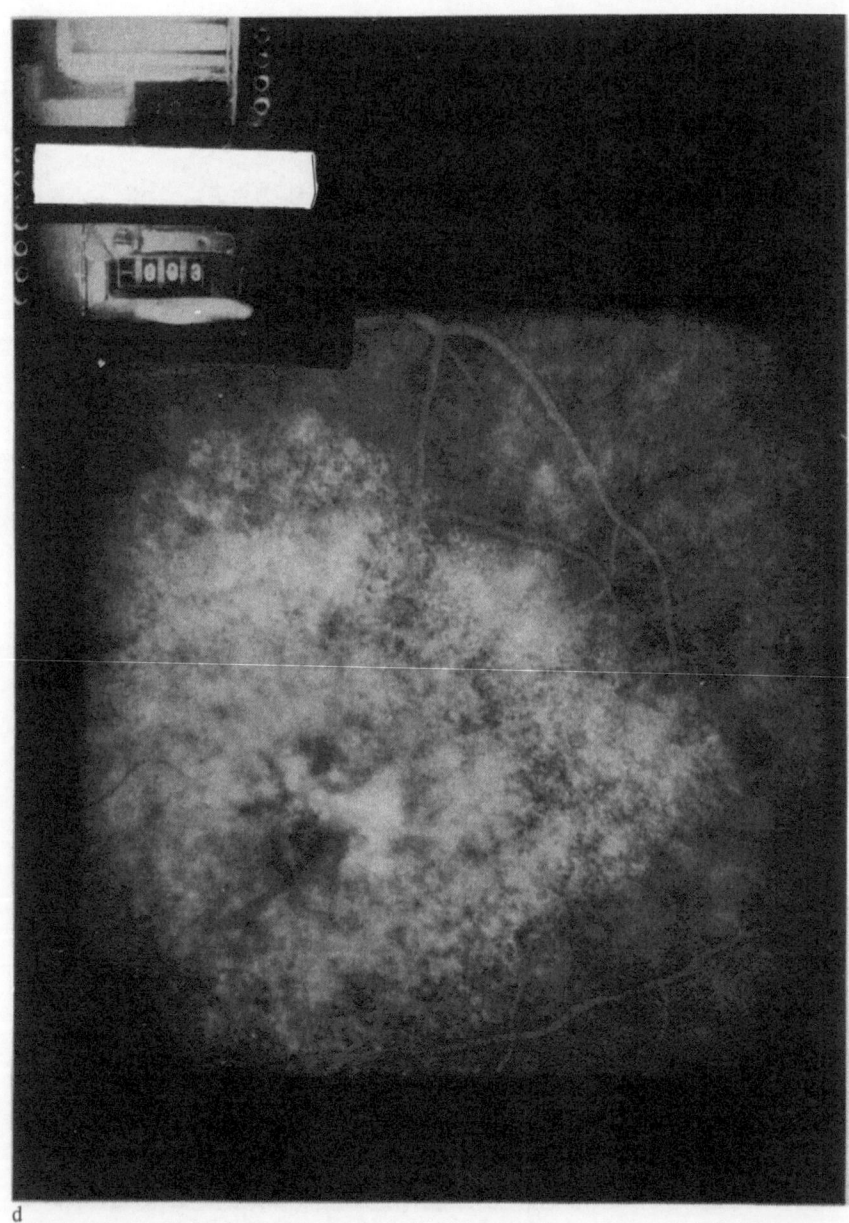

d

One 10-year-old girl was referred to me because she and her mother had both macular abnormalities. The girl had vision of 0.4 in both eyes and some evidence of cystoid macular oedema. Fluorescein angiography showed a classic pattern of leaking perimacular capillaries (Fig. 4). The ERG was completely normal, but the EOG was somewhat affected. There was no signs of pars planitis. Het mother had a visual acuity of 0.1 in both eyes. She demonstrated an atrophic macular degeneration in both eyes. Fluorescein angiography showed atrophy of the retinal pigment epithelium centrally and some leakage of perimacular retinal capillaries (Fig. 5). The ERG was normal, but the EOG was definitely disturbed (RE 1.56, LE 1.71).

The parents of the proband did not have a consanguineous marriage and the grandparents were not alive anymore. Nevertheless the inheritance pattern seems to be autosomal dominant.

Another young girl appeared to have a similar abnormality, while her mother also had leaking perimacular capillaries. A brother of the mother, however, had extensive atrophic macular degeneration with leaking retinal capillaries. This pedigree is being examined in our Institute together with Dr. PINCKERS.

The young girl was an 11-year-old girl with a delicate macular oedema, with fine radiating streaks due to leaking perimacular capillaries in both eyes (Fig. 6).

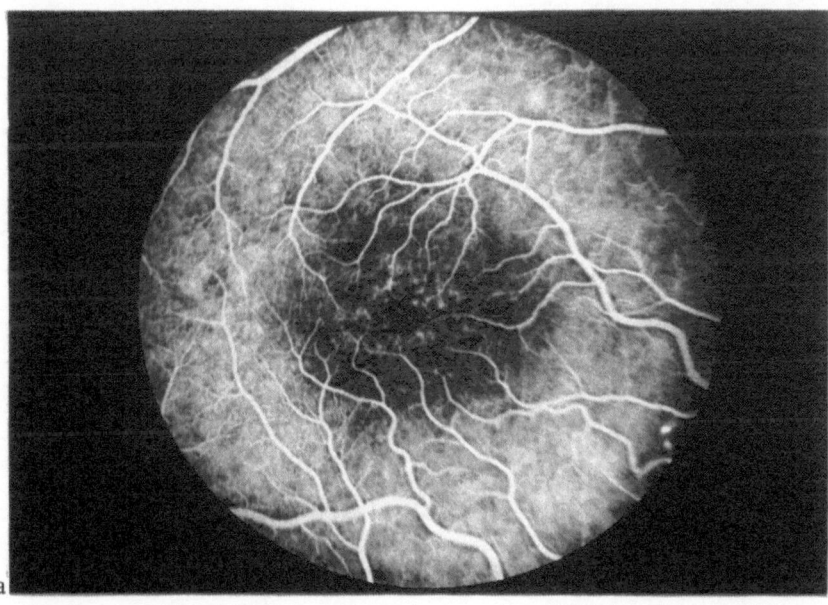

Fig. 6. Dominant cystoid macular oedema in a 11-year-old girl, showing leaking perimacular capillaries and some fluorescein leakage in and around the disk (a, b, c, d).

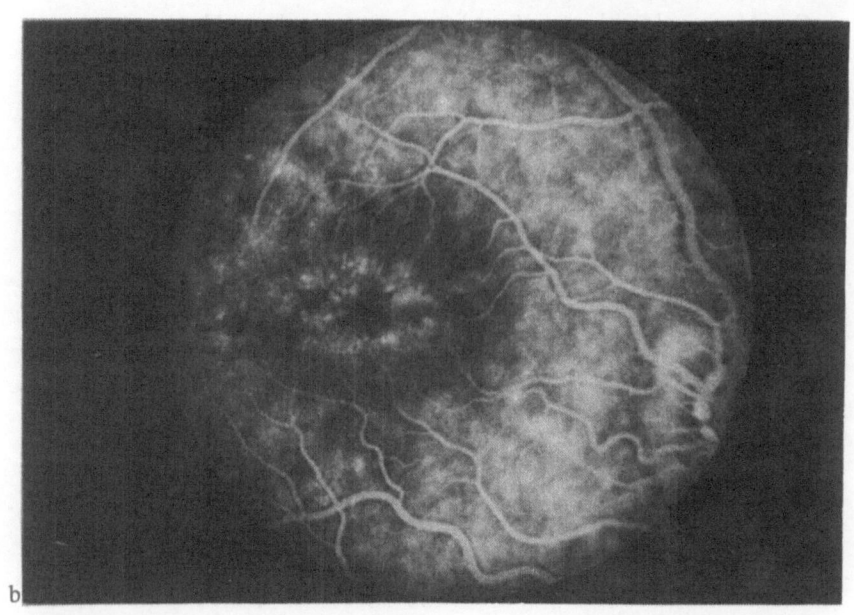

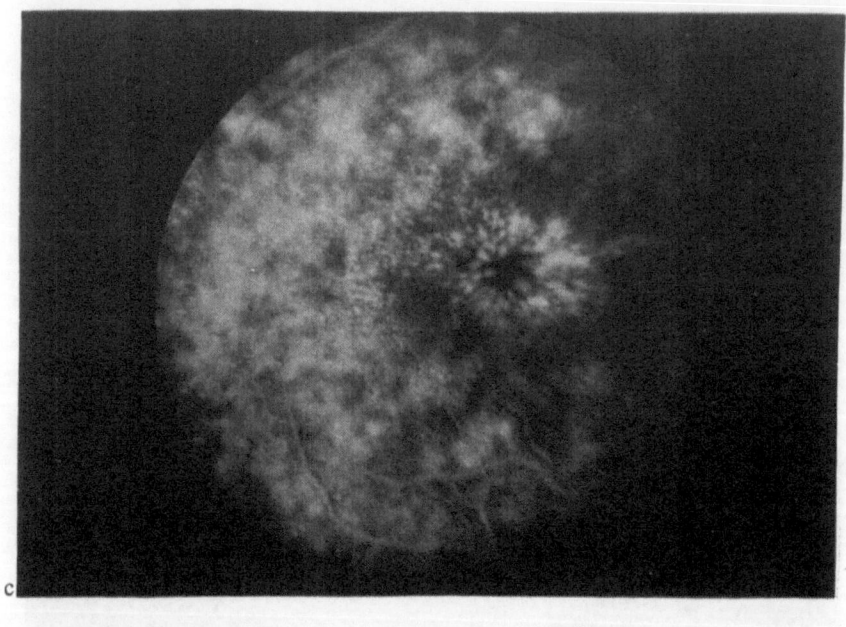

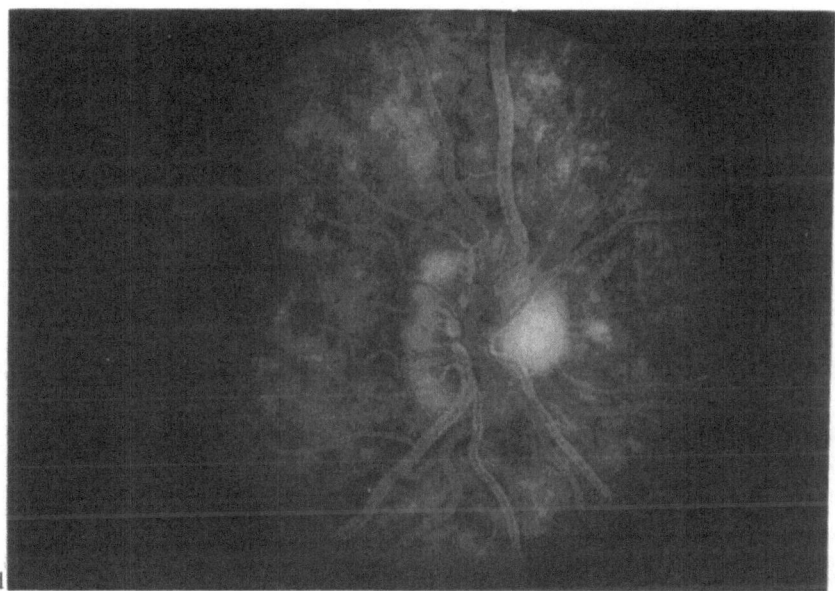

d

There was a left esotropia since age one and a high hyperopia of S + 9 = C–1 x 15° in the right eye and S + 9 = C–1 x 165° in the left eye. Her visual acuity was 0.8 in the right eye and 0.25 in the left eye. ERG and EOG have been normal throughout the years while colour visoin was also normal. Apart from whitish punctate vitreous opacities and some disk drusen there were no obvious changes in the eyes.

Her mother, a 33-year-old woman, who also had a high hyperopia of S + 8.75 in the right eye and S + 9.50 in the left eye, also demonstrated leaking capillaries in the perimacular area and around the disk (Fig. 7). The grand-father of the proband had poor vision throughout his life. A 32-year-old uncle of the proband had a mild hyperopia (S + 4.75 and S % 3. =) and very poor vision with atrophic macular degeneration and many leaking retinal capillaries in the posterior pole of the eye (Fig. 8).

Although leaking perimacular capillaries are by no means the only abnor-malities seen in these patients, they nevertheless are a striking and pre-dominant finding.

It may be that the leaking capillaries are secondary in nature on the basis of primary retinal abnormalities. This has also been seen in retinitis pigmen-tosa, where cystoid macular oedema is by no means a rare finding (Fig. 9). It may be that toxic degeneration products cause the capillaries to leak or it may be due to defective oxygenation. Some patients also showed some whitish punctate opacities in the vitreous body without an associated posterior cyclitis. The high hyperopia and the abnormal EOG together with a normal ERG are furthermore interesting features, that are difficult to understand.

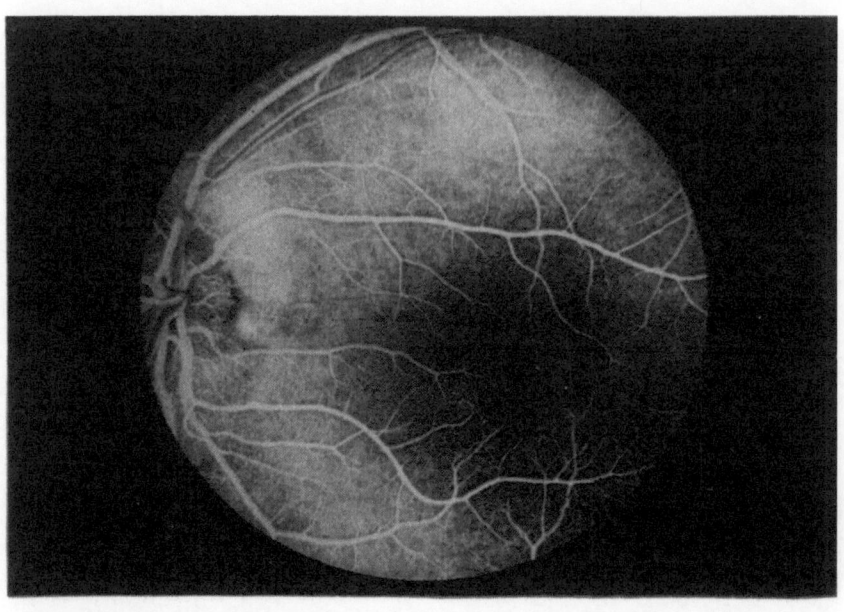

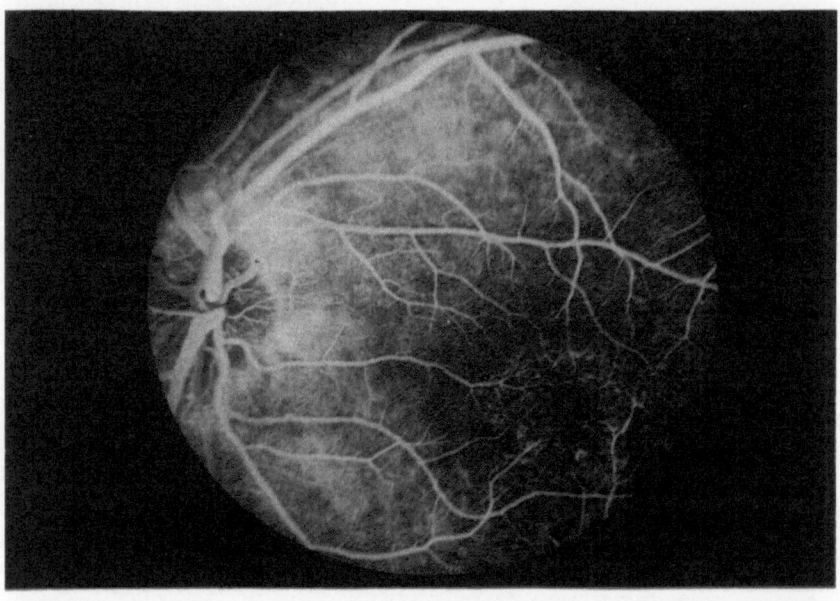

Fig. 7. Dominant cystoid macular oedema in a 33-year-old woman, showing leaking capillaries in the macular area, in the posterior pole and around the disk. This woman is the mother of the 11-year-old girl, whose fundus pictures are depicted in Fig. 6.

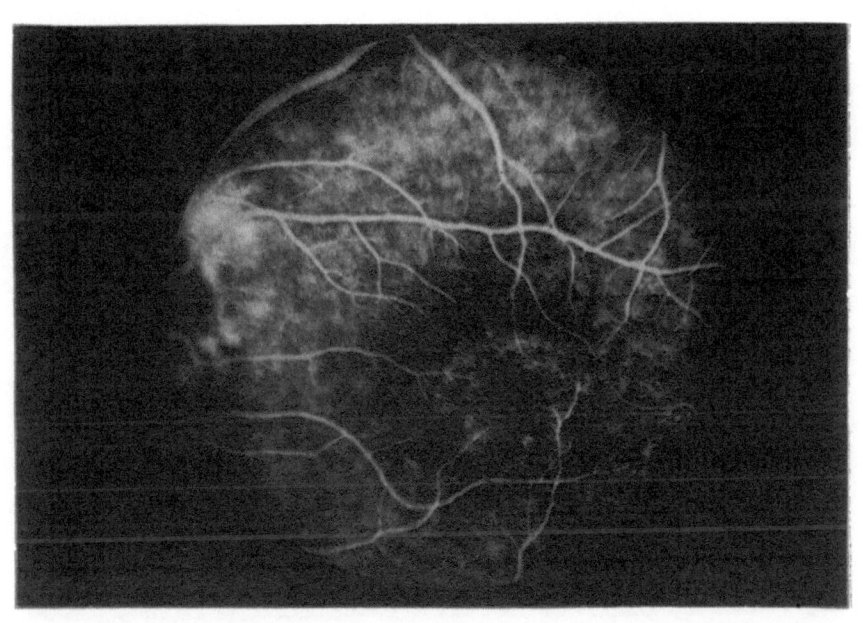

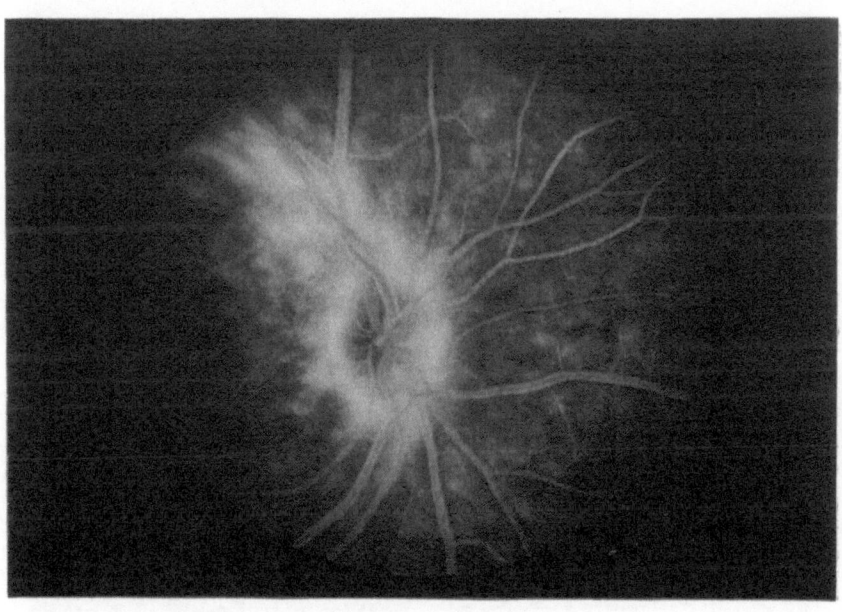

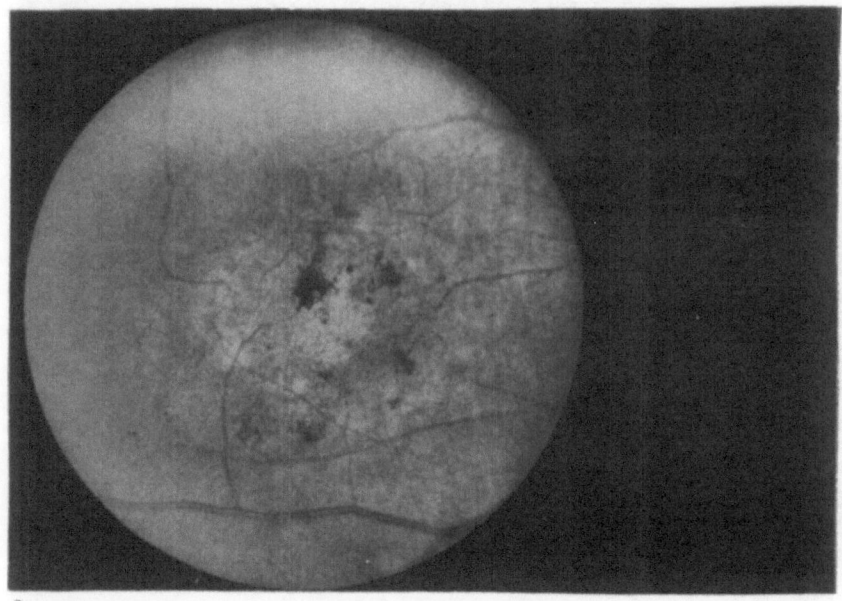

a

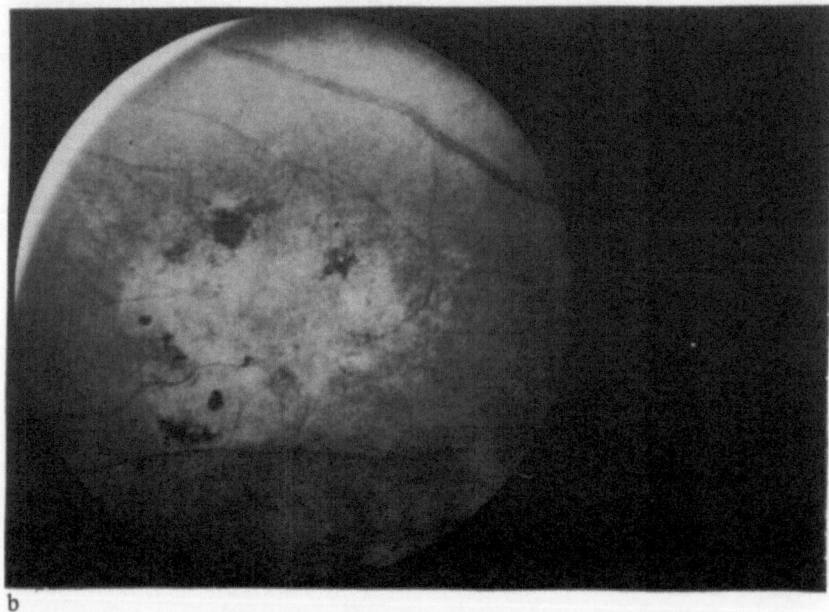

b

Fig. 8. Atrophic macular degeneration with leaking capillaries centrally (cd) and flecks (e) and leaking capillaries around the disk (f) in a patient who is member of a family with dominant cystoid macular oedema. It may be that the central leaking capillaries are part of the choriocapillaries, and not of the retina.

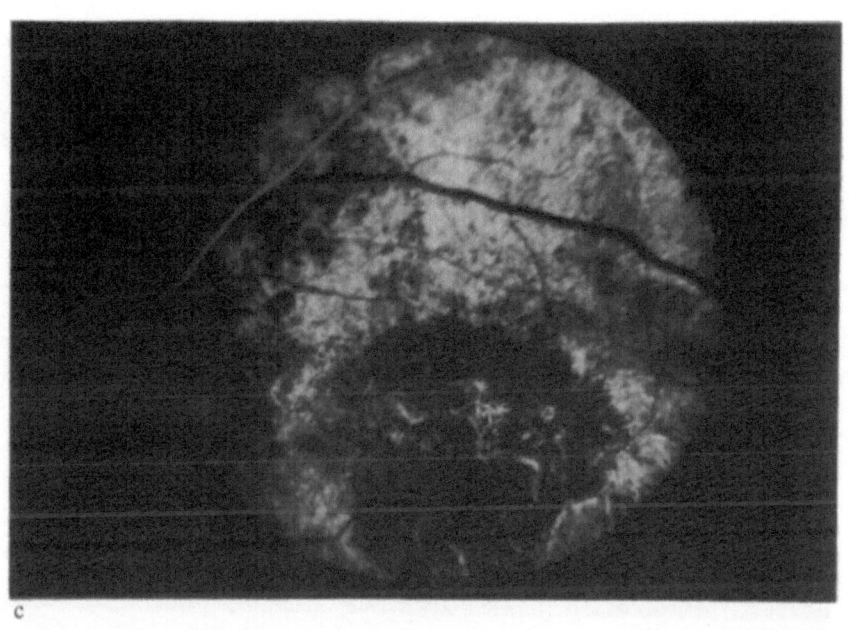

c

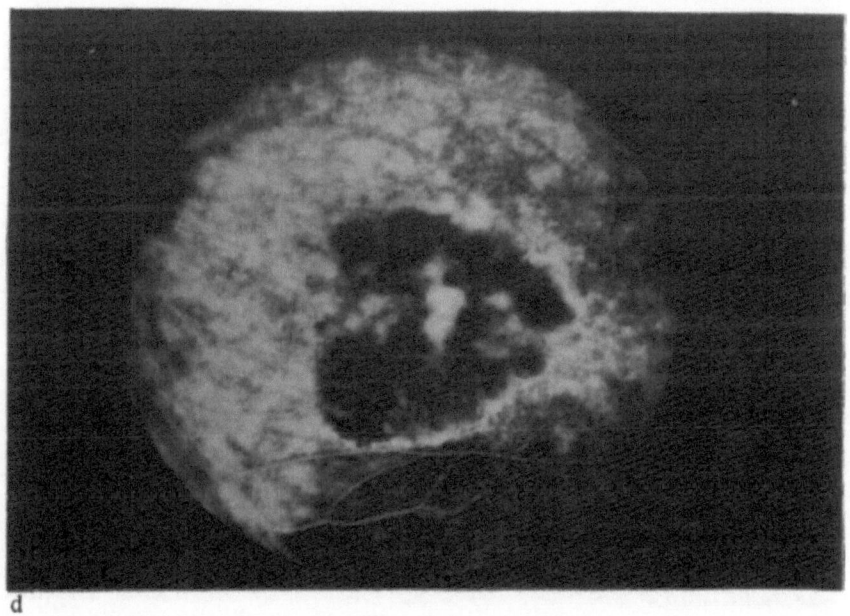

d

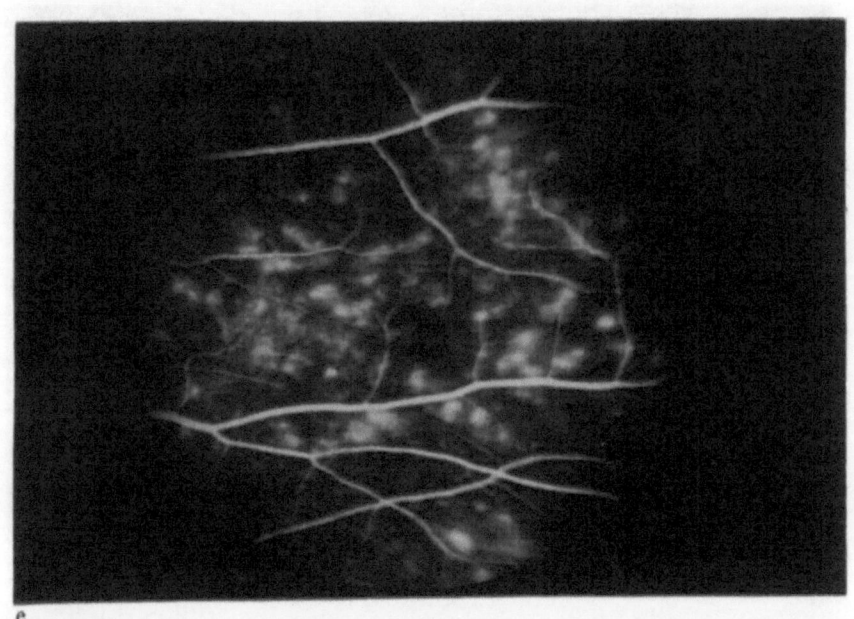

e

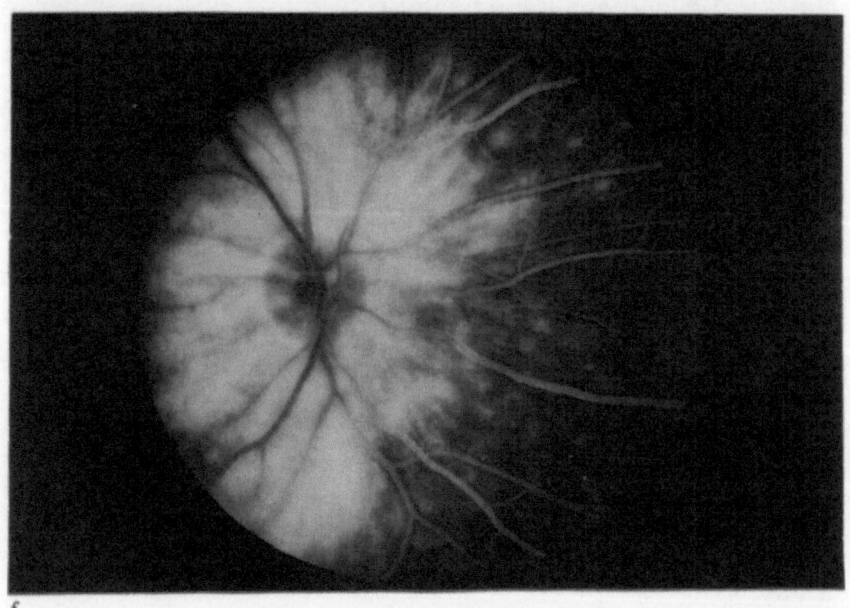

f

306

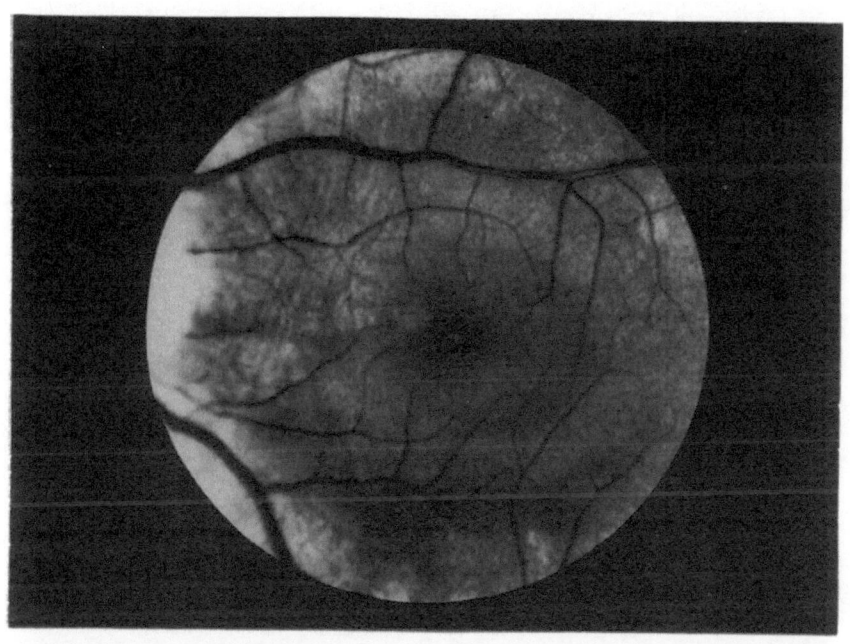

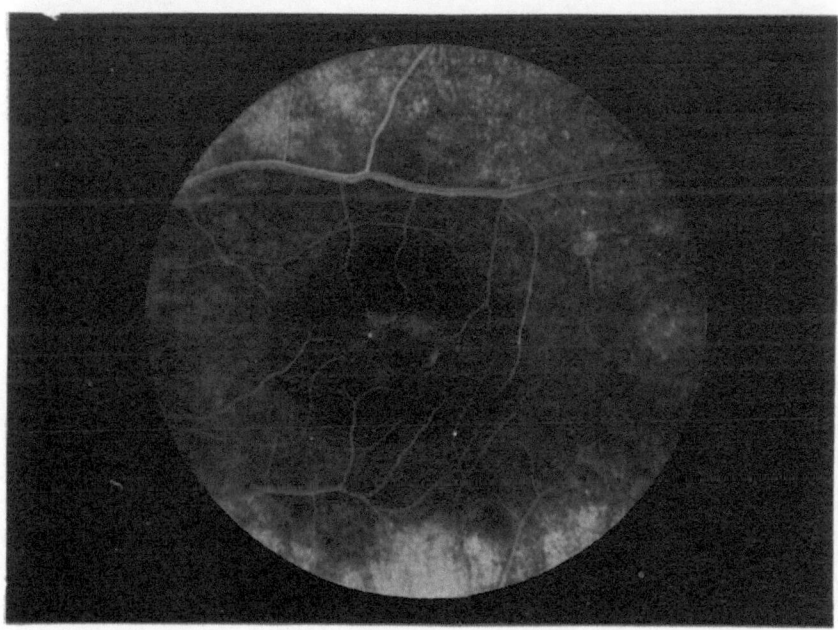

Fig. 9. Cystoid macular oedema due to leaking perimacular capillaries in a patient with retinitis pigmentosa (rod-cone dystrophy) (abcd).

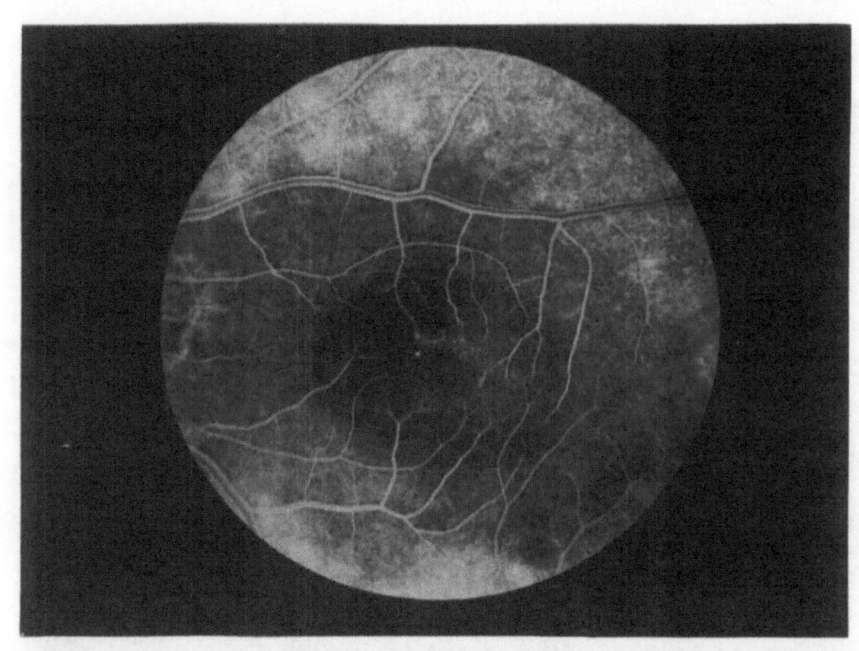

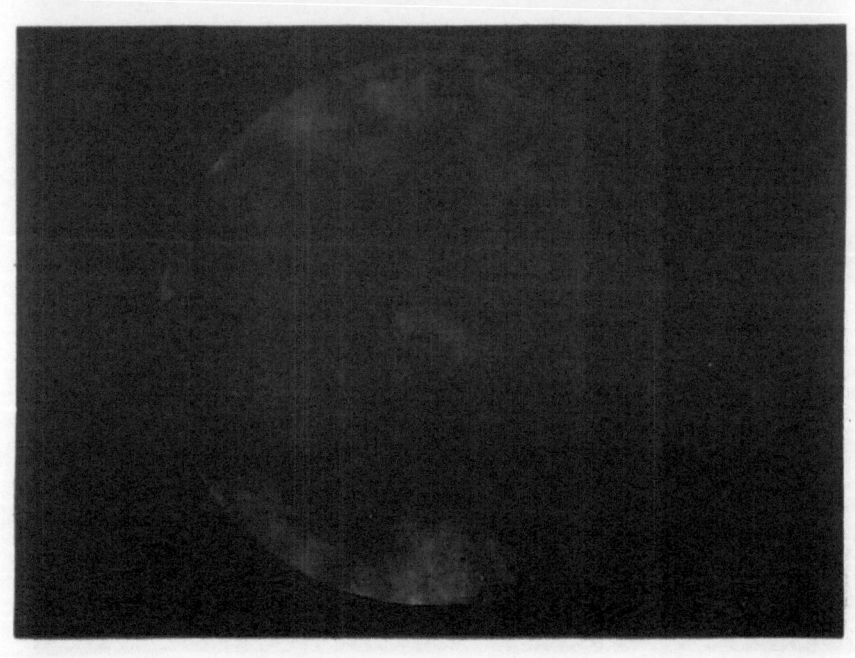

More details regarding these pedigrees will be presented elsewhere (DEUTMAN, PINCKERS & AAN DE KERK). So far, though, dominant macular oedema appears to be a rather specific type of macular dystrophy that deserves to be separated from other dominant macular dystrophies (DEUTMAN, 1974).

3. STARGARDT'S DISEASE

Stargardt's disease *(atrophic macular dystrophy with fundus flavimaculatus)* This autosomal recessive condition is not too rare. However, together with Dr. P. BOS from Amsterdam I have seen an interesting patient who combined the features of Stargardt's disease in both eyes and Coats' disease in her right eye (Fig. 10).

Retinal function studies were completely compatible with Stargardt disease. Certain areas of the congenital teleangiectasia (Coats) were treated by photocoagulation (Fig. 10).

Visual acuity is still 0.4. in the right eye and 0.1 in the left eye.

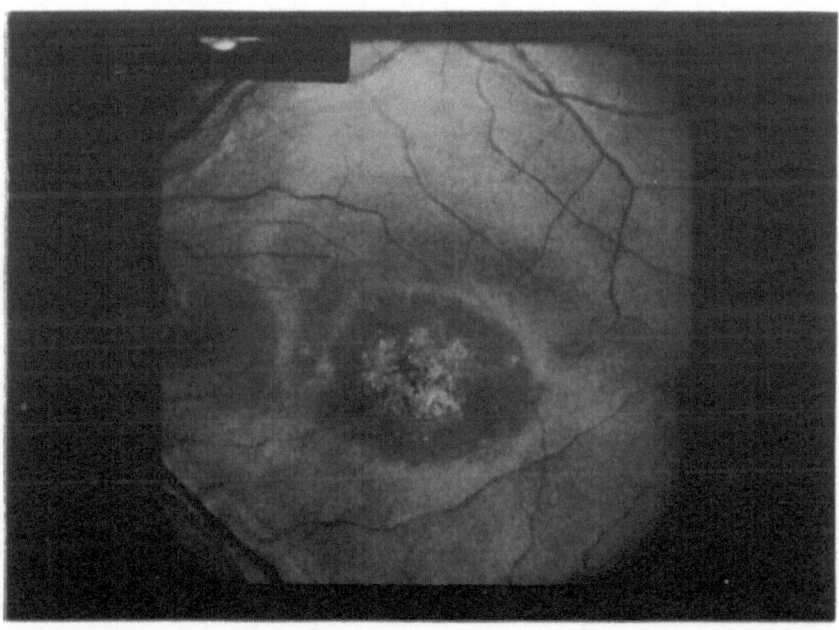

Fig. 10. Patient with Stargardt's disease (atrophic macular degeneration with fundus flavimaculatus) in both eyes (abc) and Coats' disease in her right eye only (de).

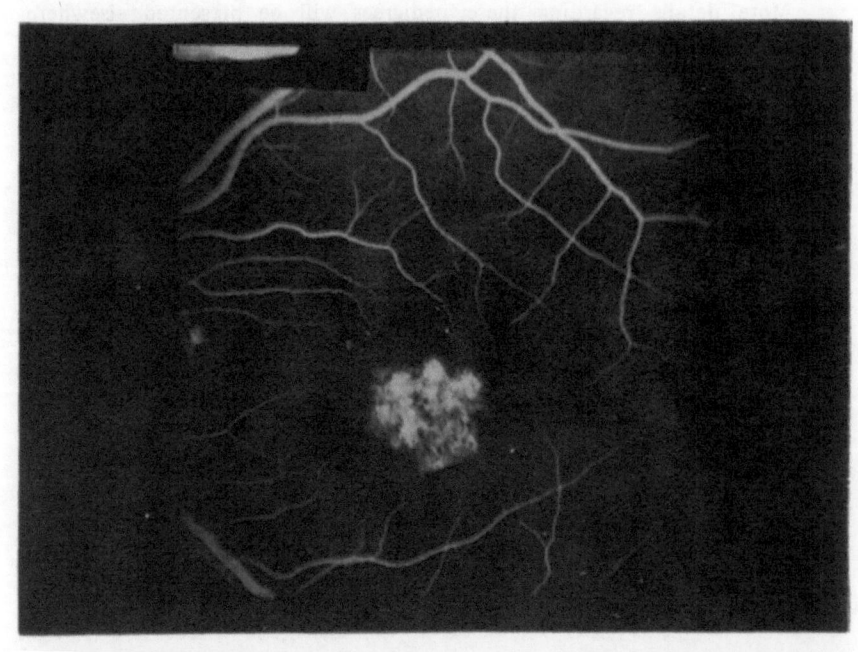

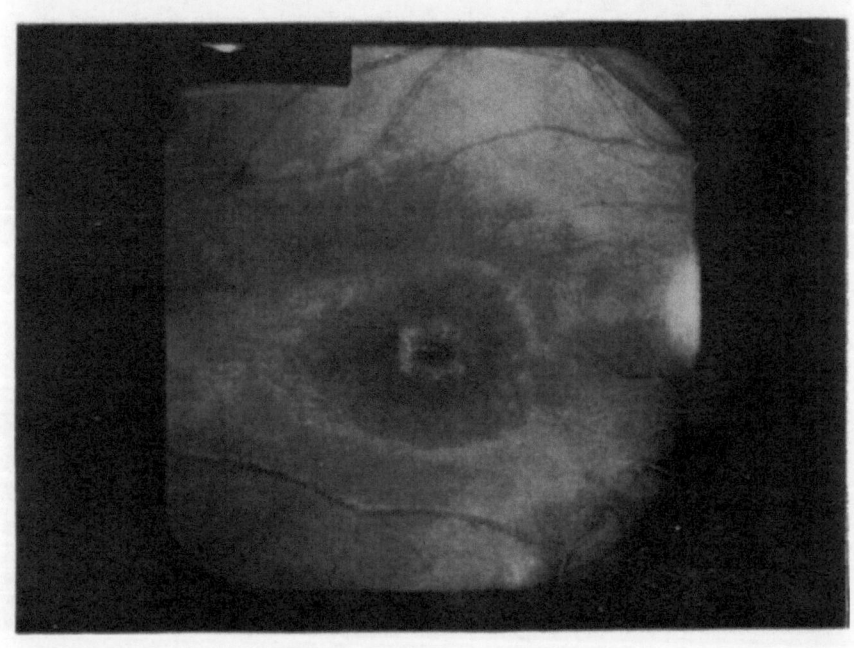

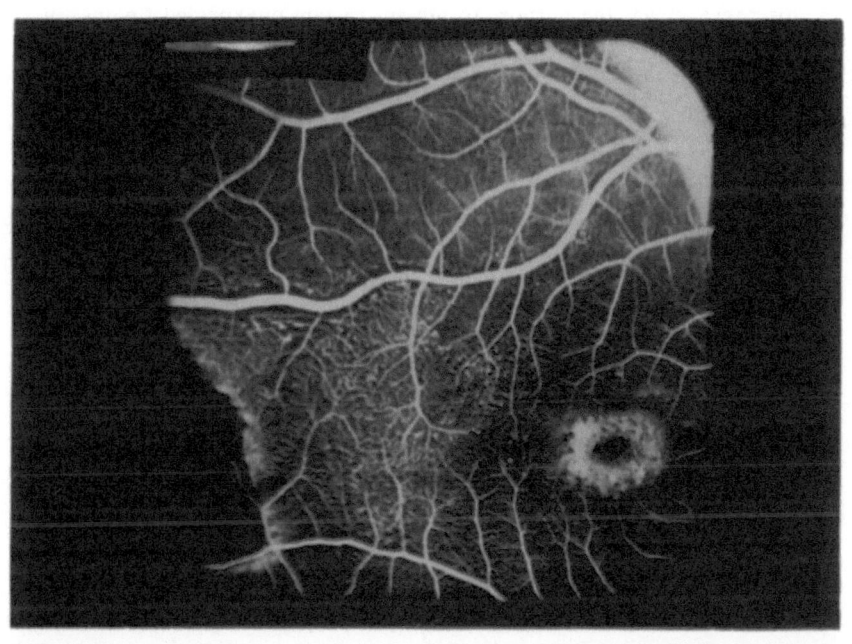

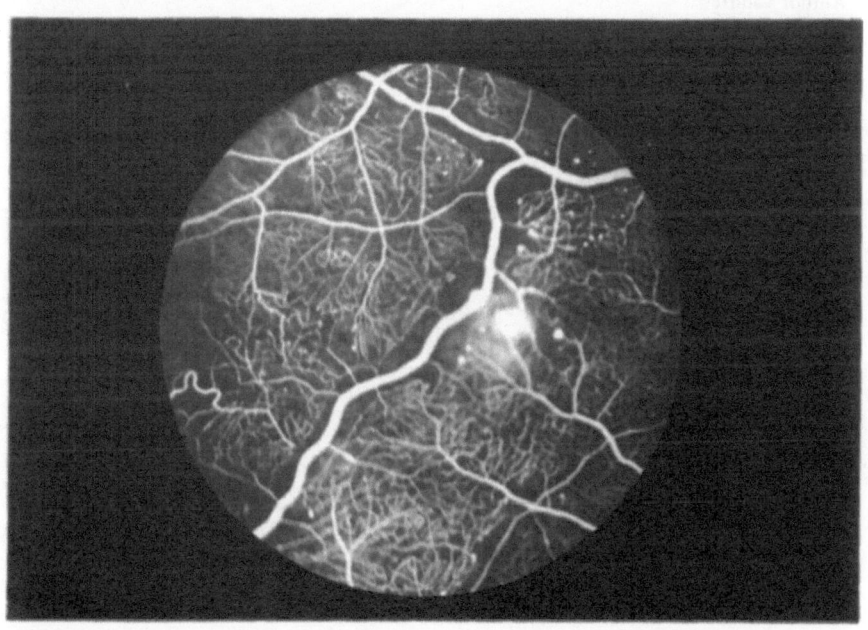

In this paper it was the purpose to present certain unexpected findings in hereditary macular dystrophy. I am certain that by pursuing our efforts and studies, we will detect many more interesting data in this very polymorphous, but intriguing group of dystrophies of the posterior pole of the eye.

ACKNOWLEDGEMENTS

I wish to thank Mr. ALBERT AAN DE KERK who made the photographs.

REFERENCES

BENSON, W.E. KOLKER, A.E., ENOCH, J.M., VAN LOO, J.A. & HONDA, Y. Best's vitelliform macualar dystrophy *Amer. J. Ophthal.* 79: *59-66* (1975).

BRALEY, A.E. Dystrophy of the macula. *Amer. J. Ophthal.* 61: *1-24* (1966).

DEUTMAN, A.F. The hereditary dystrophies of the posterior pole of the eye. Thesis. Van Gorcum & Comp. Assen, The Netherlands, 1971

DEUTMAN, A.F. Benign Concentric Annular Macular Dystrophy. *Amer. J. Ophthal.* 78: *384-396* (1974).

DEUTMAN, A.F., PINCKERS, A. & AAN DE KERK, A.L. Cystoid Macular Oedema, dominantly inherited. *Amer. J. Ophthal.* (in press).

Key words: Macula, Cystoid macular oedema, Dystrophy, Leaking capillaries.

Author's address:
Institute of Ophthalmology
University of Nijmegen
Nijmegen
The Netherlands

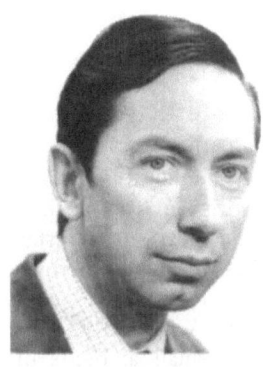

LIPIDS IN TISSUES OF THE EYE XIV.
CORNEOSCLERAL LIPIDS DURING
AGEING AND IN ARCUS SENILIS

RENÉ M. BROEKHUYSE

(Nijmegen, the Netherlands)

The lipid composition was studied of ageing human cornea and sclera and of arcus senilis. The composition of the two tissues was similar and is age-dependent. It was influenced by the formation of an arcus in the cornea. The lipid pattern of the arcus seemed more aged than of the centrum of the same cornea. Ageing of human cornea and sclera was characterized by an accumulation of cholesterol linoleate, by an increase in cholesterol and sphingomyelin, and by degradation of phosphoglycerides.

The pattern of lipid accumulation resembled that in ageing aorta and to a certain extent that in atherosclerosis.

INTRODUCTION

The intriguing phenomenon of arcus senilis attracted research on its nature at the beginning of this century. Although it was claimed that the arcus was a form of calcareous degeneration (LEBER, 1908) or that it consisted of hyaline concretions (FUCHS, 1891), other laboratories showed that lipid deposition was the major abnormality (TAKAYASU, 1901; PARSONS, 1903). Staining and solvent-extraction of sections demonstrated that lipids accumulated also in senile sclera (KREKELER, 1923) and it was supposed that this process would develop parallel to the formation of arcus senilis (LOEWENSTEIN, 1940). Sudanophilia of the sclera consisted of red dots between the laminae while cells appeared normal (COGAN & KUWABARA, 1959). In arcus senilis, Descemet's membrane seemed to be involved as well, although the limbus region was spared. Histologically, sclera and cornea showed a deposition of fat interrupted by the relatively fat-free zone of the vascular limbus and paravascular regions about the emissaria in the sclera (COGAN, 1960). Lipid deposits in the inner layers of the sclera of normal eyes were found even at 40 years of age. At a higher age, an increasing deposition was detected, especially in arcus senilis (DU CHESNE, 1967). Arteriosclerosis was not always present. There was some indication that cholesterol esters accumulated in the cornea as well as in sclera (ANDREWS, 1962).

These findings correspond with statistical data about the occurrence of the arcus DUKE-ELDER & LEIGH, 1965):

15% in men between   40-44 years of age
59% ,,   ,,   ,,   40-60 ,,   ,, ,,
80% ,,   ,,   ,,   60-69 ,,   ,, ,,
90% ,,   ,,   ,,   70-80 ,,   ,, ,,
100% ,,   ,,   older than   80 ,,   ,, ,,

These figures are not surprising, because it has been frequently observed in clinics that incidence of arcus senilis is associated with the occurrence of high concentrations of cholesterol in blood. High concentrations are especially common in old age. For these reasons, arcus has intrigued atheroma specialists for more than a hundred years.

Using the cornea as a model of the arterial intima, WATERS (1965) studied the phenomenon experimentally by injecting small amounts of serum from hypercholesterolaemic hyperlipaemic rabbits into the cornea of rabbits. After 9 to 13 days massive lipid-containing fibrocytic foam-cellular plaques had formed. The stromal reactions reproduced many of the morphological features of small atherosclerotic plaques in man. Corneal tissue reactions were virtually eliminated by removing lipid from the sera prior to injection. WATERS concluded that such lesions depended on the lipid of the lipoprotein in the serum. Indeed, the lipids of the hyperlipaemic serum were retained and typical reactions developed. However, the properties of the lipoproteins may themselves play an important role in certain human pathological conditions (see below).

Similar tests with hyperlipaemic serum from rabbits injected with the detergent Triton WR-1339 produced opacities that cleared faster and better than those initiated by the hyperlipaemic serum from cholesterol-fed animals (SILVER et al., 1965). Although several controls were included, they evoked more questions than answers. The true composition of lipid deposits in arcus senilis was not available for comparison and it was (and remains) uncertain which biochemical changes of the corneal and arterial connective tissues precede and accompany pathological phenomena in hypercholesterolaemia.

In order to study the detailed lipid composition of the cornea and sclera during the life-span and in arcus senilis, these tissues were further examined in our laboratory (BROEKHUYSE & KUHLMANN, 1972; BROEKHUYSE, 1972, 1975, 1976). The results will be discussed below.

RECENT DATA ABOUT ARCUS SENILIS AND AGEING CORNEOSCLERAL TISSUE

The major phospholipids in human sclera are sphingomyelin, phosphatidylcholine and phosphatidylethanolamine, constituting about 90% of total phospholipids (BROEKHUYSE, 1972). In the ageing sclera, a gradual continuous shift occurs in the proportional distribution of these lipids (Fig. 1). The main shift is in the percentage of sphingomyelin, which increases from 20 to 50% between the ages of 3 and 68 years. The percentages of the other phospholipids decrease linearly over the same period. At an early age (between 3 and 17 years), no lysophospholipids can be found. However from 24 years, varying amounts of lysophosphatidylcholine (3.9-19.5%) and lysophosphatidylethanolamine (4.0-9.9%) occur in human sclera. Senile sclera contains the highest percentages of these lipids.

A similar shift has been found for the phospholipid concentrations (Fig. 2). The sphingomyelin concentration increases from 0.45 to 1.30 μg/mg wet wt. between 3 and 68 years of age. The increase is almost entirely compensated a decrease in the other phospholipids. Hence, the total phospholipid content increases only slightly during life (2.25-2.60 μg/mg wet wt. The concentrations of free fatty acids, free cholesterol and triglycerides increase (0.30-1.17, 0.81-1.49, and 0.60-1.65 μg/mg wet wt. respectively. Monoacyl and diacyl glycerol are present in trace amounts. The cholesterol esters show the most marked change in concentration, 0.16-3.70 μg/mg wet wt. (factor 23). Until about 33 years of age, change is minimal, but thereafter becomes very rapid. This contributed most to the increase in total lipids of the human sclera during life: 4.1-10.6 μg/mg wet wt. or from 0.41-1.06% (w/w).

Gas chromatography revealed that in the phospholipids only slight changes in fatty acid pattern occur with age. However, in phosphatidylcholine, and especially in the cholesterol esters, the linoleate content increases (respectively, 8-12% and 10-40%). Cholesterol palmitate and stearate decrease (21-11% and 21-1% respectively).

Our present data (BROEKHUYSE, 1976; this article, Table 1) confirm

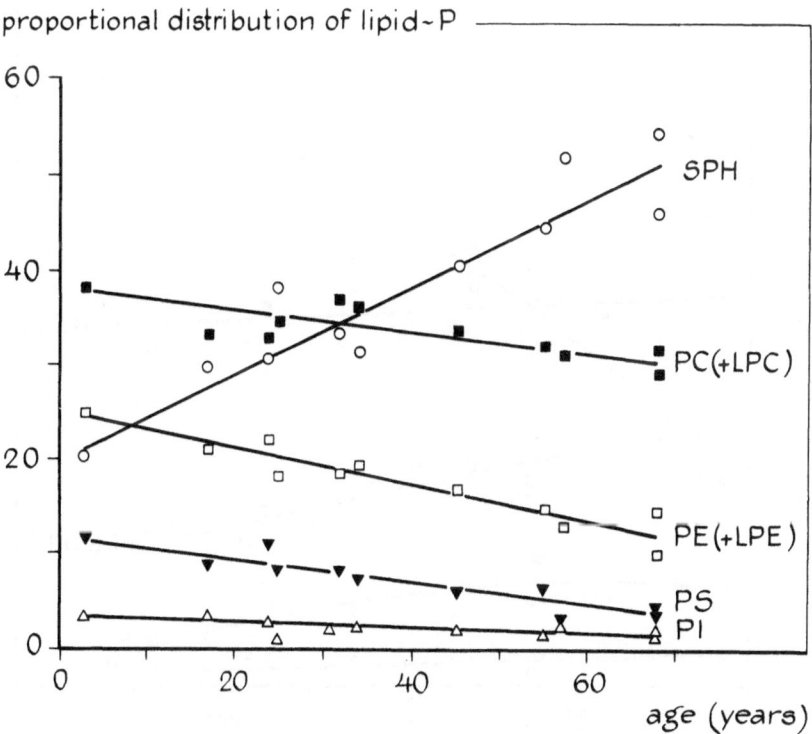

Fig. 1. Age-dependent changes in the proportional distribution of the phospholipids of human sclera. SPH, sphingomyelin; (L)PC, (lyso) phosphatidylcholine; (L)PE, (lyso) phosphatidylethanolamine; PS, phosphatidylserine; PI, phosphatidylinositol.

the high relative concentration of sphingomyelin in human cornea. The high value for neutral lipids was mainly due to high cholesterol ester concentration, as in human sclera. Table 1 shows that the central part differed from the annular outer part of the human cornea in composition in both normal and in arcus-containing cornea. Sphingomyelin increased in the outer part of both types of cornea, but especially in arcus. In both parts of the arcus-containing cornea, the total phospholipid concentration is increased markedly too, as in sclera, where sphingomyelin was the major phospholipid after 40 years of age (Fig. 1).

DISCUSSION

The various data for the corneal parts and sclera suggest that the corneal centre has a 'younger' phospholipid composition than the peripheral part. The total phospholipid and cholesterol ester concentrations in human cornea are age-dependent as in sclera (Table 1). The data show that the arcus

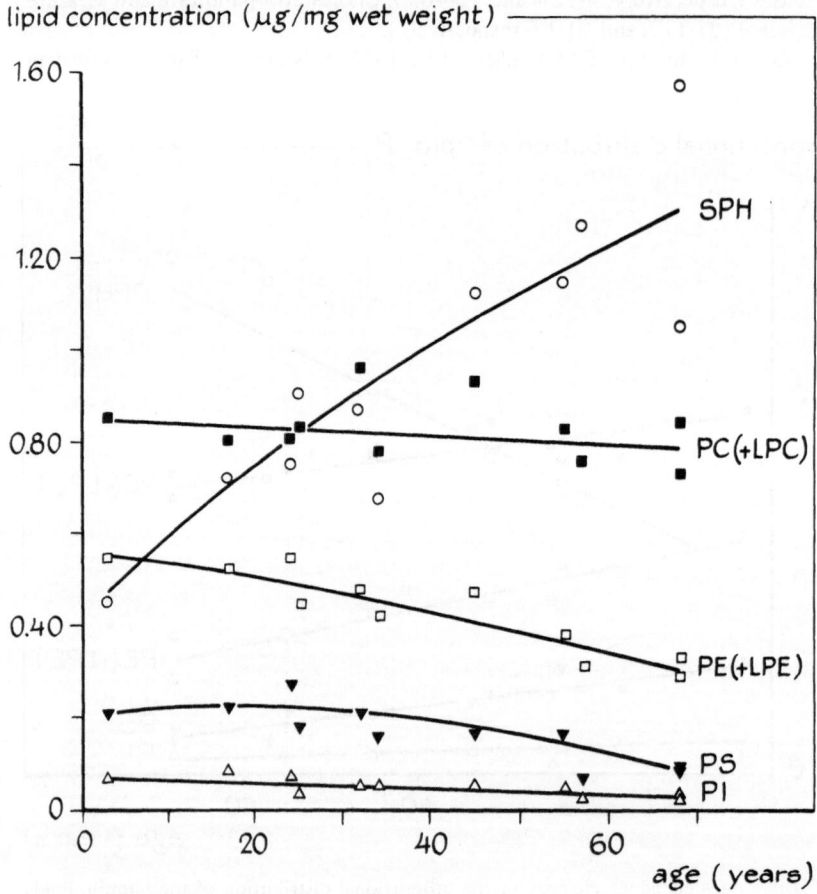

Fig. 2. Age-dependent changes in the phospholipid concentrations of human sclera. Abbreviations as Fig. 1.

316

TABLE I

Lipid composition of normal and arcus containing cornea at different ages

Age (years):	Clear human corneas				Human corneas with arcus				Bovine corneas	
	21	34	70		69		73		0.3	6
			c.p.[a]	p.p.[b]	c.p.	arcus[b]	c.p.	arcus		
Sphingomyelin	15	18	33	39	32	42	32	40	14	19
Phosphatidylcholine	44	41	32	36	34	29	33	30	61	53
Phosphatidylethanolamine	26	29	18	12	21	17	20	14	16	18
Phosphatidylinositol	6	5	8	7	2	3	5	4	2	2
Phosphatidylserine	7	6	5	5	6	6	6	6	7	7
Lysophosphatidylcholine	1	–	–	–	2	–	3	4	–	–
Lysophosphatidylethanolamine	–	1	3	2	1	2	2	1	–	–
Phosphatidic acid	–	–	1	–	2	1	–	1	–	–
Total phospholipid (mg/g wet wt.)	1.4	1.1	0.8	1.3	1.7	3.2	1.1	3.4	1.4	1.8
Cholesterol (,, ,, ,,)	0.2	0.3	0.3	0.4	1.0	1.5	1.2	1.6	0.3	0.3
Cholesterol esters (,, ,, ,,)	0.5	1.0	0.3	1.4	1.8	2.2	2.0	2.5	0.4	0.4
Number of corneas per extract	2	2	5		6		5		22	13

[a] c.p. = central part; [b] p.p. = peripheral (annular) part; weight ratio c.p.: p.p. = 1 : 1.7
– = not detected

Phospholipid composition is presented in weight percents phosphorus of total lipid phosphorus recovered. Analyses were carried out as described previously (Broekhuyse, 1972), with duplicate determinations on each extract; one extract per column of results. Corneal epithelia were removed before use. Triacylglycerol and free fatty acid fractions amounted to 0.1 – 0.3 mg/g each, and squalene to 0.03 – 0.08 mg/g in all cornea tissues.

has a higher cholesterol and cholesterol ester concentration than the central part and the clear peripheral part as well. The annular arcus represents a more 'aged' cornea part in view of its lipid composition. In this respect, it more resembles the sclera of the same age.

Although it has been suggested that accumulation of cholesterol esters by itself is the cause of the opacity of the arcus, it is more likely that high total lipid concentrations make the tissue opaque. The supposition that the extracted lipoidal material originates mainly from the epithelial cell membranes (FELDMAN, 1967) is not supported by Table 1, because all analysis was on epithelium-free corneas. In fact, histological staining (COGAN & KUWABARA, 1959) points to lipid accumulation in stroma and Descemet's membrane. It is not known whether gangliosides are involved in the arcus. FELDMAN (1967) reported them to be present in normal cornea in a higher proportion of total lipids (16%) than in brain (11%). The patterns of age--dependent changes of the various lipid concentrations in the human sclera are strikingly similar to those in aorta and, as far as can be seen from recent reports, also with changes in certain other connective tissues. BÖTTCHER & WOODFORD (1962) and ROUSER & SOLOMON (1969) established that sphingomyelin increased steadily with age in normal aorta in grossly sclerotic aorta. In grossly sclerotic aorta, ROUSER & SOLOMON found that sphingomyelin was not greatly elevated. They obtained a pattern of straight lines for the phospholipid percentages of normal aorta similar to that in our study of sclera. Moreover, the proportional distribution of the various phospholipids at corresponding ages closely resembled those in sclera. In aorta lipids, SMITH et al. (1967) found age-dependent changes in the concentrations of cholesterol esters, phospholipids, triglycerides and free cholesterol, which are also similar to our results. The marked increase in cholesterol linoleate is another point of resemblance.

The findings for aorta seemed unique, until analysis by CROUSE et al. (1972) of various connective tissues revealed that dense connective tissues 'trap' esterified cholesterol. A 5 to 10-fold increase in cholesterol esters was found over the whole life-span, whereas free cholesterol rose more slowly, as in aorta and sclera. In the skin too, high concentrations of cholesterol esters are present, though no influence of ageing could be demonstrated (HSIA, 1971). A hitherto unknown component of sclera is the hydrocarbon squalene, which was identified by gas chromatography (BROEKHUYSE, 1972). Squalene was present in a concentration about equal to that of cholesterol. Hence, it seems to be one of the major neutral lipids in sclera, as it is in the surface lipids of skin (HSIA, 1971) and to a lesser extent of aorta (STEFANOVITCH & KAJIYAMA, 1970).

The origin of the high sphingomyelin concentrations is obscure. PORTMANN & ALEXANDER (1970) found increased synthesis and uptake from serum of sphingomyelin in atherosclerotic aorta of squirrel monkeys. The lipid accumulation in ageing sclera and cornea resembles that in the intima of aorta, both in chemistry and morphology. The decreasing number of cells in senile sclera seems to exclude intracellular synthesis of large amounts of cholesterol esters. These components occur perifibrously and may originate from serum. The increase in cholesterol linoleate, the major cholesterol ester of serum, supports this assumption. This data for sclera support the corresponding theory for aorta, which is more difficult to prove because choleste-rol esters could be synthesized in situ. However, extracellular intima lipid contains cholesterol linoleate and intracellular lipid contains cholesterol oleate as the dominant sterol ester. Other data too implicate β-lipoprotein from serum as donor of the cholesterol linoleate (SMITH, 1968). It is un-certain whether this lipid deposit in connective tissue must be considered 'normal'. The close correlation between severity of atherosclerosis and age makes it difficult to differentiate between lipid that accumulates as a result of the disorder and lipid that accumulates as a result of a 'normal' aging process.

The severity of arcus is closely related to the concentration of cholesterol or β-lipoprotein in serum. For that reason, a pronounced arcus is always found in hypercholesterolaemia. In 'normal' persons, however, the arcus usually consists of a slight opacity. Noteworthy is the extremely low inci-dence of coronary disease in Bantu, though corneal arcus is quite common among them (DAVIDSON & KOLBE, 1965). In them, in contrast to people from industrial countries, there was no association between arcus and serum cholesterol. LEMP (1973) has reviewed the incidence of arcus in Bantu and other races and its relationship to systemic disease has recently appeared. His conclusions agree with my previous supposition based on the studies of lipids from ageing cornea and sclera. Corneal arcus in the elderly is probably a reflexion of 'normal' ageing processes.

In corneas of cholesterol-fed rabbits, RODGER (1971) found lipid deposits infiltrating the keratocytes. In the deeper stromal layers, lipid droplets turned to solid crystals. These crystals consisted of cholesterol or cholesterol esters. Some of the droplets consisted of cholesterol, as well as phospholipids, but mostly as esters. Triacylglycerols were increased around the blood vessels in the periphery.

Lipid accumulation in cornea and sclera is closely related to that of atherosclerosis. Research on ocular lipids may help to elucidate the patho-genesis of atherosclerosis. This disorder is being studied in man, experi-mental animals and tissue cultures in many laboratories, and much of the attention is focused on the plasma lipoproteins. Immunoelectrophoresis has shown that the concentration of lipoprotein in normal intima is closely correlated with plasma lipoprotein level and the two pools are in equili-brium (SCOTT & HURLEY, 1970). The amount of lipoprotein increases in early fibrous lesions and provides a reservoir from which lipid could be deposited. Knowledge about the molecular events which precede deposition and about the final molecular form in which the proteins and lipids accu-mulate is scarce. Of great importance is the detection of a cell surface receptor in human fibroblasts that binds serum low-density lipoproteins and thereby regulates cellular cholesterol metabolism. Cholesterol of these lipo-proteins is transferred into the cell, the cellular mechanism for esterification of cholesterol is stimulated, cholesterol biosynthesis is promoted and the protein component of the lipoprotein is degraded. In several patients with homozygous familial hypercholesterolaemia, the low-density lipoprotein was not bound to the cell surface and none of the functions of a receptor could be detected, perhaps because of absence of functional receptor molecules (GOLDSTEIN et al., 1975). In tissue culture, cholesterol was removed from aortic smooth muscle cells by fractions of high-density apolipoprotein (STEIN et al., 1975) suggesting the great importance of the plasma lipoproteins as 'effector' molecules and to their specific interaction with connective tissue cells. Undoubtedly these findings will influence thinking about the problem of arcus senilis and the phenomena of ageing of the corneo-scleral tissue.

REFERENCES

ANDREWS, J.S. The lipids of arcus senilis. *Arch. Ophthalmol.* 68: *264-266* (1962).
BOTTCHER, C.J.F. & WOODFORD, S.P. Chemical changes in the arterial wall associated with atherosclerosis. *Fed. Proc.*, Suppl. 11, 21: *15-21* (1962).
BROEKHUYSE, R.M. Lipids in tissues of the eye VII. Changes in concentration and composition of sphingomyelin, cholesterol esters and other lipids in aging sclera. *Biochim. Biophys. Acta* 280: *637-645* (1972).
BROEKHUYSE, R.M. The lipid composition of aging sclera and cornea. *Ophthalmologica* 171: *82-85* (1975).
BROEKHUYSE, R.M. & KUHLMANN, E.D. Lipids in tissues of the eye VI. Sphingomyelins and cholesterol esters in human sclera. *Exp. Eye Res.* 14: *111-113* (1972).
BROEKHUYSE, R.M. & DAEMEN, F.J.M. The Eye. In: Lipid metabolism in mammals. (F. SNYDER, Ed.), Plenum Press, in the press (1976).
COGAN, D.G. Some aspects of fat in degeneration. In: The transparency of the cornea. (DUKE-ELDER, S. & PERKINS, E.S., eds.) Blackwell Scientific Publications, Oxford, pp. 149-163 (1960).
COGAN, D.G. & KUWABARA, T. Arcus senilis. *Arch. Ophthalmol.* 61: *553-560* (1959).
CROUSE, J.R. GRUNDY, S.M. & AHRENS, Jr., E.H. Cholesterol distribution in the bulk tissues of man: variation with age. *J. Clin. Invest.* 51: *1292-1296* (1972).
DAVIDSON, J.C. & KOLBE, R.J. Arcus senilis and ischaemic heart disease. *Lancet* 1: *707* (1965).
DU CHESNE, J. Fettgehalt und Morphologie der menslichen Sclera in den verschiedenen Alterstufen. Thesis, Leipzig (1967).
DUKE-ELDER, S., & LEIGH, A.G. Diseases of the outer eye. Cornea and sclera. In: System of ophthalmology., Vol. 8, Pt. 2. (S. DUKE-ELDER, ed.) C.V. Mosby Co. St. Louis (1965).
FELDMAN, G.L. Human ocular lipids: their analysis and distribution. *Survey of Ophthalmol.* 12: *207-250* (1967).
FUCHS, E. Zur Anatomie der Pinguecula. *Von Graefes Arch. Ophth.* 37 (Pt. 3) *143-191* (1891).
GOLDSTEIN, J.L., DANA, S.E., BRUNSCHEDE, G.Y. & BROWN, M.S. Genetic heterogeneity in familial hypercholesterolemia: evidence for two different mutations affecting functions of low-density lipoprotein receptor. *Proc. Nat. Acad. Sci.* 72: *1092-1096* (1975).
HSIA, S.L. Potentials in exploring the biochemistry of human skin. In: Essays in biochemistry (P.N. CAMPBELL, ed.) Vol. 7, pp. 1-38, Academic Press, New York, (1971).
KREKELER, F. Die Struktur der Sclera in den verschiedenen Lebensaltern. *Arch. Augenheilk.* 93: *144-150* (1923).
LEBER, T., cited in Vosius,A. Lehrbuch der Augenheilkunde (Ed. 4), Leipzig & Wien, F. Deuticke, p. 422.
LEMP, M.A. Cornea and sclera. *Arch. Ophthalmol.* 90: *408-422* (1973).
LOEWENSTEIN, A. Lipoid droplets in the episclera as a regular change with age. *Ophthalmologica* 100: *345-350* (1940).
PARSONS, J.H. Arcus senilis. *Roy. Lond. Ophth. Hosp. Rep.* 15: *141-155* (1903).
PORTMAN, O.W. & ALEXANDER, M. Metabolism of sphingolipids by normal and atherosclerotic aorta of squirrel monkeys. *J. Lipid Res.* 11: *23-30* (1970).
RODGER, F.C. A study of the ultrastructure and cytochemistry of lipid accumulation and clearance in cholesterol-fed rabbit cornea. *Exp. Eye Res.* 12: *88-93* (1971).

ROUSER, G. & SOLOMON, R.D. Changes in phospholid composition of human aorta with age. *Lipids* 4: *232-234* (1969)

SCOTT, P.J. & HURLEY, P.J. The distribution of radio-iodinated serum albumin and low-density lipoprotein in tissues and the arterial wall. *Atherosclerosis 11: 77-103* (1970).

SILVER, M.D. WEIGENSBERG B.I. & MCMILLAN, G.C. Hyperlipemic sera in the rabbit's cornea. *Arch. Path. 80: 171-176* (1965).

SMITH, E.B., The origin and significance of the changes in the lipids of vascular tissue with age. *J. Atheroscler. Res.* E8: 197-199 (1968).

SMITH, E.B., EVANS, P.H. & DOWNHAM, M.D. Lipid in the aortic intima. The correlation of morphological and chemical characteristics. *J. Atheroscler. Res.* 7: *171-186* (1967).

STEFANOVICH, V. & KAJIYAMA, G. Squalene and cholesterol in normal rabbit aorta. *Atherosclerosis* 11: *401-403* (1970).

STEIN, Y., GLANGEAUD, M.C., FAINARU, M. & STEIN, O. The removal of cholesterol from aortic smooth muscle in culture and Landschutz ascites cells by fractions of human high-density apolipoprotein. *Biochim. Biophys. Acta* 380: *106-118* (1975).

TAKAYASU, M. Beiträge zur pathologische Anatomie der Arcus senilis. *Arch. Augenheilk.* 43: *154-162* (1901).

WATERS, L.L. Corneal stromal reactions in rabbits following injection of hyperlipemic and of delipidized homologous serum. *Am. J. Pathol.* 47: *51-59* (1965).

Key words: Cornea, lipids, ageing, arcus senilis, cholesterol, phospholipids, Sclera, lipids, ageing, cholesterol, phospholipids, Atherosclerosis, Lipoproteins, Hypercholesterolemia.

Author's address:
Institute of Ophthalmology
University of Nijmegen
Nijmegen. The Netherlands

SYSTEMATIC ECHO–OPHTHALMOGRAPHY

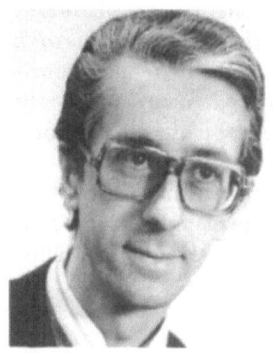

JOHAN M. THIJSSEN & G.-J. KOOMEN

(Nijmegen, the Netherlands)

Echography, or ultrasonic diagnosis, has already proved to be of great value in ophthalmology. The examination technique is simple, not very discomforting to a patient and without danger of direct or cumulative traumatic effects. One wonders therefore why so few clinics actually apply the technique routinely. The first reason may be that the interpretation of an echogram is much more difficult than the simplicity of the technique would suggest. Hence a thorough knowledge of the physical backgrounds and of the pitfalls and artifacts is indispensable (cf. THIJSSEN, 1971, 1972, 1973, 1974, THIJSSEN & OTTO, 1971, THIJSSEN & GOMMERS, 1975, THIJSSEN & KOOMEN, 1975). The second reason may be that the pieces of equipment commercially available have different amplifier and filtering characteristics which produce a variety of echographic wave-forms. Fortunately, in ophthalmology an initiative of OSSOINIG (cf. OSSOINIG, 1971) has resulted in a strictly standardized ultrasonic apparatus (Kretz Technik, 7200 MA) that is used all over the world. So in ophthalmology at least we have the opportunity to compare the results from one clinic with those of another, and what may be of even greater importance to learn from each other's experience.

The general indications for an echographic examination are:

a) opacity of ocular media, whether other intraocular pathology or traumatology are suspected or not

b) intraocular tumor: confirmation, localization and differential diagnosis

c) biometry: e.g. for the calculation of the refractive power of an implant lens

d) orbital lesions

These indications are not absolute and they never exclude other diagnostic techniques. It is a matter of case history which technique prevails and which other techniques are used to extend or to confirm the results.

The principal visualization techniques of echography are the A-scan and the B-scan. In the A-scan the information is one-dimensional, i.e. along the axis of the emitted sound beam, and the echoes are displayed on an oscilloscope screen. The time of an echo with respect to the emission time of the sound reveals the depth information, and the magnitude of an echo shows the acoustic properties of an inhomogenity within the tissue. The A-scan is therefore more suitable for exact dimensional measurements, for the demonstration of movements of structures (e.g. vascularities) and for tissue differentiation. The B-scan produces a two dimensional (sonar) picture in which amplitude information is 'translated' to brightness, though to a limited extent. The main characteristic of the B-scan is the two-dimensionality of the picture so that anatomical structures and pathology are clearly shown in a sagittal cross section. The B-scan is therefore more suitable for a *topographic* display of pathological structures.

We divide the echographic examination into four different aspects that depend on the clinical case and take place either independently, or in a step by step decision scheme. The four aspects will be discussed now and illustrated by clinical data.

1. BIOMETRY

Exact measurement of the dimensions of the eye ball and the ocular media can be useful in deciding the cause of the refractive error. In our clinic the main question for this so-called *functional biometry* is to calculate the refractive power of a lens implant (cf. THIJSSEN, 1975). The A-scan picture of such an examination is shown in Fig. 1. A kind of sclera lens with a water basin is placed at the eye of a patient. The ultrasound probe is therefore acoustically coupled to the eye by a fluid and causes no indentation of the cornea. The left wave in Fig. 1 stems from the emission pulse itself. Following from left to right are the cornea echo, both lens echoes and the posterior pole echo, which is followed by an irregular echopattern of the orbital tissues. The rectangular waveform in the lower part of the figure is a calibration signal, that is used to calibrate the exact distance between the various echoes.

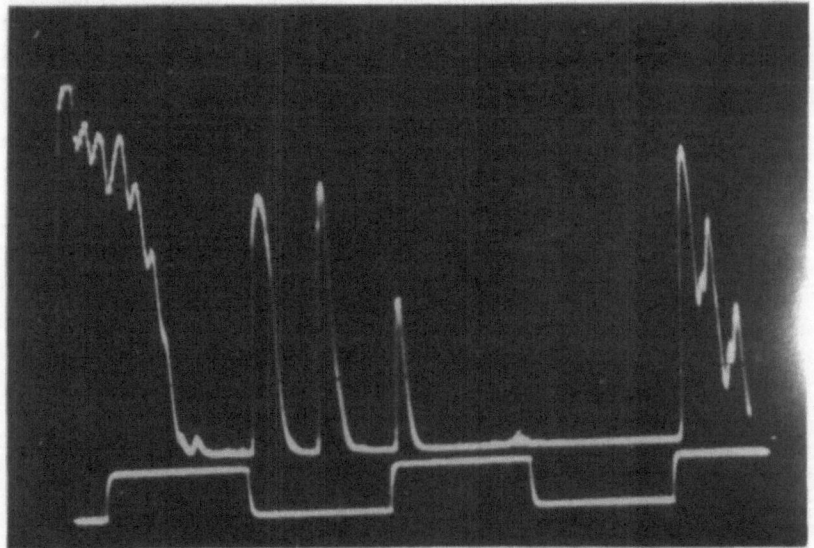

Fig. 1. Biometry: A-scan echogram along central eye axis by using a water filled sclera lens. Echoes from left to right: emission pulse, corneal echo, lens echoes, posterior pole echo followed by orbital fat echoes. Lower trace: calibration pulse (20 microsec.)

An illustration of *anatomical biometry* is reproduced in Fig. 2, which shows in the lower part an A-scan trace from a direct application of the probe to the eye and made from the equator through the centre of the eye. The upper part shows a trace of another equatorial application of the probe, but now the posterior wall echo (right) is clearly displaced to the left (15 mm instead of 21) thus demonstrating the indentation due to the presence of a plombe after retinal detachment surgery.

2. TOPOGRAPHIC ECHOGRAPHY

Fig. 3 is a B-scan picture of both eyes of a patient with a funnel shaped retinal detachment. A striking feature of the topography of retinal detachments is clearly demonstrated, i.e. the attachment of the retina to the globe at the blind spot.

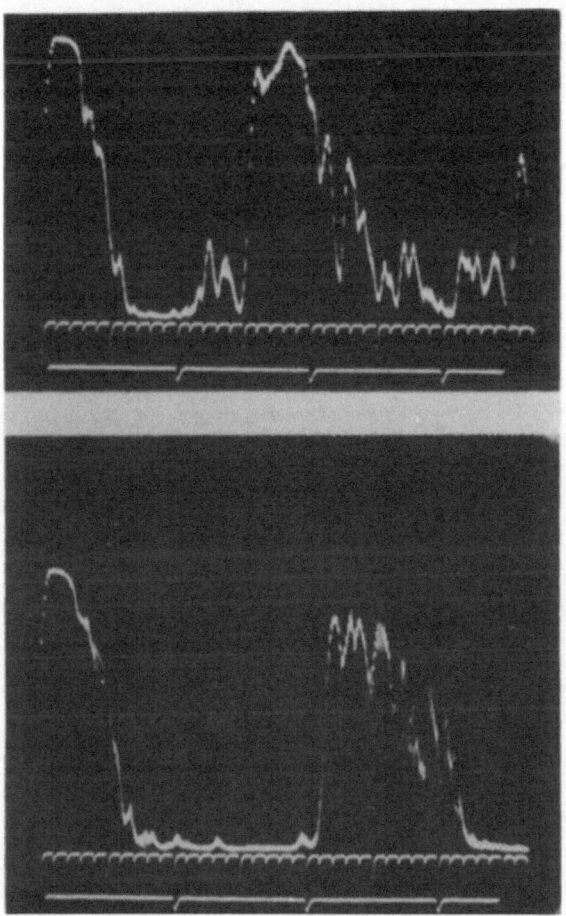

Fig. 2. Biometry: Lower part: direct application at equator, directed through center. Diameter 21 mm. Upper part: same eye, directed at plombal indentation. Diameter 15 mm.

325

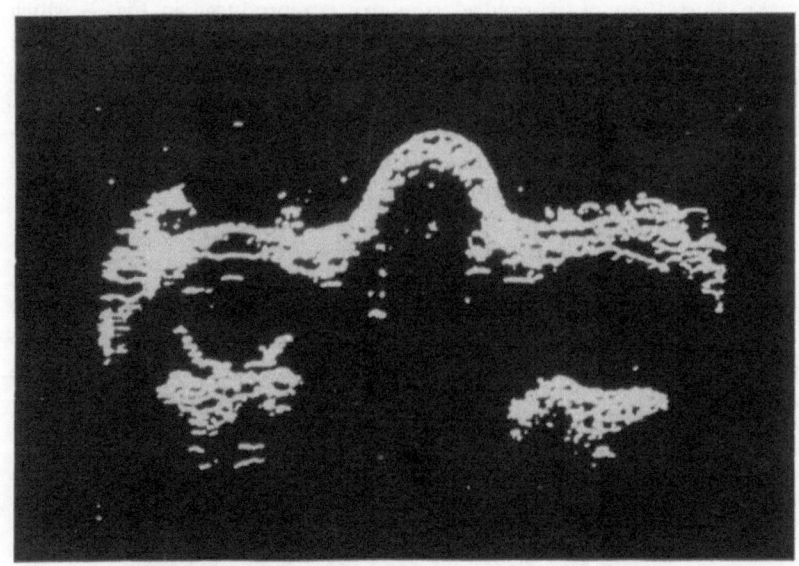

Fig. 3. Topographic echography: Left: (right eye) funnel shaped retinal detachment. Right: (normal eye, looking temporally).

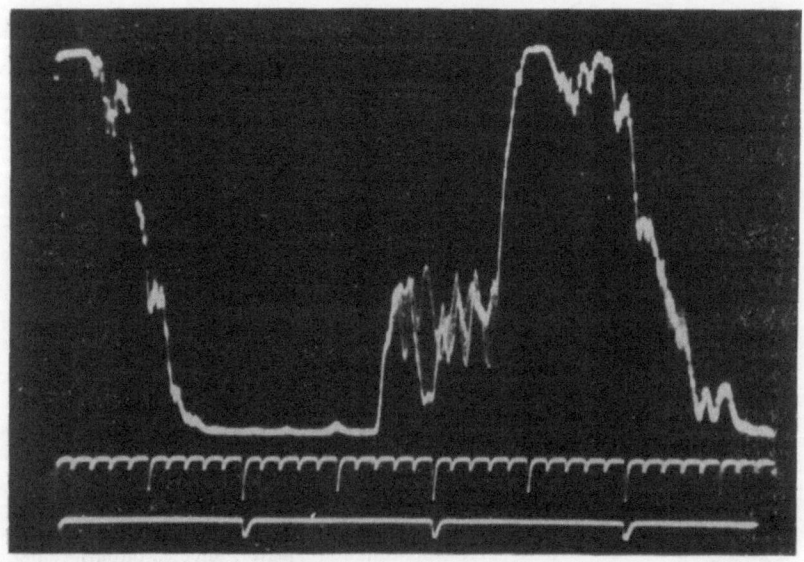

Fig. 4. Kinetic echography: Moving echo. before posterior wall echo. Subchoroidal fluid.

3. KINETIC ECHOGRAPHY

The movement of pathological structures relative to the normal anatomy can be spontaneous, as in the case of a highly vascularized lesion, or induced as for example after an eye movement. The latter kind of movements may be used in the differential diagnosis of vitreous membranes v. retinal detachments. Fig. 4 shows an A-scan picture of an eye containing a subchoroidal lesion of unknown nature. As can be seen all echoes are sharply depicted except the small ones just anterior to the posterior wall echo. The unsharpness indicates rapid movements within the pathology.

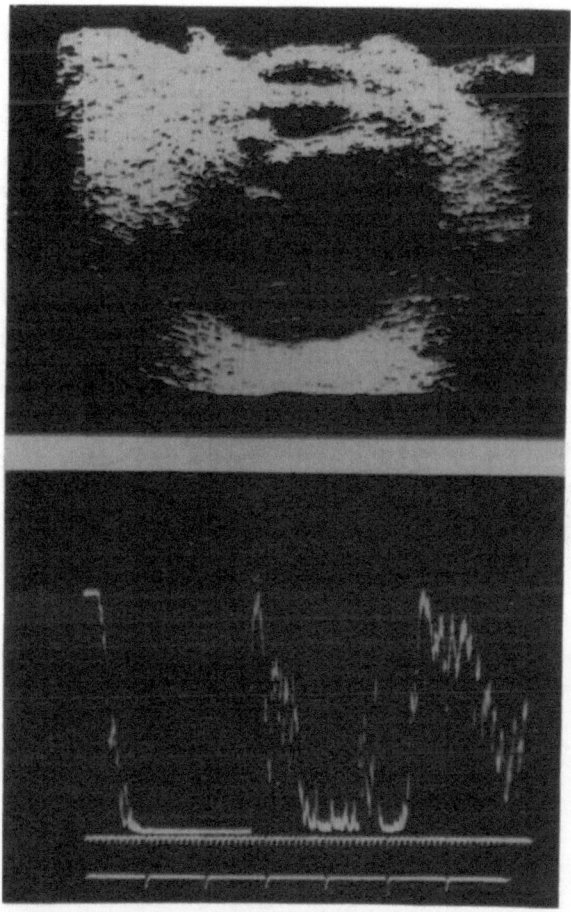

Fig. 5. Quantitative echography: Lower part: A-scan, made with water bath (first 28 mm) directed through limbus and center of the globe. Low magnitude echoes from vitreous haemorrhage, membrane spikes 60% magnitude. Upper part: B-scan through horizontal meridian, vitreous membrane.

4. QUANTITATIVE ECHOGRAPHY

The next figures show the procedure used to differentiate various kinds of lesions by considering the magnitude of the echoes, the texture of the echopattern and the ultrasound attenuation within the lesion. It is therefore clear that to be able to use the possibilities of echography fully in tissue differentiation the three other aspects of echography described above should also be incorporated in the decision process.

The next figures were all taken from the same patient at various stages of the disease. The patient consulted our out-patients clinic for unclear reasons very irregularly, so that the disease could develop extensively as the last picture shows. The upper part of Fig. 5 displays a B-scan picture of the left eye through the horizontal meridian. A membrane like structure is depicted,

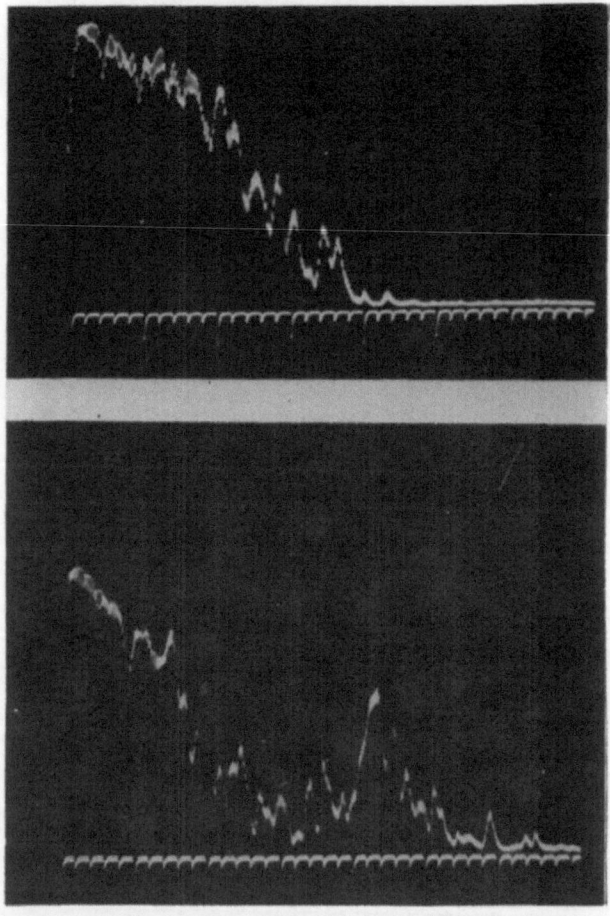

Fig. 6. Patient of Fig. 5, after 1 year. Both A-scan traces from application at the upper nasal side of the eye lid, directed into the orbit and bypassing the globe. Upper: healthy side. Lower: abnormal echoes low to medium magnitude, low attenuation, no border spikes.

which according to the A-scan examination (lower part) was a vitreous membrane accompanied by a vitreous haemorrhage.

One year later the intraocular conditions appeared to be unchanged but we found a clear indication of orbital pathology as is seen in Fig. 6. The A-scan traces were made para-ocularly, through the upper eye lid by directing the probe from the upper nasal position into the orbit. The upper trace was obtained from the healthy (right) eye, the lower one from the left eye. The latter trace shows that the normal orbital echopattern is interrupted by a low reflective and less attenuating tissue without clear border echoes. From these quantitative aspects we concluded that the presence of either a lymphoma, a sarcoma, or a meningioma was likely.

Nine months later the patient reappeared at our clinic and then she had an extreme exophthalmus and severe ophthalmoplegia. The echographic findings at that time are shown in Fig. 7 together with 2 sketches of a front view and sagittal cross section through eye ball and orbit. The B-scan is

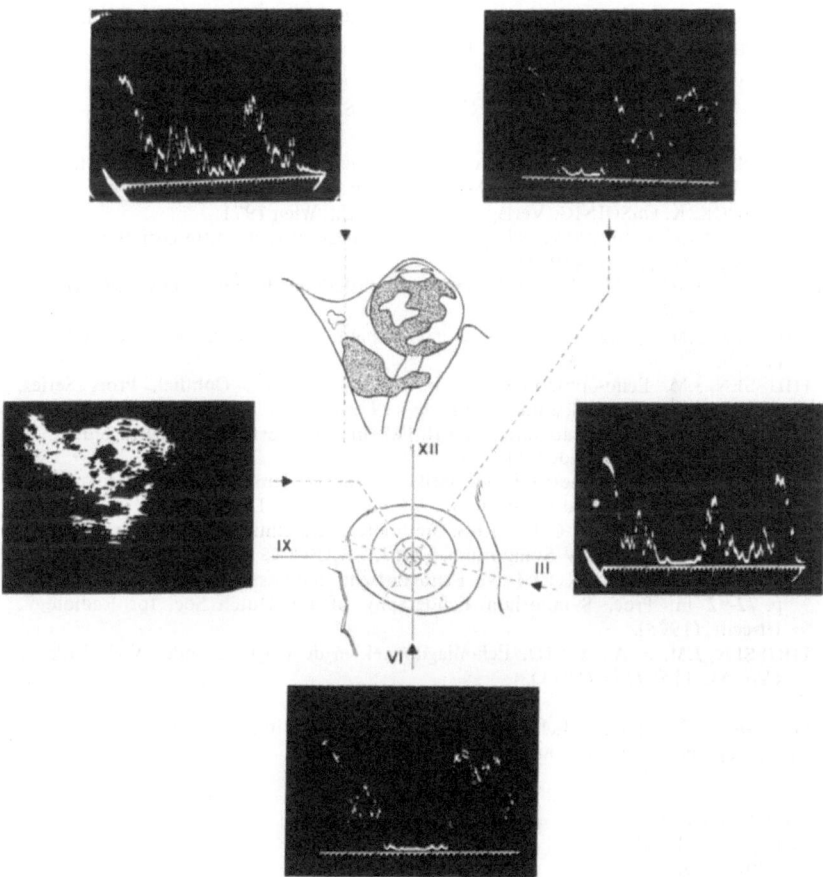

Fig. 7. Patient of Fig. 5 after 21 months. Sketched cross section corresponds to B-scan. Arrows indicate direction of A-scan traces. Proven sarcoma.

shown in the middle left picture and it demonstrates a solid mass in the vitreous humour, which is depicted white due to inhomogenities in the process, whereas the vitreous is homogeneous black. On the contrary the process is depicted black in the orbit which indicates echoes of smaller magnitude than those from the orbital fat. The A-scan trace at the upper left is taken parabulbar as indicated in the cross section and it displays a large mass characterized by an irregular texture and medium to low echo magnitude. The 3 other A-scan pictures were made by transocular applications of the probe. The intraocular solid mass appears here as a medium size amplitude and low attenuation pattern with high boundary spike (upper right). The middle right picture simultaneously shows the intra- and extraocular patterns. According to the scheme of OSSOINIG (1974) and our own experience we concluded that either a pseudotumor, or a sarcoma was present. Examination of the process after enucleation revealed a reticulo-sarcoma of the orbit which had penetrated into the globe.

In future we hope to refine the echogram interpretation by means of computer analysis of echotraces and we trust that a wider spread of this valuable diagnostic technique will increase clinical experience which is necessary to consolidate present knowledge.

REFERENCES

OSSOINIG, K.C. Grundlagen der echographischen Gewebsdifferenzierung. I. Teil. pp. 155-168. II. Teil. pp. 419-439 in: Ultrasonographia Medica, Vol. I. Eds. J. BÖCK, K. OSSOINIG. Verlag Wiener Med. Ak., Wien 1971.
OSSOINIG, K.C. Quantitative echography – the basis of tissue differentiation. *J. Clin. Ultrasound*: 2, *33-46*, (1974).
THIJSSEN, J.M. A new B-scan system for ophthalmic diagnosis. *Ophthal. Res.* 2: *285-294*, 1971.
THIJSSEN, J.M. Ultrasonic diagnostics in Ophthalmology. *Ophthalmologica*, 165: *517* (1972).
THIJSSEN, J.M. Echo-ophthalmology. p. 273-318 in: Doc. Ophthal. Proc. Series, vol. 3, Ed. H. HENKES, Junk, Den Haag, (1973).
THIJSSEN, J.M. Echo-oculografie. p. 148-187 in: Diagnostiek met Ultrageluid. Ed. W. PLATE, Stafleu, Leiden, (1974).
THIJSSEN, J.M. The emmetropic and iseikonic implant lens: computer calculation of the refractive power and its accuracy. *Ophthalmologica*, 171: *467-486*, (1975).
THIJSSEN, J.M. & P.A.M. GOMMERS. Methodical and clinical aspects of echo-oculography. Proc. SIDUO V Symposium, Eds. J. FRANÇOIS & J. GOES, Gent, (1975).
THIJSSEN, J.M. & C.J. KOOMEN, Echografische toepassing in de Oogheelkunde. p. 72-92 in: Proc. Symposium Echography of the Dutch Soc. for Radiology. Utrecht, (1975).
THIJSSEN, J.M. & A.J. OTTO. Echodiagnostiek in de Oogheelkunde. *Ned. Tijds. v. Geneesk.* 115: *1117* (1971).

Key words: Echography, Echo ophthalmography, Quantitative echography, Topographic echography, Kinetic echography, Biometry.

Author's address:
Biophysics Laboratory
Institute of Ophthalmology
University of Nijmegen
Nijmegen, The Netherlands

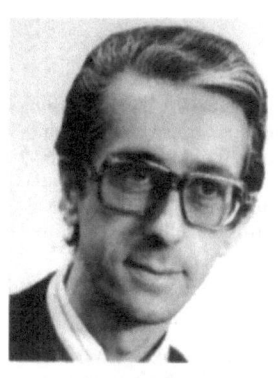

INVARIANCES OF THE CONE–DOMINATED E.R.G. (TREE SHREW AND MAN)

J.M. THIJSSEN & H.J. TERLAAK*

(Nijmegen, The Netherlands)

INTRODUCTION

The genus Tupaia is generally considered to be standing at the base of primate phylogenetic development (cf. HAFLEIGH & WILLIAMS, 1966; SCHWAIER, 1973). Therefore, correlation of electrophysiological data of the visual system of this animal with human vision and its electrophysiological properties should be more or less straightforward. The retina of the tree shrew contains a single type of photoreceptors, i.e. cones (SAMORAJSKI et al., 1966). The presence of spurious rod-shaped cones was found by these authors in a fraction of 5%. Whether these receptors are really rods, or not, is not sure (see also DIETERICH, 1969), but for a study of the electroretinogram such a small fraction will not interfere with the photopic responses of the cones. Moreover, careful analysis of the ERG data from dark adapted conditions did not reveal any indication of the presence of the response of rods (TERLAAK, 1975; TIGGES et al., 1963).

A study of the ERG of the tree shrew, therefore, should be comparable to the investigation of the human fovea, apart from colour dependence. According to POLSON (1968) the tree shrew is a deuteranope whereas the human fovea has tritanopic vision. A small difference in spectral sensitivity may therefore be expected (cf. TIGGES et al., 1963).

We measured the response to short flashes of varying intensity and at different levels of light adaptation (cf. TERLAAK, 1975). From these so-called stimulus-response curves increment threshold curves could be constructed which according to e.g. BIERSDORF (1965) are analogous to psychophysical increment threshold curves. The stimulus response curves are also used to study the presence of a particular invariance in the shape of the ERG wave form. Furthermore the responses to stimulation with constant energy light flashes of varying duration were compared to data of critical flicker fusion (CFF) measurements, and a second type of invariance was examined. In order to illustrate the relevance of the data of the shrew for human electrophysiology some results of experiments with human subjects have been added. These experiments were inspired by the data obtained from tree shrew and the results may lead to useful procedures for clinical examinations.

---

* Now at the Department of Neurology.

METHODS

Preparation

The animals were given an intramuscular injection of atropine (0,3 mg/kg) during halothane anaesthesia. After placing the animals in a stereotaxic apparatus the halothane was removed from the oxygen-nitrous oxide mixture (30%, 70%, respectively) and the animals were paralysed by an injection of galamine triethiodide (28 mg/hour). The artificial respiration was stabilized at 5% CO_2 in the expired air (cf. TERLAAK et al., 1975). The pupil of the eyes was dilated by dropping atropine sulphate on to the cornea.

Recording

Both eyes of an animal were provided with a contact lens containing a silver/silver chloride wire. One of the lenses was blackened, the electrode of which served as a reference. The lenses were kept in place by means of the negative pressure from a tube filled with saline solution (Fig. 1A).

The ERG was derived differentially from the electrodes in the contact lenses. Earthing was provided by a subcutaneous electrode in one of the hind legs. The signal was amplified by an amplifier with a pass band of 0.2-250 Hz. While stimulating with short light flashes a computer of average transients (CAT) was used to improve the signal to noise ratio of small responses. With sinusoidal stimulation the ERG response passed a lock-in amplifier system (Vector voltmeter, cf. FRICKER, 1971; PADMOS & NORREN, 1971). By this means it was possible to maintain a fixed response level, or alternatively to measure amplitude and phase with respect to the sinusoidal stimulation.

The light sources consisted of unfocussed and fast phosphor cathode ray tubes (Ferranti). The spectrum of the phosphor almost coincided with the spectral sensitivity of red human cones. The light could be modulated electronically either sinusoidally (0-99% modulation depth), or flashed. The light was projected at a diffuse screen subtending 80 degrees visual angle.

Light intensities were expressed in photopic trolands using the human spectral sensitivity and taking into account the small size of the eye of the tree shrew. The ERG response to flashes was measured according to the scheme in Fig. 1B. The amplitude of the x-wave was taken relative to the peak of the a-wave.

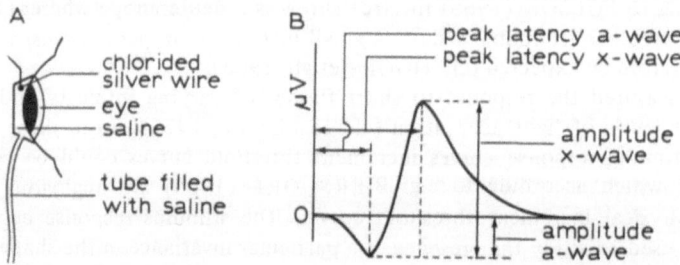

Fig. 1A. Contact lens electrode.   Fig. 1B. Data calculated from the ERG.

RESULTS

The ERG responses to a short (1 msec) flash and to a relatively long flash (50 msec) are shown in Fig. 2. The peak latencies of the a-wave are of the order of 20 msec, and of the x-wave 35 msec. These short latencies are typical for a cone ERG response (cf. ARDEN & TANSLEY, 1955; NYE, 1968). The response to the 50 msec flash consists of two parts: a normal

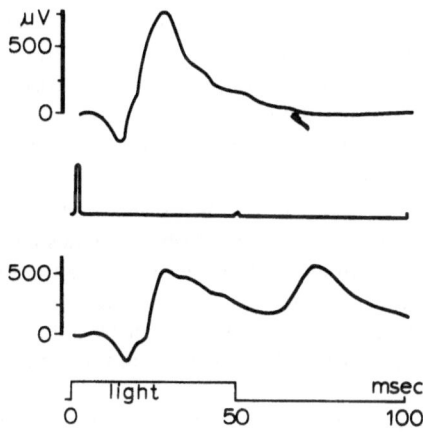

Fig. 2. Upper part: ERG obtained from 1 1 msec flash. Lower part: ERG from a 50 msec flash of equal energy.

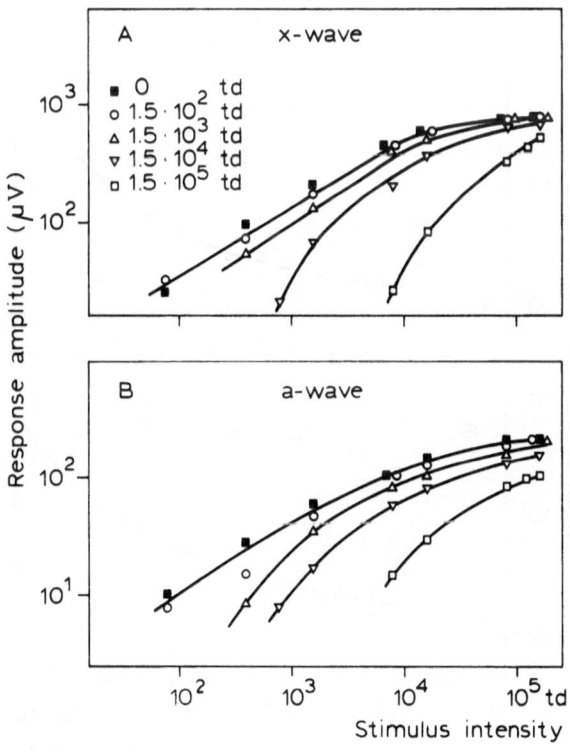

Fig. 3. Stimulus-response curves for the x-wave-(A) and the a-wave-(B) amplitude. Background illumination as a parameter.

ERG after the onset of the light and a positive wave after the offset. Since both flashes contain equal light energies, it follows from this result that a long flash will evoke a smaller response than a very short flash. This property will be used to measure the critical duration (CD), which is defined as the longest duration of a flash that yields the same response as a very short one of equal energy (= duration x intensity).

Stimulus v. response curves are shown in Fig. 3. As can be seen, the curves tend to be straight lines at low flash intensities and they saturate at high levels. The main influence of the level of adaptation is to shift the response curves to the right and to increase the curvature. The range of stimulus intensities from which a response can be obtained without saturation is rather large; approximately 3 log units in the dark and at low adaptation levels.

The stimulus v. response curves can be used to construct increment threshold curves. The latter being defined as a plot of the flash intensity that evokes a response equal to a particular threshold level v. adaptation level. The procedure is to determine the points on the curves of e.g. 25 μV response level and to read the corresponding flash intensities. In this way at every adaptation level the increment threshold flash is defined and then plotted versus the various adaptation levels. Increment threshold curves resulting from this procedure are plotted in Fig. 4. As can be seen the

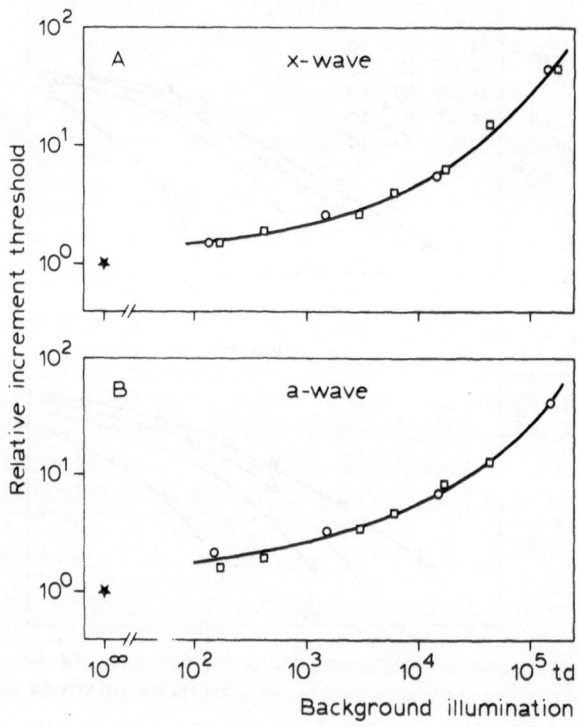

Fig. 4. Increment threshold v. background illumination for the x-wave (A) and the a-wave (B). Response threshold 100 μV and 25 μV, respectively.

threshold curve starts from an almost horizontal part at low adaptation levels and gradually reaches a slope of 45 degrees. The latter observation indicates a proportionality which is the so-called 'Weber law' known from psychophysics. Hence, the increment threshold curve of the ERG displays qualitatively the same relationship as the human perceptive curve.

The stimulus response curves can also be used to display still another and very important property of the cone ERG. Fig. 5A shows that the relationship of the amplitude of a-wave versus x-wave is a straight line when plotted logarithmically. This property not only holds true at a particular adaptation level, but the points from all the five adaptation levels fall along a single line. It will be clear that this result reveals a very fundamental characteristic of the retina which will be discussed later on. We repeated the experiment with four other animals and as can be seen in Table I the slope of the curves is mostly of the order of 1. The average x-wave to a-wave ratio appears to be 4.3. Hence on average the x-wave is 4 times as large as the a-wave.

We also carried out a few experiments with human subjects to investigate the universality of the result. The adaptation field subtended 180° by using an adaptometer sphere (HORSTEN et al., 1959; THIJSSEN et al., 1974). The stimulus was obtained from a Xenon flash tube covering a 10° visual angle. We found that the responses to white flashes did not yield the invari-

Table I

ANIMAL	SLOPE	x/a-RATIO
C3	1.00	3.7
F6	1.10	4.7
F7A	1.06	3.6
F7B	1.04	4.6
H6	1.30	4.8

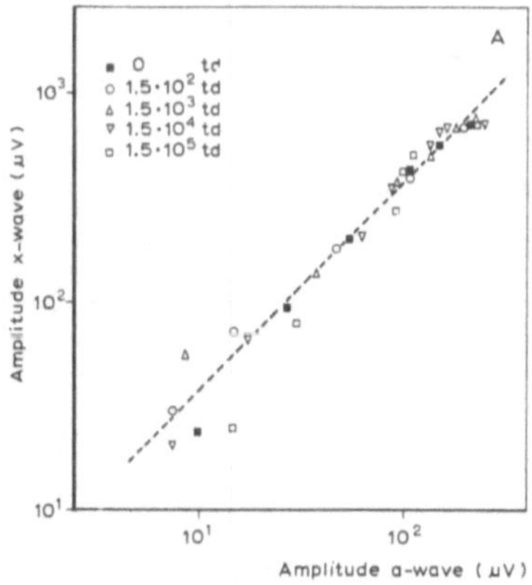

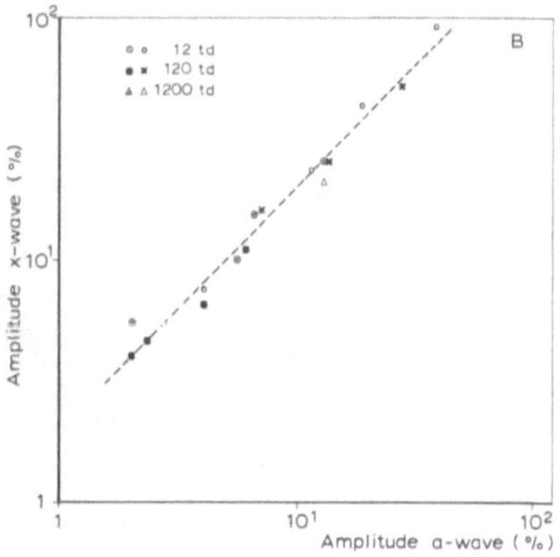

Fig. 5A. X-wave amplitude v. a-wave at various adaptation levels for the tree shrew. Broken line indicates proportionality: invariance of the x/a ratio.

Fig. 5B. Same plot for two human observers. 100% equals 100 μ V approximately.

335

ance of the x/a ratio when changing the adaptation level. By using a red filter (Wratten 92) the invariance was present, as can be seen from Fig. 5B.

As is known the visual system will follow higher frequencies of flickering light stimulation the higher the adaptation level. This is expressed in the dependency of the CFF on adaptation level. In psychophysics the CFF is defined as the upper frequency limit of the perception of flicker. The operational definition for the CFF of ERG responses will be the upper frequency limit whereby the response reaches a particular fixed level. Since the ERG response generally is not a simple sinusoid we have used the first harmonic component only. This means that we filtered the response in such a way that mainly the component of a frequency equalling the stimulation frequency was measured. It may be added that in our definition of CFF the light modulation was fixed at 100% depth. The data from three animals are shown in Fig. 6. The straight part of the curve can be characterized by the slope value of 28 Hz/log unit, which means that by changing the adaptation level with one log unit a change of the CFF results amounting to 28 Hz.

Theoretically the CFF and the above defined critical duration (CD) should display analogous behaviour in dependency on adaptation level. This can be explained by the assumption that the time constants in the visual system change. As can be seen from Fig. 7 the CD becomes shorter the higher the adaptation level, but since we have plotted the inverse of the CD the plot goes upwards. The straight line of Fig. 7 yields a reasonable fit to the data. The dashed line has been drawn through CFF data corrected for the change of the relative increment threshold in depency on the adaptation level (Fig. 4). The corrected data reveal the changes in time constants only, and therefore they are to be preferred instead of the original curve (Fig. 6).

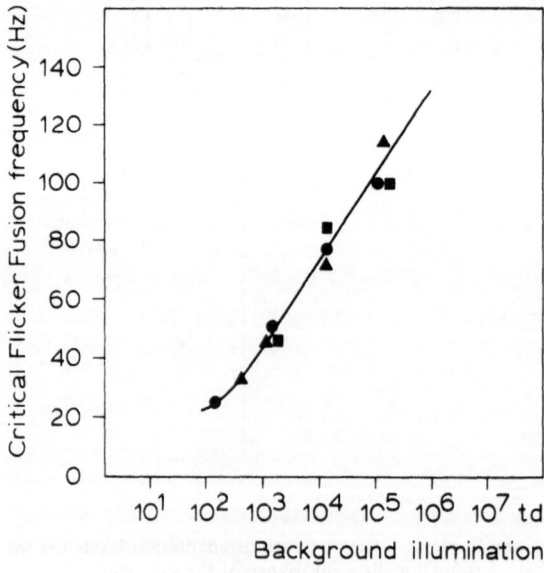

Fig. 6. Critical flicker frequency (CFF) v. adaptation level. Symbols indicate three different animals.

The parallelism of the lines in Fig. 7 illustrates another fundamental invarience as will be discussed later on.

DISCUSSION

The ERG recordings, as shown in Fig. 2, are typical for the cone system. The latencies of the a-wave and x-wave peaks are short compared to those of the rod dominated ERG (cf. BROWN, 1968), and the response at the offset of the light stimulus is positive going. The latter phenomenon can be explained by relatively short time constants of the receptor potential. The presence of high frequency wavelets with a period time of 7 msec (140 Hz) is obvious only at high stimulus energies. Moreover, no more than two or three wavelets are visible which coincide with the x-wave. This observation does not agree, however, with the results of NYE (1968) who found for the pigeon ERG more wavelets with a period time in the range of 10 to 15 msec.

The stimulus response curves of Fig. 3 closely resemble the curves measured by BOYNTON & WHITTEN (1970) and BARON & BOYNTON (1970), for the cone late receptor potential and the local ERG response of cynomolgus monkeys. At high adapting luminances the steeper slope at the lower flash intensities is explained by these authors to the contribution of the steady potential generated by the adapting light. The importance of measuring a whole response curve at a particular adaptation level for clinical

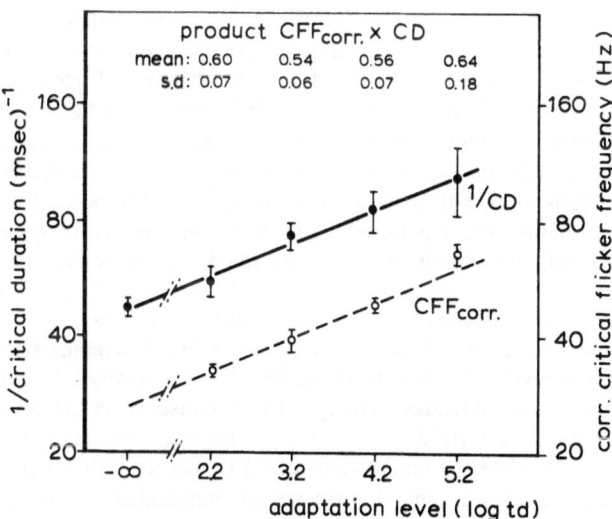

Fig. 7. Plots of 1/critical duration and CFF_{corr} v. adaptation level. Lines are drawn parallel indicating invariance of the product $CD \times CFF_{corr}$.

measurements'has already been stressed by GOURAS (1970). The argument is that the actual value of the response at a particular stimulus setting may be partially influenced by absorption and scattering in the ocular media, but the saturation level of the response always indicates whether the retina is functioning normally or not. It may be remarked that this statement is valid only by using Ganzfeld stimulation.

The human psychophysical increment threshold curve for foveal stimulation displays a proportionality with backgrounds of an intensity higher than 10^2 to 10^3 trolands. As can be seen from Fig. 4 the ERG increment threshold curves for tree shrew are shifted by one log unit to the right as compared to the data for man (cf. BOYNTON & WHITTEN, 1970). An explanation for this difference is not obvious, since the saturation level is reached at a level identical with the monkey cone potential (BOYNTON & WHITTEN, 1970) which displays a reasonable correspondance to human psychophysics. A possibility may be that the psychophysical result is influenced by the choice of the stimulus area.

The relationship between a-wave and x-wave (Fig. 5) displays a striking feature i.e. a proportionality, not only at a particular background level but from dark to the highest level used. The invariance of the proportionality constant means that the shape of the ERG as a whole is maintained, whereby the amplitudes of the responses of the receptor cells and the cells in the inner nuclear layer change by a same factor. Although the ERG is a summation of potentials from both cell layers it will be clear that the response of the inner nuclear layer is activated by the receptor cells. Therefore, it may be concluded that adaptation effects are primarily expressed in the receptor responsiveness.

The clinical value of the proportionality could be the differentiation between receptor layer pathology versus inner nuclear layer pathology (cf. LITH, 1973), since it can be expected that the proportionality constant will change both by an increase in the time constants of the inner nuclear layer potential, and by a decrease in magnitude. No change will occur in case of receptor pathology. The results of Fig. 5A and Table I may be influenced by the kind of stimulus light source we used. As can be seen from Fig. 5B the human ERG reveals analogous properties when a red filter is placed before the Xenon flash lamp. This situation is comparable to the set-up for the tree shrew experiments, i.e. a coloured flash favouring one cone system. The human data may be explained if it is assumed that either the three cone systems have different properties or alternatively that by using red light stimulation the rod contribution is more effectively excluded.

The critical fusion frequency as depicted in Fig. 6 depends strongly on the adaptation level (cf. GRIND et al., 1973, for a survey). As previously noted this behaviour indicates a change of time constants in the system. The straight part is characterized by a 28 Hz per log unit change of the adaptation level. HICK (1957) found a value of 25 Hz per log unit for the Human ERG, which indicates a general property of mammalian cones. It may be mentioned that for the evaluation of clinical CFF data it is essential to maintain very strict adaptation conditions.

The correction of CFF data has been carried out by means of connecting the so-called 'De Lange'-curves (threshold modulation amplitude v. frequency curves) at the high frequency side by a 'high frequency asymptote' and thereafter shifting the CFF points upwards with an appropriate factor found in the increment threshold curves (Fig. 4). This procedure yielded the second invariance displayed in Fig. 7, which is given by the product of critical duration to CFF. Analogous data are known for human psycho-physics (ROUFS, 1972). It may be concluded from this invariance of the ERG that the localization of the effects of adaptation on the time constants of the visual system is at a very early stage, perhaps even the receptor cell layer.

SUMMARY

The electroretinogram of a tree shrew (Tupaia chinensis) has been investigated and, in some respects, compared to the human photopic ERG. The retina of tree shrews contains only cones, hence cone specific aspects of the primate ERG can be clearly demonstrated. The present analysis revealed two invariances. Firstly: the ratio of x-wave to a-wave amplitudes is invariant while changing stimulation and adaptation light intensities or both. The proportionality constant for tree shrew was found to be 4.3. The human photopic ERG appears to reveal the invariance only if the rod system is completely inactive, which can be favoured by using red light stimulation. The proportionality constant for the human ERG appeared to be 2.0.

A second invariance was found when at various adaptation levels the so-called critical time duration, CD (integration time) for flash evoked ERG responses was compared to the critical flicker frequency, CFF, after correction of the latter for the changes in incremental sensitivity. Then, the product of CD times CFF_{corr} is independent of the adaptation level and it equals on the average 0.6. This figure found for the tree shrew's ERG is very similar to the value of 0.5 obtained from psychophysical measurements of human foveal vision.

ACKNOWLEDGEMENTS

The authors wish to thank Professor Dr. *A.J.H. Vendrik* for his valuable suggestions, Drs. *P. van Well* for his experimental assistance, and *W. Braak-huis*, *J. Bakker* and *H. Kokke* for their technical assistance. This work has been supported by the Netherlands Organization for the Advancement of Pure Research (Z.W.O.) via its Biophysics Foundation.

REFERENCES

ARDEN, G.B. & K. TANSLEY. The spectral sensitivity of the pure-cone retina of the grey squirrel (sciurus carolinensis leucotis.) *J. Physiol.* 127: *592-602* (1955).

BARON, W.S. & R.M. BOYNTON. The primate electroretinogram: an indication of photoreceptor activity. *Vis. Res.* 14: *495-501* (1974).

BIERSDORF, W.R. Electrical measurements of increment thresholds in the human eye. *J. Opt. Soc. Amer.* 55: *454-455* (1965).

BOYNTON, R.M. & D.N. WHITTEN. Visual adaptation in monkey cones: recordings of late receptor potentials. *Science* 178: *1423-1426* (1970).

BROWN, K.T.
The electroretinogram: its components and their origins. *Vis. Res. 8: 633-677.* (1968).

DIETERICH, C.E. Die Feinstruktur der Photorezeptoren des Spitzhörnchens. (Tupaia glis) . *Anat. Anz.* 125, (suppl.): *305-312* (1969).

GOURAS, P. Electroretinography: some basic principes. *Invest. Ophthal.* 9: *557-570* (1970).

GRIND, W.A. V.D., G.-J. GRÜSSER, & H.U. LUNKENHEIMER. Temporal transfer properties of the afferent visual system. Psychophysical, neurophysiological and theoretical investigations. P.p. 431-573. In: Handbook of Sensory Physiology, Vol. VII/3 A, ed. R. Jung. Springer, Berlin 1973.

HAFLEIGH, A.S. & C.A. WILLIAMS. Antigenic correspondence of serum albumines among the primates. *Science* 151: *1530-1535* (1966).

HORSTEN, G.P.M., H.H.A. HÖTTE & J. E. WINKELMAN. Method of electroretinographic examination. *Ophthalmologica* 137: *3-6* (1959).

LITH, G.H.M. VAN. Electro-ophthalmology. pp. 257-270. In: Doc. Ophthal. Proc. Series Vol. 3 ed. H.E. Henkes. Junk, The Hague, 1973.

NYE, P.W. An examination of the electroretinogram of the Pigeon in response to stimuli of different intensity and wavelength and following intense chromatic adaptation. *Vis. Res.* 8: *679-696* (1968).

POLSON, M.C. Spectral sensitivity and color vision in Tupaia glis. Thesis, Indiana University, 1968.

ROUFS, J.A.J. Dynamic properties of vision. I. Experimental –, II. Theoretical relationships between flicker and flash thresholds. *Vis. Res.* 12: *261-292* (1972).

SAMORAJSKI, T., J.M. ORDY & J.R. KEIFE. Structural organization of the retina in the tree shrew (Tupaia Glis). *J. Cell. Biol.* 28: *489-504* (1966).

SCHWAIER, A. Breeding tupaias (Tupaia belangeri) in captivity. *Z. Versuchtierkunde* 15: *255-271* (1973).

TERLAAK, H.J. Electrophysiological investigations into luminance coding in the retina of a tree shrew (Tupaia chinensis). Thesis, Nijmegen University, 1975.

TERLAAK, H.J., J.M. THIJSSEN & A.J.H. VENDRIK. A method for prolonged electrophysiological experiments with a tree shrew (Tupaia chinensis). *Z. Versuchtierkunde* 17: *195-204* (1975).

THIJSSEN, J.M., A. PINCKERS & A.J. OTTO. A multipurpose optical system for ophthalmic diagnosis. *Ophthalmologica* 168: *308-314* (1974).

Key words: Tree shrew, Human E.R.G., Cone E.R.G., Critical flicker frequency (CFF), Critical time duration (CD), Invariances (ERG).

Author's address:
Biophysic Laboratory
Institute of Ophthalmology
University of Nijmegen
Nijmegen, the Netherlands

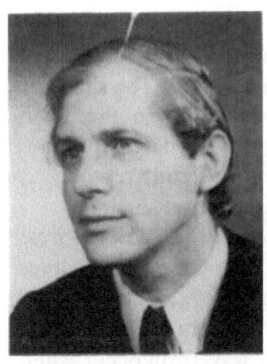

MULTIVARIATE ANALYSIS OF THE ELECTRORETINOGRAM

L. DAAN VAN HOEK & J.M. THIJSSEN

(Nijmegen, the Netherlands)

The electrical response of the retina depends on a variety of stim.lation parameters. Moreover the duplex nature of the human retina and the involvement of several cell layers in the generation of the waveform can give an ambiguous interpretation of the ERG.

The method commonly used to evaluate an ERG is to measure the magnitude and the latency of the peaks by means of visual inspection or by using a computer program (cf. POTTS et al., 1971, 1972). Another way of tackling the problem is to determine the parameters of a mathematical model of the retinal processes underlying the ERG response (cf. THIJSSEN et al., 1974a).

The method for dealing with the duplexity of the retina is to choose the adaptation level carefully at which the ERG is being evoked. This can be achieved by using a 'Ganzfeld' adaptation light at either scotopic, or photopic level. The stimulation light flash is adjusted to scotopic conditions with neutral density filters. Without the filters photopic stimulation conditions prevail. With these precautions it is possible to measure the retinographic response of rods and cones separately. In the intermediate range of adaptation and stimulation conditions a compound response will be evoked, which depending on, e.g., the colour of the stimulating light flash will be dominated by the rod system or the cone system. The details of our equipment have been previously described (THIJSSEN et al., 1974b).

VAN HOEK recently introduced a multivariate technique for evaluation of Visual Evoked Responses (VER) recorded at the skull (cf. VAN HOEK, 1974a, b, 1975). This statistical method is particularly suitable for numerical evaluation of changes occurring in complex waveforms. It produces a vectorial representation of responses, in which a vector is characterized by 2 to 4 numbers. The vectorial space is formed by a set of basic vectors which are uncorrelated (orthogonal) components accounting for the maximal share of signal power. These components are called principal components, hence the commonly used term 'principal component analysis'. An individual response vector is expressed in fractions of the principal components in such a way that the length of it stands for the root-mean-square value of the complete response waveform, and the direction of the vector is a measure of the shape of the waveform.

We have applied the multivariate analysis technique to ERG-data. The results of a pilot experiment serve as an example. White, red and blue flashes were used to evoke the ERG's. In addition, the eye of the subject was light adapted by a white background of 2-200 cd/m². In order to decrease the variability of the responses 20 individual ERG's were averaged. The shape of the 2 principal components of the set of ERG's are given in Fig. 1. In principal component I the photopic (i.e. cone) response apparently dominates, whereas in principal component II the scotopic (i.e. rod) response is greater. These principal components account for 94% of power.

The vectorial representations of the ERG's are given in Fig. 2. Each circle is located at the endpoint of a vector of an ERG. The connecting curves indicate the dependence of the ERG on the flash intensity, as described in the legend. These curves deviate only slightly from straight lines. This means that only slight distortions of the shape of the ERG waveform occur when increasing the flash intensity. The shape of the ERG's apparently depends greatly on the adapting background intensity and the colour of the evoking flash, since the direction of the vector varies considerably. This variation of shape is well known and is generally ascribed to the relative variation of the balance between rod and cone contributions in the ERG. Blue test flashes as well as a low background intensity may favour the rod contribution to the ERG (curves 1, 2). For red test flashes hardly any variation of shape of the ERG can be observed (curves 5, 6, 7). Apparently these ERG's all have a predominant cone contribution. For the white and blue test flashes the relative contribution of rods v. cones depends considerably on the background intensity (curves 1-4).

The vectorial diagram indicates that the shape of the ERG can yield a good measure of the photopic vs scotopic nature of the ERG. The shape can be quantified by the direction of a vector, which is expressed as an angle. From the point of view of clinical fundamental physiology this plot tells us

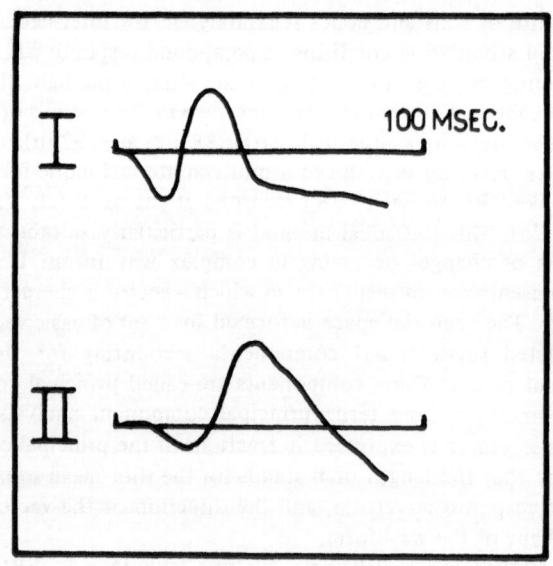

Fig. 1. The 2 principal components of a set of E.R.G. responses (see legend of Fig. 2).

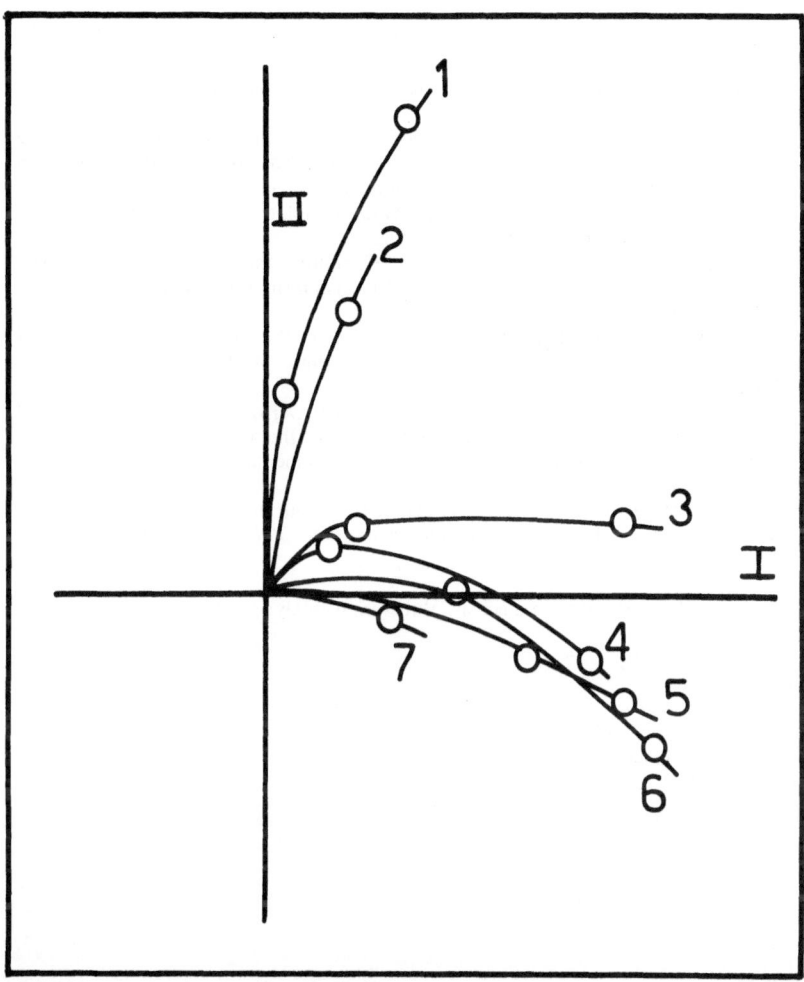

Fig. 2. Vectorial diagram of a set of ERG-responses.
The circles indicate the endpoints of the ERG-vectors, which start at the origin. The (principal) axes correspond to the principal components of Fig. 1.
Curve 1: Blue test flashes, background luminance   2 cd/m²

2: white ,,	,,	,,	,,	2	,,
3: blue ,,	,,	,,	,,	20	,,
4: white ,,	,,	,,	,,	20	,,
5: red ,,	,,	,,	,,	2	,,
6: red ,,	,,	,,	,,	20	,,
7: red ,,	,,	,,	,,	200	,,

that the ERG for these experimental conditions can be sufficiently described by 2 processes, i.e. the scotopic and the photopic, for only these 2 principal components contribute significantly.

REFERENCES

HOEK, L.D. VAN Multivariate vectorial analysis of the visual evoked response. *Kybernetik* 15: *65-72* (1974a).

HOEK, L.D. VAN Luminance and color components in the V.E.R. In: Proc. of the XIth ISCERG Symposium, E. Dodt & J.T. Pearlman, eds., pp. 303-306. Documenta Ophthalmologica Proc. SEries IV. Dr W. Junk, The Hague (1974b).

HOEK, L.D. VAN Multivariate evoked potential correlates of color and luminosity processing. Thesis, Univ. of Utrecht (1975).

POTTS, A.M., BUFFUM, D. & BENNET, S.E. Computer- assisted analysis of the electroretinogram. In: Proc. of the VIIth ISCERG Symposium. D. Basar & Bengisu, eds. pp. 340-354, Univ. of Istanbul (1971).

POTTS, A.M. INOUE, J., BUFFUM, D. & FRITZ, K.J. The morphology of the human E.R.G. In: Proc. of the VIIIth ISCERG Symposium. A. Wirth, ed., pp. 170-181, Pacini, Pisa (1972).

THIJSSEN, J.M. MUNCKHOF, W.M. VANDEN & BRAAKHUIS, W.J.M. Analysis and synthesis of the scotopic ERG (rabbit). In: Proc. of the XIth ISCERG Symposium. E. Dodt & J.T. Pearlman, eds., pp. 75-83. Documenta Ophthalmologica Proc. Series IV. Dr. W. Junk, The Hague (1974).

THIJSSEN, J.M. PINCKERS, A. & OTTO, A.J. A multipurpose optical system for ophthalmic electrodiagnosis. *Ophthalmologica* 168: *208-214* (1974).

Key words: Electroretinogram analysis, Multivariate analysis (ERG), Principal component analysis (ERG).

Authors' address:
Biophysics Laboratory
Institute of Ophthalmology
University of Nijmegen
Nijmegen, the Netherlands

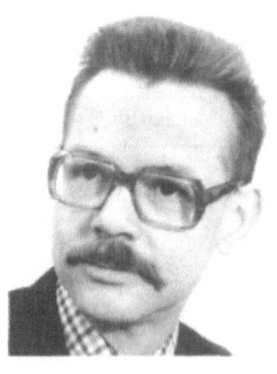

THE LIGHT-SENSITIVE NEGATIVE COMPONENT IN CLINICAL ELECTROOCULOGRAPHY

A. PINCKERS

(Nijmegen, The Netherlands)

In 1974 we studied the flat electrooculogram (EOG), Lp/Dt x 100 < 1.00, divided it into 4 subtypes and added to these the reversed polarity group. Reversed polarity and paradoxical curve (type IV) only occur in uniocular diseases; it was shown that both subtypes are the result of contralateral influence by the normal eye (PINCKERS & THIJSSEN, 1974).

The types II (Iv ≥ Dt > Lp) and III (Lp < Dt; Lp absent?) can be found in both eyes simultaneously; therefore contralateral influence can be excluded. The types II and III show a large light-sensitive negative component, the light-sensitive positive component being absent (type II) or reduced (type III).

In clinical EOG virtually no attention is paid to the light-sensitive negative component because the EOG mostly is judged by means of the Arden-ratio; the Initial value (Iv) or Base value is taken into account sometimes. In this study the presence of a light-sensitive negative component in our clinical material is summarized, in flat EOG and also in EOG's with a Lp/Dt ratio ≥ 1.00.

MATERIAL AND METHOD

I reviewed a total of 1950 EOG recordings, the technique being described elsewhere (THIJSSEN, PINCKERS & OTTO, 1974). Firstly, I gathered the flat EOG types II and III (PINCKERS & THIJSSEN, 1974). Then EOG-recordings with a markedly light-sensitive negative component combined with a Lp/Dt ratio ≥ 1.00 were listed; excluded are EOG's with a potential fall of 50 μV or less, EOG's suspected for irregular eye-movement of the patient and finally patients in which, as a sequence of turning on the adaptation lights at the 12th minute, tearing occurred.

RESULTS

The flat EOG type II and III were found in 33 cases (1.7%); they are summarized in Table I.

TABLE I

Flat EOG (Lp/Dt < 1.00)

Disease	Number of patients	
	type II (Iv ⩾ Dt > Lp)	type III (Lp < Dt; Lp absent?)
Tapetoretinal degeneration	9	4
Choroidal atrophy	1	2
Stargardt	2	1
Retinopathia diabetica	1	2
Rheumatoid arthritis	–	4
Cystoid macular edema	–	2
Haemangioma chorioideae	1	–
Retrolental fibroplasia	1	–
Retinal detachment	–	1
Cryocoagulation ciliary body	1	–
Perforatio bulbi	1	–

TABLE II

Presence of light-sensitive negative component

	number of patients	normal Lp/Dt ratio	subnormal Lp/Dt ratio
I *MACULAR DISEASES*			
Stargardt (Flavimaculatus)	16	0	16
Vitelliform	3	0	3
Dominant autosomal	6	3	3
Dominant autosomal cystoid	3	1	2
Cerebroretinal	3	0	3
Doyne	1	0	1
Senile	6	0	6
Cystoid edema	1	0	1
Central serous retinopathy	1	1	0
Pigmentepithelium defects	4	3 (local)	1 (gyrate)
Not specified	17	5	12
II *MYOPIA*			
(Macular involvement)	13	4	9 (2 Wagner)
III *RHEUMATOID ARTHRITIS*			
No medication	6	3	3
Hydroxychloroquin	22	12	10
Chloroquin	6	2	4
Indomethacin	1	0	1
Bull's eye (Intoxication)	4	1	3
IV *UVEITIS*	6	2	4

A markedly light-sensitive negative component in EOG's with an Lp/Dt ratio of $\geqslant$ 1.00 was seen in 138 patients, that is in 7.0% of our EOG recordings. These were arbitrarily classified in 4 groups; in each group we also noted the Arden-ratio; the Lp/Dt ratio is considered normal if Lp/Dt x 100 $\geqslant$ 180 (PINCKERS & THIJSSEN, 1969). The results are summarized in Table II.

For the remaining 19 patients the diagnoses were: dense nuclear cataract (13), periphlebitis retinae (1), juvenile retinoschizis (1), senile retinoschizis (1), chorio-retinal coloboma (1), occlusion of macular arteriole (1) and melanoma of choroid (1).

DISCUSSION

The light-sensitive potential of the EOG consists of at least two components: a slow positive component with a culmination time of approx. 9 min. and a more rapid negative component with a culmination time of 1 to 2 min. (KOLDER & NORTH, 1967). The negative component persists during light adaptation and can be found in normal subjects (KOLDER 1967; ARDEN & KELSEY 1962 a, b; FRANÇOIS et al. 1957) but manifests itself clearly when the positive component is absent (FRANÇOIS & DE ROUCK 1973). As pointed out (PINCKERS & THIJSSEN, 1974) there is no measurable contralateral influence in these cases. In Fig. 1 the left eye has a pronounced light-sensitive negative component, resulting from a diabetic retinopathy: over the evise crated right orbit we measured a reversed polarity; this illustrates that a negative component occurs in uniocular diseases; moreover, our example demonstrates that even the electrical field of a diseased eye spreads over to the contralateral orbit. It seems that the negative component is, compared to the positive one, more resistent to damage. According to this the sequence of ultimate EOG deterioration is: type III → type II → type I; in type III there is discernable some light-peak, in type II there is only a light-sensitive negative component, while in type I there is no longer any light-sensitive component at all (Fig. 2). In uniocular disease contralateral influence by the normal eye can cause a paradoxical curve (type IV); if the light-insensitive potential is very low we can find potential reversal during the light-adapted phase (Imaizumi, 1964); finally, if the diseased eye has no potential of its own, the result of contralateral influence is a totally reversed registration.

From a clinical point of view the just described sequence of ultimate EOG deterioration is acceptable. The question arises, what happens in early stages of EOG pathology? Is it merely a diminishing light-peak or does the 'appearance' of a negative component also have a clinical significance? Out of the 119 cases listed in Table II, 37 cases (31%) prove to have a normal Lp/Dt-ratio and 82 cases (69%) have an abnormal Lp/Dt-ratio. These findings could fit the resisting-to-damage theory with regard to the light-sensitive negative component. Still considering the negative component as the result of a normal (metabolic?) mechanism, its clear manifestation is subnormal or disturbed EOG's may indicate that the latency of the mechanism producing the light-sensitive positive component is delayed.

The interpretation of Table II is very difficult. It seems that the light-sensitive negative component appears predominantly in diseases which can affect the posterior pole of the eye. At first glance the rheumatoid arthritis group is out of place. We must, however, remember the fact that in rheumatoid arthritis the EOG is subnormal in about 20%. I found this percentage in patients before any treatment was given, in patients treated with hydroxychloroquine or chloroquine and even if there were signs of an intoxication (PINCKERS & V.D. EERDEN, 1973). This means that rheumatoid arthritis sui generis can affect the EOG. It is also known that during an active phase of the rheumatoid process the EOG can be temporarily disturbed (KOLB 1965). Uveitis and macular edema are not uncommon ocular manifestations of rheumatoid disease; therefore the presence of rheumatoid arthritis in Table II is not unexpected.

In gathering the material for this paper I noticed that there were patients in whom the negative component was clearly manifesting itself constantly during several years. Furthermore I happened to find it in two or three members within some affected families.

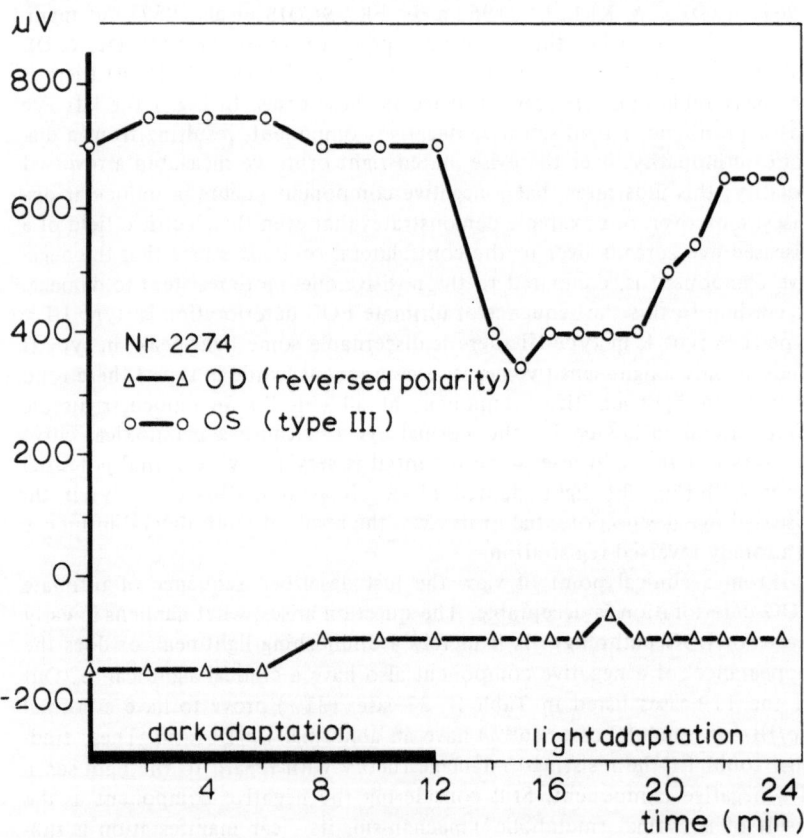

Fig. 1. Combination of a type III flat EOG (left eye) and a reversed polarity type (right orbit) demonstrating the occurrence of a negative light-sensitive component in uniocular diseases.

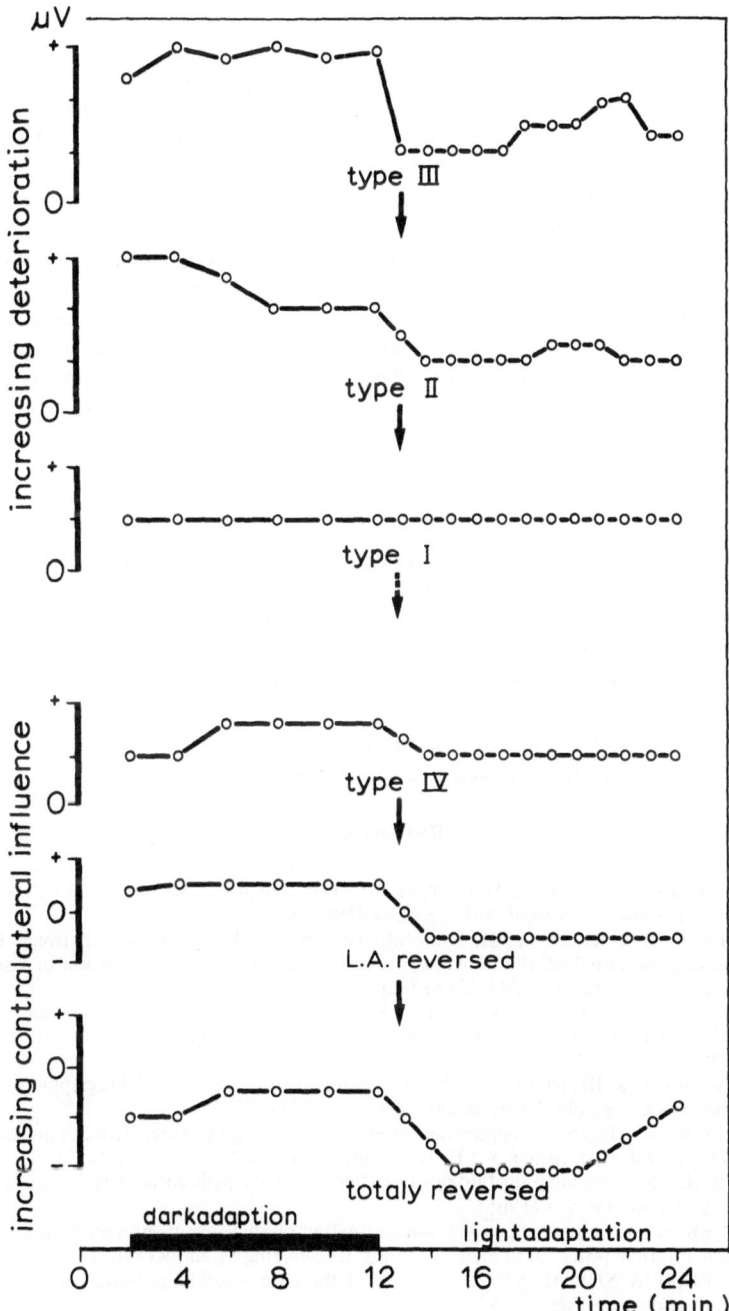

Fig. 2. Sequence of ultimate EOG deterioration, including contralateral influence.

CONCLUSION

The light-sensitive negative component of the EOG is present in normal as well as in diseased eyes. In cases with a relatively well preserved light-peak a fairly pronounced negative component is somehow related to ocular pathology, especially to diseases affecting the posterior pole. Perhaps in the future we shall be able to demonstrate that a marked negative component is a sign of changes in the mechanisms that produce the light-peak.

In flat EOG the light-sensitive negative component seems to be more resistent to choroido-retinal damage than is the positive component.

In some patients, not listed in Table I or II, with diminished visual acuity from onknown cause the EOG shows a clearly distinguishable negative component and a normal Lp/Dt ratio. The study of these patients probably can help us to understand something more of both the light-sensitive components.

SUMMARY

The author gives a summary of clinical EOG's with a marked light-sensitive negative component. As a result, a scheme of sequence of ultimate EOG deterioration (flat type with Lp/Dt ratio < 1.00) is presented. EOG's with an Lp/Dt $\geqslant 1.00$ and a fairly pronounced negative component were encountered in diseases affecting the posterior pole of the eye. It may be possible that in these cases the negative component is more resistent to damage; also a delayed and/or diminished light-peak producing mechanism could facilitate the registration of the negative component.

REFERENCES

ARDEN, G.B. & KELSEY, J.H. Changes produced by light in the standing potential of the human eye. *J. Physiol.* 161: *189-204* (1962a).

ARDEN, G.B. & KELSEY, J.H. Some observations on the relationship between the standing potential of the human eye and the bleaching and regeneration of visual purple. *J. Physiol.* 161: *205-226* (1962b).

FRANÇOIS, J., VERRIEST, G. & DE ROUCK, A. L'électro-oculographie en tant qu'examen fonctionnel de la rétine. *Progrès en ophthalmologie.* Vol. VII: *1-67* (1957).

FRANÇOIS, J. & DE ROUCK, A. Valeur comparative de l'électro-rétinographie et de l'électro-oculographie. *Ann. Oculist.* 206: *235-243* (1973).

IMAIZUMI, K. The clinical application of electro-oculography. Proc. IIIrd Symposium, 311-326. Ed. H.M. Burian & J.H. Jacobson. Pergamon Press, New York. (1964).

KOLB, H. Electro-oculogram findings in patients treated with antimalarial drugs. *Brit. J. Ophthalm.* 49: *573* (1965).

KOLDER, H. Automatic recording and evaluating oscillations of indirectly measured corneo-retinal potential in man. *Med. Res. Engineering* 5: *26-29* (1967).

KOLDER, H. & NORTH, A.W. Oscillations of the corneo-retinal potential in animals. *Ophthalmologica (Basel)* 152: *149-160* (1967).

PINCKERS, A. & THIJSSEN, J.M. The A-criterion in electro-oculography. Proc. VIIthe ISCERG symposium. 284-288. Ed. D. Basar, Instanbul (1969).

PINCKERS, A. & V.D. EERDEN, J. La polyarthrite rhumatoide et les antipaludéens de synthèse. *Ann. Oculist. (Paris)* 206: *305-309* (1973).

PINCKERS, A. & THIJSSEN, J.M. Flat type electro-oculogram. *Acta Ophthal.* 52, *429-440* (1974).

THIJSSEN, J.M. PINCKERS, A. & OTTO, A.J. A multipurpose optical system for ophthalmic electrodiagnosis. *Ophthalmologica (Basel)* 168: *308-314* (1974).

Key words: Electro-oculogram, Light-sensitive negative potential, Macular involvement

Author's address:
Department of Ophthalmology
University of Nijmegen
Nijmegen, the Netherlands

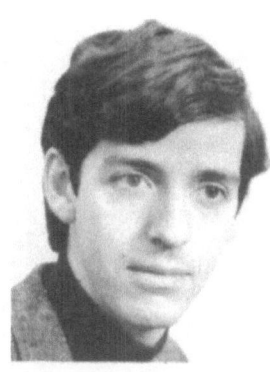

CYSTOID MACULAR EDEMA A SIGN WITH MANY CAUSES

J.G.A. NOTTING

(Nijmegen, The Netherlands)

Since GASS & NORTON (1966) described the biomicroscopic and fluorographic picture of cystoid macular edema (CME) and papilledema following cataract extraction (Irvine-Gass syndrome) many authors have reported the same symptoms in a variety of other diseases (see Table).

TABLE

Causes of cystoid macular edema

Vascular	:	· central retinal vein occlusion
		– branch vein occlusion
		chronic ischemic retinopathy
		· diabetic microangiopathy
		Coats' disease (retinal telangiectasis)
Inflammatory	:	– idiopathic retinal periphlebitis
		– uveitis (especially peripheral uveitis)
		chronic rheumatoid arthritis
Traumatic	:	· after cataract extraction (Irvine-Gass syndrome)
		after other kinds of intra-ocular surgery (e.g. trabeculectomy)
		after retinal detachment surgery
		· after X-ray irradiation
		vitreous traction (perforating trauma, macular puckering)
		·· long standing detachment of the macula caused by central serous retinopathy, disciform degeneration or malignant melanoma
Toxic:	:	topical epinephrine
	(	systemic griseofulvin)
Degenerative	:	– retinitis pigmentosa
		· dominant macular dystrophy
	(–	senile degeneration)
Idiopathic		

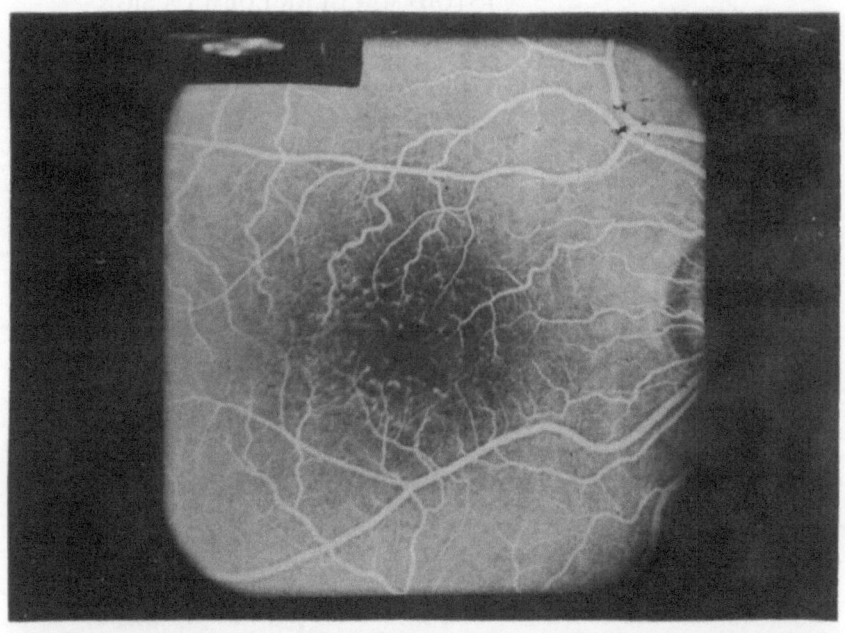

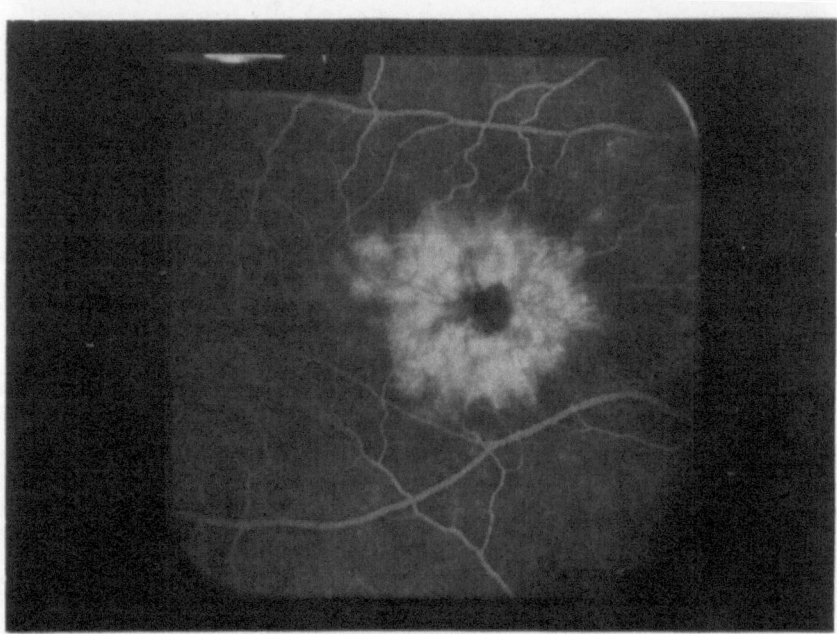

Fig. 1. Male aged 58. Corrected vision OD 0.4, OS 0.1. Not many fusiform capillary dilatations in the macular area (a, OD 28 seconds after dye injection). From these dye leakage occurs in a great number of symmetrically distributed cystoid spaces (b, OD· and c, OS 5 minutes after dye injection). In this case no underlying ocular or systemic disease could be established.

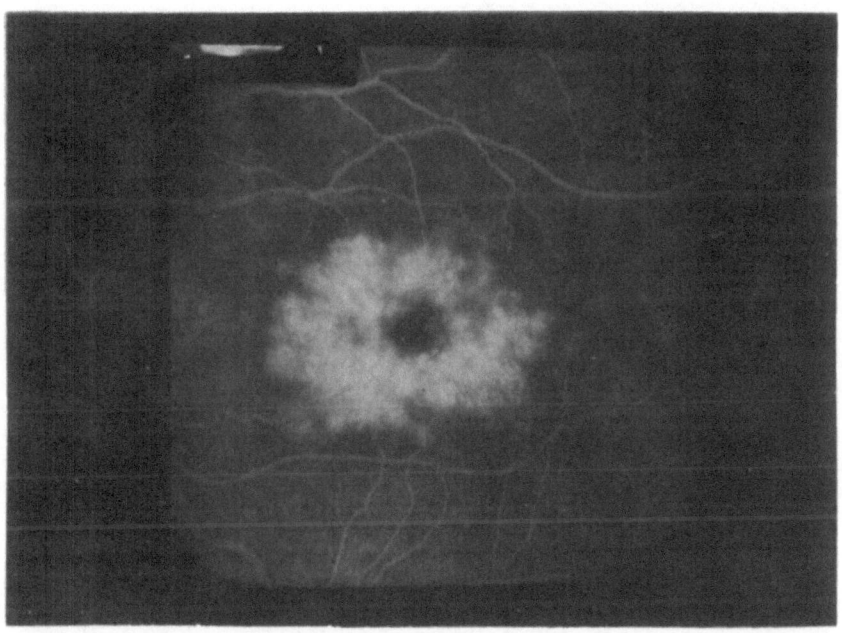

The cystoid nature of CME is perfectly illustrated by fluorescein angiography (Fig. 1b, c) but it can also be suspected when the retinal surface shows a delicate wrinkled or honey-comb appearance — best seen in red free light — as VOGT (1918) already mentioned. The cystoid spaces are also easily visible in biomicroscopic fundus examination (BANGERTER, 19 45). In a less developed picture however fluorography is essential for the dia no-sis. The fluorescence pattern is well known: retinal capillary dilatatio in the macular area (Fig. 1a, 4a, 7a) from where gradual dye leakage o(rs (BONNET, 1972). Histopathologic examination supports the view that o-rescein accumulates in cystoid spaces in the outer plexiform (Henle's) layer and inner nuclear layer (NEWSON et al., 1972). The distribution of cystoid spaces is responsible for the typical flower-like fluorescence pattern in the late phase (Fig. 1b, c, 3, 5a, 7b). Some degree of papilledema (sometimes with small haemorrhages) is frequently seen together with CME. (Fig. 2 gives an extreme example). In most cases an enhanced diffusion of dye into the vitreous and aqueous can be noted even in the absence of cells and/or flare.

Vision decrease varies from slight or none to severe, and is generally reversible unless formation of a lamellar hole has taken place. The therapy and prognosis depend on the character of the underlying disease. The table summarizes the possible etiologies of CME (confirmed by fluorography) based upon the classifications given by FFYTCHE & BLACH (1970) and FRANÇOIS et al., (1972).

355

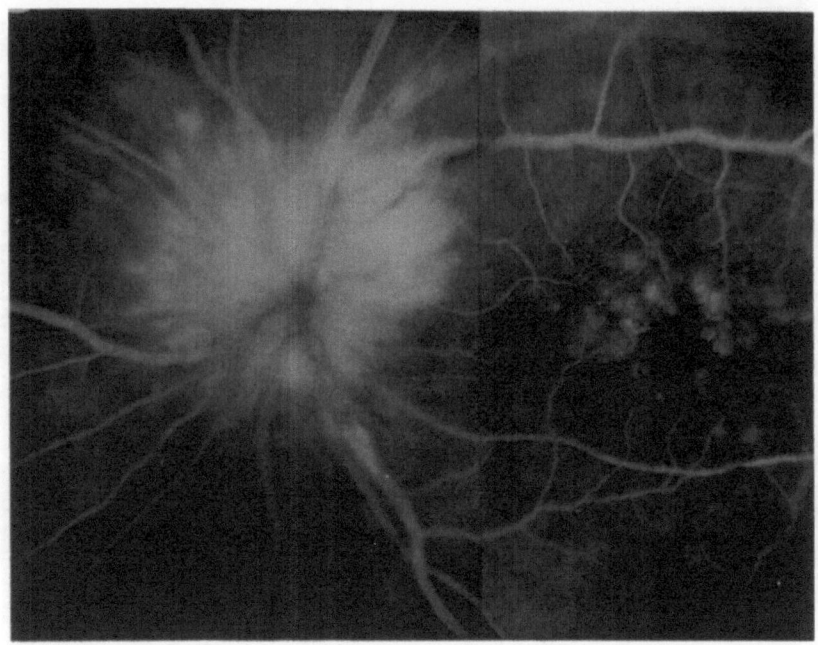

Fig. 2. Female aged 79. Three months after cataract extraction in the left eye the corrected vision fell from 1.0 to 0.05. In this case the papilledema is more impressive than the macular edema (one minute after dye injection).

Vascular:

- CME is present in many cases of *central vein occlusion* or *branch vein occlusion* with involvement of the macular area (BANGERTER, 1945; WISE & WANGVIVAT, 1966; GASS, 1968). We observed – as have OOSTERHUIS & SEDNEY (1975) – a marked reduction of CME and improvement of vision after photocoagulation (preferably by means of argon laser) in the area of the occluded branch. One of our cases of central vein occlusion showed complete spontaneous regression of a typical CME in 4 months, but vision remained unaltered.
- arterial hypertension and *chronic ischemia* due to retinal artery disease or chronic glaucoma can be a cause of macular edema (BANGERTER, 1945; GASS 1968); in some of these cases a true picture of CME may develop (FLYTCHE & BLACH, 1970).
- *diabetic microangiopathy* is frequently complicated by CME (GASS, 1968) (up to 25% of cases, LÜLLWITZ, 1973). In our material we often found the cystoid edema present in part of the macular area only or even excentric, related to the localization of the microangiopathy.
- in *Coats' disease* (retinal telangiectasis) (SPITZNAS et al., 1975) we also find CME in the part of the macular area where the vascular anomalies are located. Sometimes angiomatous malformations in the temporal periphery can lead to CME as well (WISE & WANGVIVAT, 1966; GASS, 1968).

356

Inflammatory:

- the association between *idiopathic retinal periphlebitis* (retinal vasculitis) and CME is mentioned in the literature, though not documented by fluorography(BANGERTER, 1945; DUKE-ELDER, 1967). Recently we saw a patient with bilateral idiopathic periphlebitis demonstrating a frank CME in her left eye (Fig. 3).
- other forms of *uveitis* (iridocyclitis, chorioditis, chorioretinitis) BANGERTER (1945), GASS (1968), FFYTCHE & BLACK (1970), FRANÇOIS et al. (1972), LÜLLWITZ (1973) especially *peripheral uveitis* are frequently accompanied by CME (WELCH et al., 1960; PRUETT et al., 1974) and often the diagnosis is only made after careful investigation in unexplained cases of CME. We have seen a few patients showing a marked reduction of CME after parabulbar corticoid aministration. In another patient the diagnosis could not be verified initially by fluorography: only half a year later we found a clear fluorographic picture of CME.
- during the last year we saw two patients with *chronic rheumatoid arthritis* in our clinic, both with a fluorographically demonstrable CME (one of them is shown in Fig. 4), but without other signs of ocular inflammation or other possible causes of CME. GASS (1968) describes two patients with collagen vascular disease and (fluorographic) macular changes, though not typical CME. From these cases we feel that a

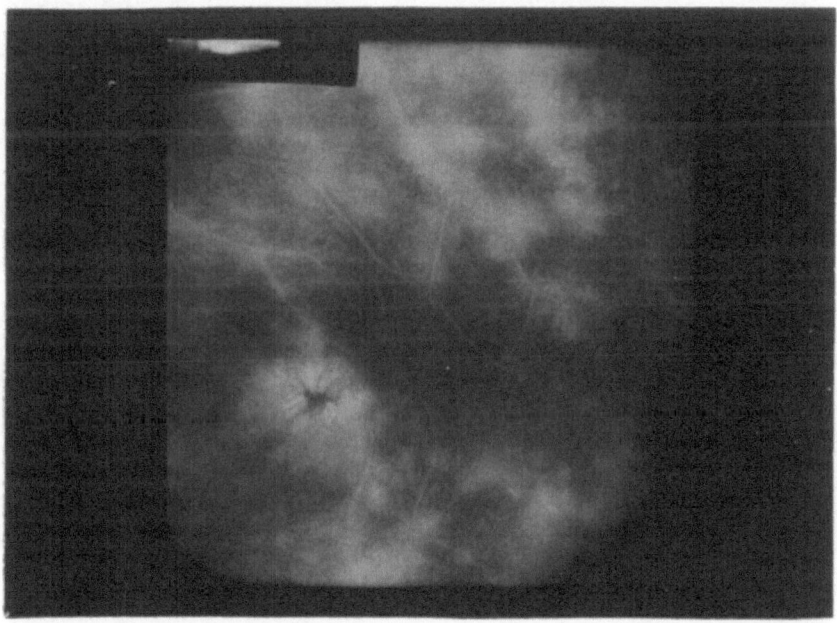

Fig. 3. Female aged 20. Idiopathic retinal periphlebitis. Vision OD 1.25, OS O.5. There is extensive dye leakage from retinal capillaries and veins. The picture shows the typical CME in the left eye 4 minutes after dye injection.

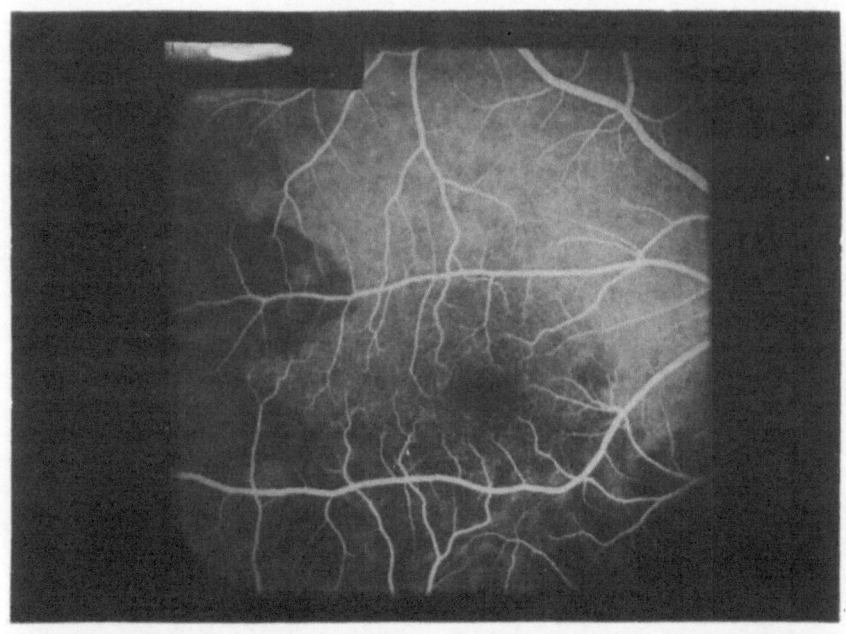

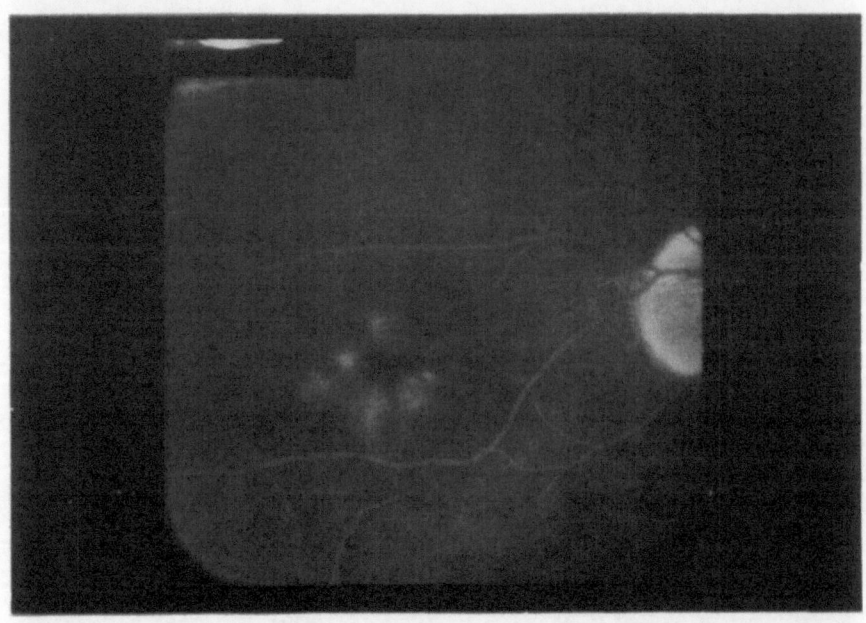

Fig. 4. Female aged 74. Chronic rheumatoid arthritis. Corrected vision OD 0.6, OS 0.8. The capillary dilatations in the macular area are visible in the arterio-venous phase (a). In the late phase a slow dye diffusion occurs (b, c: right and left eye approx. 5 minutes after dye injection).

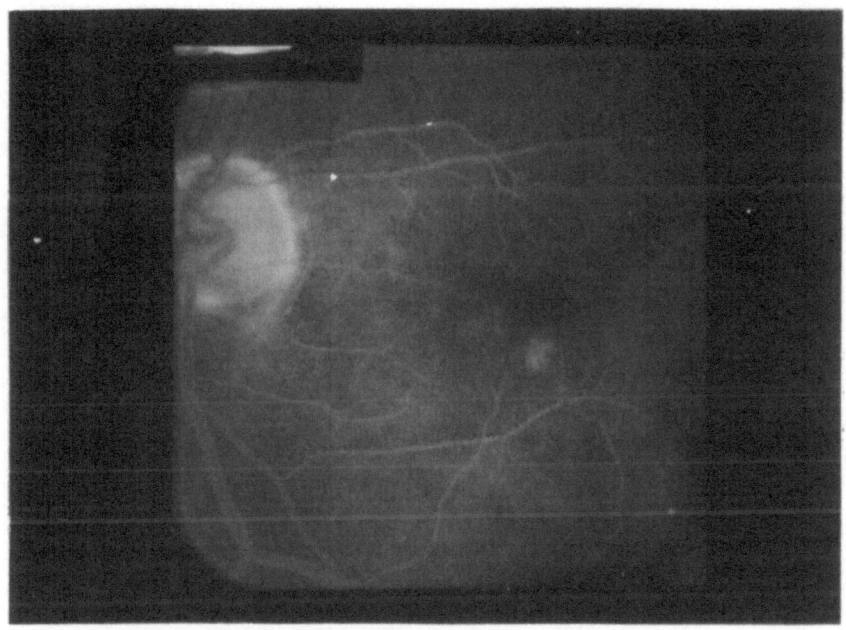

relation must exist between the rheumatoid arthritis and the occurrence of CME and suggest that every case of 'idiopathic' CME should be carefully screened for collagen disease.

Traumatic:

The macular edema following blunt trauma did not show the characteristics of CME in the few cases we were able to investigate by means of fluorography).
– CME *after cataract extraction* (Irvine-Gass syndrome) has been investigated by many authors (IRVINE, 1953; NICHOLLS, 1954; GASS, WELCH, COOPER, 1958; GASS, 1966; GEHRING, 1968, NORTON, 1969; BONNET, 1972, 1975; WEST et al., 1973; JACOBSON, DELLA-PORTA, 1974; HITCHINGS et al., 1975), but important questions have not been sufficiently answered yet: What exactly is the role of the vitreous? How can the free interval (up to 10 or even 20 years after extraction) be explained? Recently NORTON et al. (1975) concluded from a histopathologic examination that 'peripheral uveal tract and especially ciliary body inflammation seems to play an important role in effecting the pathogenesis of cystoid macular edema'. In our country the Irvine-Gass syndrome has gained much interest because of the fast growing use of intra-ocular implant lenses. Artificial lens implantations seem to show a higher percentage of CME than regular cataract extractions (an example from our clinic is demonstrated in Fig. 5), but it is felt that this complication can be largely avoided by performing an extracapsular extraction with an iridocapsular implant (BINKHORST, 1976).

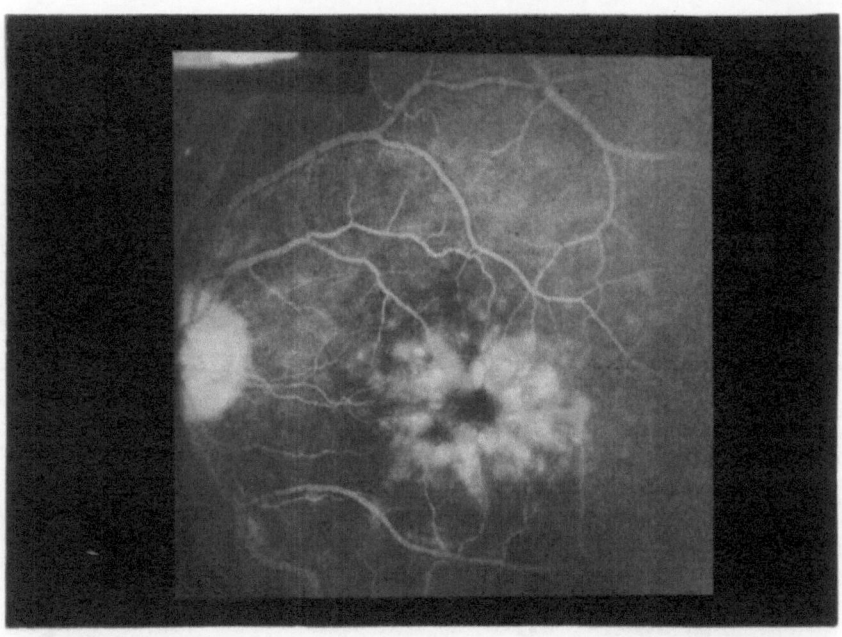

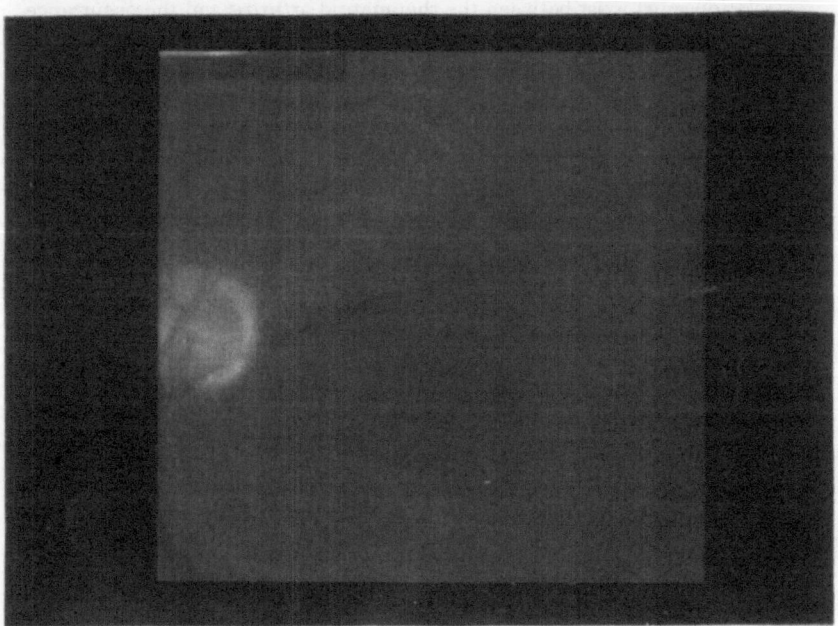

Fig. 5. Male aged 54. Seven months after implantation of an iris-cliplens in his left eye the postoperative corrected vision dropped to 0.5. Fluorography shows a clear picture of CME (a, 4 minutes after dye injection). Six months later this CME had completely disappeared (b, 7 minutes after dye injection) and the corrected vision was 1.0 again.

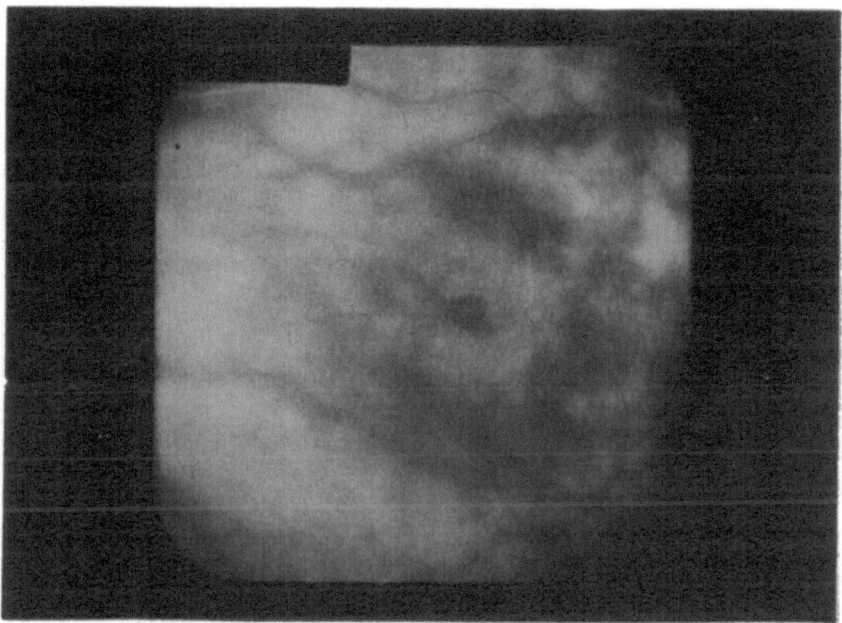

Fig. 6. Male aged 10. Retinitis pigmentosa. Vision 0.2. in both eyes. In this case there was a generalised capillary dilatation in the posterior pole with profuse dye leakage and CME. The right eye is shown $4\frac{1}{2}$ minutes after dye injection.

- CME has also been reported *after other kinds of intraocular surgery* (such as trabeculectomy, LÜLLWITZ (1973) possibly due to hypotension.
- furthermore CME is seen as a (rare) complication of *retinal detachment surgery* (RYAN, 1973).
- GASS (1968) reported two patients with CME after *X-ray irradiation*. *vitreous traction* seems to be the causative factor of CME in some cases of perforating trauma, proliferative retinopathy, macular puckering etc. (FFYTCHE & BLACH, 1970).
- *long standing detachment* of the retina in the macular area caused by central serous retinopathy, disciform degeneration or malignant melanoma can lead to CME (DUKE-ELDER, 1967; FFYTCHE & BLACH, 1970; NEWSON et al., 1972). The description of FRY & MCDONALD (1957) of CME associated with a malignant melanoma in the temporal periphery makes us wonder whether in this case a toxic factor might be responsible.

Toxic:

- KOLKER & BECKER (1968) described CME in (predominantly aphakic) patients treated with topical *epinephrine*. MICHELS & MAUMENEE (1975) demonstrated clearly initiation or aggravation of CME

361

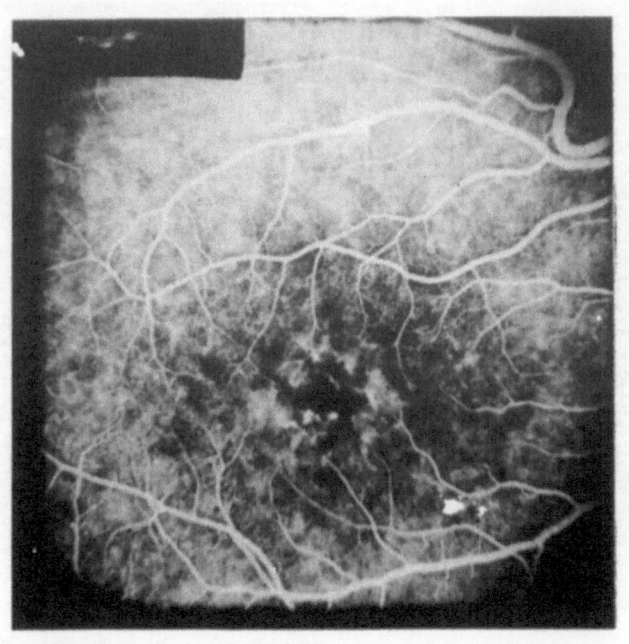

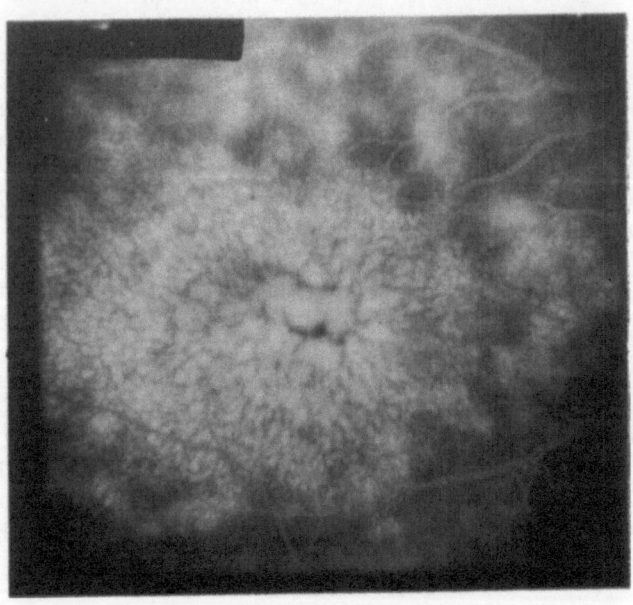

Fig. 7. Female aged 10. Dominantly inherited macular dystrophy. Leaking retinal capillaries cause the picture of cystoid macular oedema.

in aphakic eyes after the use of epinephrine drops and regression upon withdrawal of the drug.
- DELMAN & LEUBUSCHER (1963) observed macular edema after systemic administration of griseofulvin; from their description, however, it becomes not clear whether this was CME.

Degenerative:

- fluorographic evidence of CME in *retinitis pigmentosa* has been presented by a number of authors (HYVÄRINEN, 1971; FFYTCHE, 1972; FRANÇOIS et al., 1972; METGE et al., 1974). One of our cases is shown in Fig. 6.
- *senile degeneration* (BANGERTER, 1945) and chronic vitritis in patients older than 50 years (GASS, 1968) are presented as cause of CME. With regard to the available documentation this etiology still remains obscure in our opinion and we tend to classify these cases as idiopathic.
- we have examined two families with a *dominantly inherited macular dystrophy* showing a clear picture of CME (fig. 7) (to be published elsewhere) (see also in this book Deutman pp. 000).

Idiopathic:

- even after careful investigation there remain a few cases in which the etiology cannot be clarified (see Fig. 1) demanding further research. Takahashi & Uchida (1974), described an isolated case of CME in a 27-year-old male without any obvious cause.

REFERENCES

BANGERTER, A. Zur Diagnose, Differentialdiagnose und Therapie des cystoiden maculaöedems (Maculacysten). *Ophthalmologica* 109: *102-122* (1945).
BINKHORST, C.D. Pseudophakia, Intracapsular or extracapsular technique? (see elsewhere in these Proc., p. 261).
BONNET, M. Le syndrome d'Irvine-Gass I. Sémiologie clinique – II. Diagnostic différentiel – III. Anatomie pathologique. *Arch. Opht.* 32: *205-220* (1972).
BONNET, M. Les facteurs de pronostic du syndrome d'Irvine-Gass. *Ann. d'Oculist. (Paris)* 208: *275-278* (1975).
DELMAN, M., & LEUBUSCHER, K. Transient macular edema due to griseofulvin. *Am. J. Ophthal.* 56: *658* (1963).
DUKE-ELDER, S., DOBREE, J.H. Cystoid degeneration of the retina. In: System of Ophthalmology. Vol. X. Diseases of the Retina. Ed. H. Kimpton, London 10, 543-554 (1967).
FFYTCHE, T.J., & BLACH, R.K. The aetiology of macular edema. *Trans. Ophth. Soc. U.K.* 90: *637-656* (1970).
FFYTCHE, T.J. Macular oedema, *Trans. Ophth. Soc. U.K.* 92: *395-405* (1972).
FFYTCHE, T.J. Cystoid maculopathy in retinitis pigmentosa. *Trans. Ophth. Soc. U.K.* 92: *265-283* (1972).
FRANCOIS, J., DE LAEY, J.J., & VERBRAEKEN, H. L.Oedeme kystoide de la macula. *Bull. Soc. Belge d'Opht.* 161: *708-721* (1972).
FRY, W.E. & MCDONALD, P.R. Malignant melanoma in the temporal periphery associated with macular symptoms as an initial finding. *Trans. Am. Acad. Ophthalmol. Otolaryngol.* 61: *397-403* (1957).

GASS, J.D.M. & NORTON, E.W.D. Cystoid macular edema and papilledema following cataract extraction. *Arch. Ophthal.* 76: *646* (1966).

GASS, J.D.M. & NORTON, E.W.D. Follow-up study of cystoid macular edema following cataract extraction. *Trans. Am. Acad. Ophthal.* 73: *665-682* (1969).

GASS, J.D.M. A fluorescein angiography study of macular dysfunction secondary to retinal vascular disease. II. Retinal vein obstruction; III. Hypertensive retinopathy; IV. Diabetic retinal angiopathy; V. Retinal telangiectasis; VI. X-ray irradiation, catotid artery occlusion. *Arch. Ophthal.* 80: *626-631* (1968).

HITCHINGS, R.A., CHISHOLM, I.H., & BIRD, A.C. Aphakic macular edema, incidence and pathogenesis. *Invest. Ophthalmol.* 14: *68* (1975).

HYVÄRINEN, L., MAUMENEE, E., KELLEY, J. & CANTOLINO, S. Fluorescein angiographic findings in retinitis pigmentosa. *Am. J. Ophthal.* 71: *17-26* (1971).

IRVINE, R.S. A newly defined vitreous syndrome following cataract surgery. Interpreted according to recent concepts of the structure of the vitreous. *Am. J. Ophthal.* 36: *599-619* (1953).

JACOBSON, D.R. Natural history of cystoid macular edema after cataract extraction. *Am. J. Ophthal.* 77: *445-447* (1974).

KOLKER, A.E. & BECKER, B. Epinephrine Maculopathy. *Arch. Ophthal.* 79: *552-562* (1968).

LÜLLWITZ, W. Zur Klinik des Irvine-Gass Syndroms. *Dtsch. Ophth. Ges.* 73: *561-565* (1973).

METGE, P., CHOVET, M., EBAGOSTI, A., & TASSY , A. Oedème cystoïde dans la rétinographie pigmentaire. *Bull. Soc. Ophthal. Fr.* 74: *119-123* (1974).

MICHELS, R.G. & MAUMENEE, A.E. Cystoid macular edema associated with topically applied epinephrine in aphakic eyes. *Am. J. Ophthal.* 80: *379-388* (1975).

NEWSOM, W.A., IAN HOOD, C., HORWITZ, J.A., FINE, S.L. & SEWELL, J.H. Cystoid macular edema: histopathologic and angiographic correlations. A clinicopathologic case report. *Trans. Am. Acad. Ophthal. Otolaryng.* 76: *1005-1009* (1972).

NICHOLLS, J.V.V. Macular edema in association with cataract extraction. *Am. J. Ophthal.* 37: *665-672* (1954).

NORTON, A.L., BROWN, W.J., CARLSON, M., PILGER, I.S. & RIFFENBURGH, R.S. Pathogenesis of aphakic macular edema. *Am. J. Ophthal.* 80: *96-101* (1975).

OOSTERHUIS, J.A. & SEDNEY, S.C. Photocoagulation in retinal vein thrombosis. *Ophthalmologica* 171: *365-379* (1975).

PRUETT, R.C., BROCKHURST, R.J. & LETTS, N.F. Fluorescein angiography of peripheral uveitis. *Am. J. Ophthal.* 77: *448-453* (1974).

RYAN, S.J. Cystoid maculopathy in phakic retinal detachment procedures. *Am. J. Ophthal.* 76: *519-522* (1973).

SPITZNAS, M., JOUSSEN, F., WESSING, A. & MEYER-SCHWICKERATH, G. Coats' disease. An epidemiologic and fluorescein angiographic study. *Albrecht v. Graefes Arch. Ophthal.* 195: *241-250* (1975).

TAKAHASHI, H. & UCHIDA, S. A case of honey-comb macular degeneration (Primary microcystoid degeneration of the macula). *Jap. Inl. clin. ophthalmology* 28: *397-401* (1974).

VOGT, A. Weitere ophthalmoskopische Beobachtungen im rotfreien Licht: echte Netzhautfältchen, zystische Degeneration des Makula lutea. *Klin. Mbl. Augenheilk.* 61: *379* (1918).

WELCH, R.B. & COOPER, J.C. Macular edema, papilledema, and optic atrophy after cataract extraction. *Arch. Ophthal.* 59: *665-675* (1958).

WELCH, R.B. MAUMENEE, A.E. & WAHLEN, H.E. Peripheral posterior segment inflammation, vitreous opacities and edema of the posterior pole. *Arch. Ophthal.* 64: *540-549* (1960).

WEST, C.E. FITZGERALD, C.R. & SEWELL, J.H. Cystoid macular edema following aphakic keratoplasty. *Am. J. Ophthal.* 75: *77-81* (1973).

WISE, G.N. & WANGVIVAT, Y. The exaggerated macular response to retinal disease. *Am. J. Ophthal.* 61: *1359-1363* (1966).

Key words: Cystoid edema, Macula, Fluorescein angiography, Irvine-Gass syndrome.

Author's address:
Institute of Ophthalmology
University of Nijmegen
Philips van Leydenlaan 15
Nijmegen, The Netherlands